Discovering Me

A Guide to Teaching Health and Building Adolescents' Self-Esteem

Leslie Herod, M. Ed.
Turlock Junior High School
Turlock, California

Illustrated by

Meg Biddle
Biddle-Perry Studios
Monterey, California

Leslie Herod

Allyn and Bacon

Boston ■ London ■ Toronto ■ Sydney ■ Tokyo ■ Singapore

Publisher: Joseph E. Burns
Series Editorial Assistant: Sara Sherlock
Marketing Manager: Rick Muhr
Editorial-Production Service: Omegatype Typography, Inc.
Manufacturing Buyer: Julie McNeill
Electronic Composition: Omegatype Typography, Inc.

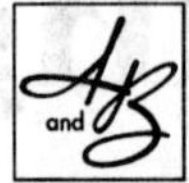

A Pearson Education Company
Needham Heights, MA 02494

Internet: www.abacon.com

Library of Congress Cataloging-in-Publication Data
Herod, Leslie.
Discovering me : a guide to teaching health and building adolescents' self-esteem / by Leslie Herod ; illustrated by Meg Biddle, Leslie Herod.
p. cm.
Includes bibliographical references.
ISBN 0-205-27474-9 (alk. paper)
1. Self-esteem in adolescence—Study and teaching (Secondary)
I. Title.
BF724.3.S36H47 1999
373.17'1—dc21 98-53704
CIP

Printed in the United States of America

10 9 8 7 6 5 4 3 2 1 03 02 01 00 99

This book is dedicated to my mother
and father and the other great teachers
who guide us in discovering our strengths.

Contents

Sexually Transmitted Diseases

Choosing a Future

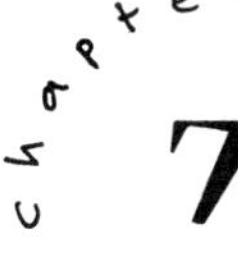

7 A Healthy Body 107

Normal Body Weights

Nutrition

Diet and Exercise

Hygiene

chapter

8 A Closer Look 122

APPENDIX: HANDOUTS

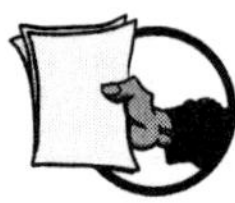

Chapter 2

Chapter 3

Chapter 4

Chapter 5

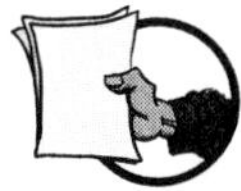

Chapter 6

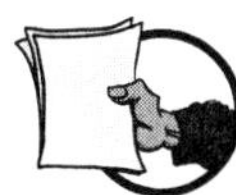

Chapter 7

Preface

Several years ago I was asked by the administration at my school to build a health curriculum for the middle school that would help students become successful, well-adjusted, informed adults. I never realized what a daunting task this would turn out to be!

I started investigating resources, went to workshops and training programs, and attended conferences until I had gained so many good ideas and materials I could not keep it all to myself. I experimented with the activities on my students and realized that I was learning, too. I was having as much fun and getting as motivated as the kids. My perspective on teaching changed. I now look forward to each encounter with students as a unique experience to share insights, and I feel privileged to watch students grow with a positive approach to life. Rather than shouldering the burden of "teaching" a group of disinterested students, I discovered the joy in providing opportunities for us all to grow and learn.

The amazing thing about these activities is that the teacher gets to watch the students become empowered. Kids enter the class with expectations, excitement, and the will to succeed because they know the topic for the lesson is *them.* Because the kids want to learn and participate, the teacher merely sets up the activity and enjoys the experience of watching his or her students succeed.

This book contains a collection of high-impact activities that you can adapt to any subject matter or use as a comprehensive Health/Life Skills curriculum. Each lesson is explained in an easy-to-understand manner with hints and follow-up ideas from experienced teachers who have used the activities. Use these activities and follow the guidelines for establishing an atmosphere of trust, connection, and respect in your classroom. Where needed, lessons provide illustrated, reproducible student handouts for the busy, overworked professional.

Most of all, keep in mind that you are not just teaching activities or lessons; you are guiding young people on their journey toward adulthood. These lessons for life will help them face their fears and replace bravado with factual information, respect, and courage. The activities in the *Discovering Me* program are designed to help you have fun with your students as you offer opportunities for them to practice the skills needed to become respected, responsible adults.

ACKNOWLEDGMENTS

I would like to thank all my students who have allowed me the privilege of sharing their transition into the world of adults. Life can be an adventure of discovery and growth. I feel honored to have shared that adventure with so many of them.

I appreciate the guidance provided by Lorrie Freitas during a period of growth in my life. I appreciated the nagging and encouragement heaped on me by my parents and those loving celestials in Biddle-Perry Studios. My appreciation goes to the following reviewers for their comments on the manuscript: Margaret Banducci, Oakdale Junior High School, Oakdale, California, and Ardith Feucht, Turlock Junior High School, Turlock, California.

A very special thank you to Ruth, my dear friend, whose support and understanding have provided the impetus I needed to make this journey.

Note to Teachers

HELPING STUDENTS BUILD SELF-RESPECT

Make your classroom a place of happiness and security for your students. Fill your lessons with humor and support so students can take risks, gain new insights comfortably, and deal with stress by allowing them to laugh and have fun. It has been proven that students retain more information when they are not under stress. Because laughter is one of the easiest ways to reduce stress, use it in large quantities. Remember that you can have a good time and still do your job!

Allow each student successes each day. Sometimes you may need to help the student recognize success. Reduce competition between students by challenging students to compete against themselves. Competition against another student results in one student succeeding at the expense of the other. Competition against oneself can only result in success as each person moves forward.

The basic elements to building self-respect are:

- Confidence, which empowers students to be assertive and choose goals that will challenge them.
- Respect, which is earned by doing worthy deeds. Respect for themselves and others builds confidence and self-actualization.
- Safety and security, which allow students to reach out further and test their limits.
- Empowerment, which gives students the feeling that they are important and of worth, enabling them to control their world rather than feeling controlled by it.

Ways to empower students include:

- Acknowledging a student's need to identify with a group of peers.
- Allowing for interaction with their peers and chances to compare choices, values, and reactions.
- Providing opportunities for students to be successful and recognize success.
- Acknowledging each student as an individual—with different needs and strengths.
- Allowing students to practice skills in a safe environment.

A teacher is an important influence on students and can make a lasting impact. You need to prepare yourself to be a positive influence each and every day!

- Leave personal problems outside the classroom.
- Remember that EVERY student is important—*look at them* and *listen to them.*
- Think of each day as a performance.
- Be prepared!
- Do affirmations. Repeat positive statements about the students, your lesson, and the day ahead rather than falling into the trap of complaining and feeling negative about the day.

The results of each lesson or activity may not always be what you would choose, but respect student choices and temper them with your experience and guidance so that the students come away from the activity with knowledge gained.

In disciplining students:

- Tell the students exactly what behavior you expect without threatening them with some ultimatum or punishment.
- Check for their understanding. Often just having the student repeat their understanding of what has been asked of them will be enough.
- Wait for them to correct the behavior and acknowledge the improved behavior.
- Retain control without threatening or arguing.

CELEBRATE YOU!

CELEBRATE YOU!

You are worth celebrating.
You are worth everything.
You are unique.
In the whole world there is only one you.
There is only one person with
    your talents
    your experiences
    your gifts.

NO ONE CAN TAKE YOUR PLACE!

You have immense potential
    to love
    to care
    to grow
    to succeed—if you believe in yourself.
It doesn't matter your age, your color, or whether your parents loved you or not.
Maybe they wanted to, but couldn't.
Let that go.
It belongs in the past.
You belong to the NOW.

It doesn't matter what you have been, the wrong you may have done,
    the mistakes you've made, the people you may have hurt.

You are okay. You are accepted.

So love yourself, and nourish the seed within you.

CELEBRATE YOU!

Begin NOW. Start anew. Give yourself a new birth.
Today.
You are you, and that is all you need to be.
You are temporary. Here today and gone tomorrow.
But today, today can be a new beginning, a new thing, a new life!
SO CELEBRATE YOU!

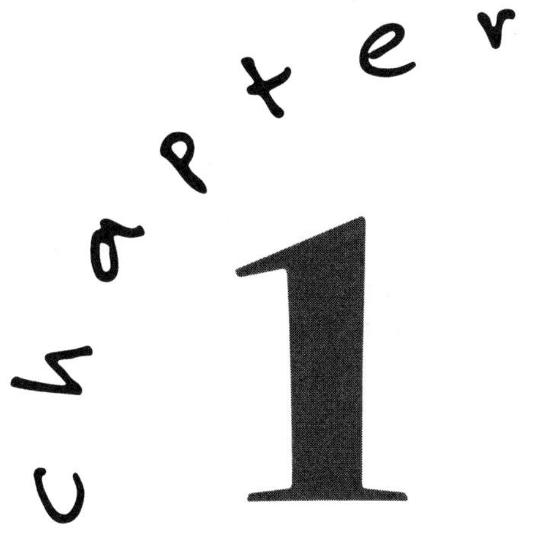

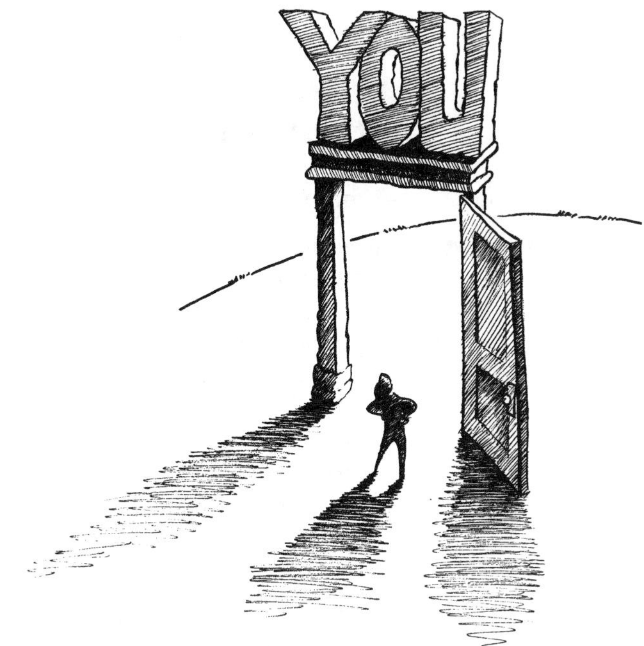

Who Am I?

Adults often look back on their teenage years with nostalgia, but very few ever want to live through those years again. For most of us, it was a time of confusion, awkwardness, and experimentation. It was a time of great friendships and exaggerated adventures. We were innocent and unconcerned about the future.

Children today experience many of those same feelings but are expected to deal with many more life-altering forces than we could have imagined. Students need to be prepared to survive the challenges of today by developing social and personal skills. This chapter provides opportunities for students to recognize and develop their values and skill levels as they confront themselves as social beings in the throes of the hormonal confusion called puberty.

activity 1 Attention Recess

time 1–2 minutes.

purpose This activity allows students to refresh their brains and wiggle, stretch, or giggle. By allowing students a short break, you will improve their ability to pay attention, which will, in turn, improve their performance. This can be revitalizing for both you and the students.

materials Imagination.

process Tell students to stand up. Have them do three jumping jacks in place, touch their toes twice, and then "high-five" a person standing next to them.

Give students a few seconds to quiet down, and then get back to your lesson. You will find that they will be much more attentive and willing to participate after their little "wake up."

hints You can do almost anything for an attention recess. Students can find a partner with eyes the same color as their own and shake hands while giving them a compliment. Students can stand up and yell out their name or birthday, sing a loud song, or untie their shoes and tie them back up. Anything that will break up the lesson and give students a bit of activity will work. It is best to keep the students near their chairs or do something that returns them to their chairs.

activity 2 Get Out of That Box

time 20 minutes.

purpose We are all locked in a box in the way we think. We often approach solutions to problems through commonly-used methods. We rarely are challenged to think beyond that confining box to solve common problems in uncommon ways. This activity will help students to think in new and creative ways. Encourage students to cooperate and collaborate to solve problems creatively.

materials Tables or desks and chairs.

process Tell students to find a partner and to sit across from that person in an arm wrestling position. Both students will use either their right or left arm, placing their elbows close together on a desk or table. The students wrap their fingers around the other's hand, getting a firm grip. It does not matter if the partnerships are made up of a boy and girl.

Tell students, "You are going to be arm wrestling. The goal of the exercise is to earn as many points as possible for each person. You get one point if the other person's hand touches the table."

Time the students for 30 seconds and let them compete without any suggestions from you. At the end of the time, ask each partnership for their combined total of points.

Repeat the directions, emphasizing that the object of the exercise is to achieve the most points possible for the partnership. Time the group for another 30 seconds.

By this time, you should have some students who have obtained a lot of points by using several different approaches to solve the problem. As you ask for scores at the end of this round, have the more successful partnerships share their secrets for success.

Time students for another 30 seconds and collect scores. By now most kids should have caught on to a solution that works well for them. Have the partnerships share their solutions with the class.

One of the most successful solutions is for both kids to offer no resistance and allow their hand to be pushed to the table. By alternating "losing" and moving quickly, the team should be able to collect many points in 30 seconds.

However, be careful about suggesting a correct way of solving the problem. Whatever works best for each team is okay.

Ask how the teams reached their solutions. Have the teams share the process they followed in reaching their solution—even if the solution was not that successful. The process of collaboration is important. Some kids will catch on and take over without discussing the solution with their partner. Other teams will talk about it and then act.

closing thoughts At the end of the activity, ask the students to tell you what they learned from this exercise. Some answers might include:

- Success comes from working together rather than fighting each other.
- Listen to the directions and think past the old way of solving a problem.
- Think of unusual ways to solve common problems.
- Sometimes the ideas that seem weird will work best.
- Don't be afraid to try an idea.
- Don't look at other people to find ways to solve problems. Rely on your own abilities.

hints This is a great icebreaker activity and gives the students a chance to let off steam. It helps them think creatively and build confidence in their problem-solving abilities. This activity can also be used as a lead-in for lessons calling for collaboration and cooperation.

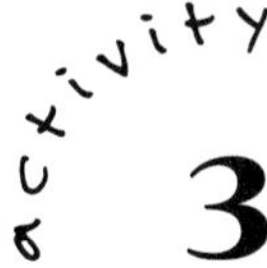

3 Halitosis Golf

time 20 minutes.

purpose This activity challenges students to work together to solve problems as a group. It develops and reveals leaders, imaginative people, and the workers—all necessary parts in a group effort to solve a problem.

This activity will also give students the opportunity to solve problems in new and creative ways. It provides another way of getting students to think beyond the most obvious solution to a problem.

materials Ping-Pong balls, paper cups, masking tape, and tables.

process Tape the paper cups to the edge of the table, in the center. I will sometimes put two tables end-to-end or in the shape of an "L" to increase the challenge. Place students in groups of four or five.

Have the students place themselves randomly around the table, and tell them that they are to get the Ping-Pong ball from the starting point at one end of the table to the cup at the other end of the table. Then tell them that they can't use their hands!

The ball must go into the cup for a group to win. The only time that students may use their hands is to pick up the ball from the floor, but the ball must be placed back at the starting point. Allow for creativity!

As groups accomplish the task, tell them that they came in first or second and that they should continue to see how many times or ways they can accomplish the task. Try to allow time for each team to be successful.

discussion When all teams have finished, have students sit down. Ask them to discuss their methods of accomplishing the task. Ask questions such as:

- How did you get the ball into the cup?
- Did you have an individual who became the leader? Who was that person? Why did you listen to that person and not to someone else?
- Who came up with the best ideas?
- What were some of the methods you tried that did not work? Why didn't they work for you?
- Can you accomplish this task if group members are not cooperating and helping? Why or why not?

hints This activity is another good icebreaker. It is hard to sit back and not become an active participant in this activity. I have used this on the first day of class and it really gives the students an opportunity to relax and enjoy each other and your class.

Make sure that you have some signal to bring the activity to a close so that students will return to their seats and quiet down for the discussion. At first glance, it may look like you are out of control while the students are trying to get the ball into the cup because of the noise level and the excitement. Allow them this freedom! Remember, a student will learn best when emotionally involved—let it happen.

Watch each group and help them identify their leaders, workers, and problem solvers. Remind students that each task they work on has different requirements, which rely on different talents used in different ways. Each student is needed to accomplish the task before the group.

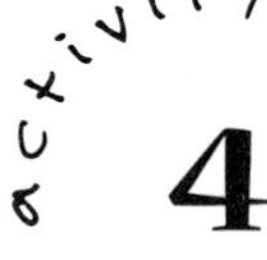

4 A Business Handshake

time 5–10 minutes.

purpose This activity teaches students the correct way to shake hands formally. Learning this skill will give students confidence and improve first impressions when they are looking for employment or trying to impress a new acquaintance in a formal setting.

materials None.

process Discuss the importance of a first impression when looking for employment. Discuss the types of clothing that would be appropriate for interviews for various jobs.

First impressions are important because they are difficult to overcome. For example, applying for a job is usually not the time to assert your rebellious nature by wearing a nose-to-ear chain.

A handshake is the first physical contact another person has with you, so it is almost as important as the visual impression. Demonstrate the correct way to perform a business handshake. Present your right hand and firmly grasp the other person's hand so that the "V" between the thumb and index finger meets the same area on the other person's hand. Wrap the fingers around the other person's hand, look the person in the eye, and shake the hand briskly once or twice.

Emphasize eye contact. Looking a person in the eye demonstrates confidence and equality.

After students practice with a partner near them, have them walk around the room and collect four or five "good" business handshakes. Have students return to their seats when they are finished.

closing thoughts Have everyone sit down and then ask if anyone found a really good handshake during their quest. Allow the person to tell who had a good handshake and why that handshake was so good. Ask if the student would have been tempted to hire the other person based on that handshake alone.

hints You can vary this activity by allowing students to share their own personal "secret" handshakes with the rest of the class. Allow the gang student to present the secret handshake used between members or let the jock present the "correct" way to do a high five. You can even make up a handshake just for your class to make them feel special.

Acknowledging other methods of greeting validates and recognizes members of the class who are sometimes overlooked. It won't hurt to learn all the subculture greetings.

activity 5 Individual Recognition

time A few seconds.

purpose This is an excellent way to recognize and honor students who do something of worth. You can recognize polite behavior, an improved assignment, or being a great kid. Emphasize the student's inherent worth.

materials Two good hands and a bit of energy.

process Use your student list to choose a student to recognize for the day. Find something positive about that student that can be applauded by the rest of the class. Begin each day by announcing the student to be applauded and the reason for his or her recognition, and have the class applaud that student.

If a student is shy and does not want to be recognized or is absent, have a second student in mind so that you don't miss a day for recognition. Check the person's name in your gradebook or student list so that you make sure each student is applauded on a regular basis and that no student is missed. If a student is absent, make sure that the class applauds him or her when the student returns and welcomes that student back.

Respect the student's right to pass. However, as recognition is accepted and they all become comfortable with it, you may call on that person again.

activity 6 Cooperative Creature

time 45 minutes.

purpose This activity allows students the opportunity to work together to build a "creature" out of the strengths of each individual in their group. Students learn to work together and to look for positive traits in other people. This is often a very affirming activity.

materials Large pieces of butcher or poster paper, crayons or markers, and a clock or watch with a second hand.

process Have the students get into groups of four or five people.

Tell students that they are going to create a picture of a creature using only the best parts of each of the individuals in their group. All the students in the group will have one minute to draw what they consider their best trait.

Every 60 seconds, the marker or crayon is passed to another person in the group to continue the construction of the creature. There should be no talking or coaching from the students waiting their turn to draw.

After each person has had at least two turns to draw, have the entire group work together to complete the drawing by connecting each of the contributions into one form.

When the drawings are complete, have each group present their creature to the rest of the class. A speaker from the group will explain each trait and who contributed that characteristic.

hints These drawings can be used as decoration around the room or as a banner for those groups as they work together on other projects. As a follow-up activity, have students collectively write a story about their creature.

activity 7 Share a Story

time About 5 minutes.

purpose This activity allows each student to feel recognized and to build attachments to other students in the class.

materials A watch or clock with a second hand.

process Have students sit in groups of four or five.

Tell each group that you need one person to volunteer. If there is no volunteer, pick a person from each group and tell them that they are going to be happy they were chosen. (This is a great way to get students to volunteer in the future.) Tell the groups that the volunteer gets to pick who is going to share first.

Give students 30 seconds to think about the funniest thing that has ever happened to them. Time the 30 seconds for thinking. Then tell the students that each person in the group will have 45 seconds in which to tell the others about that funny incident.

The first person will relate their story while the teacher times the 45 seconds. *No one* else should be talking but person number one. At the end of the time, give the storyteller a round of applause and go to person number two. Continue in this manner until all the funny stories have been told.

Additional topics might include:

- my favorite relative
- my favorite animal story
- the neatest gift you would like to give someone
- my favorite vacation
- my favorite ride at an amusement park
- my scariest moment
- something I have done of which I am very proud
- my best friend
- a quick autobiography
- my greatest success
- my happiest moment

hint If students are unable to think of something, tell them to make up a story. This takes the pressure off them, and they often share something of relevance or at least get caught up in the moment. What they are sharing is not as important as having the group's attention and being recognized.

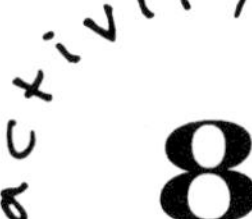

8 Zoom!

time About 10–20 minutes.

purpose This activity allows students to solve a problem creatively as a group and to recognize all the people in the group as valuable contributors to a solution for a common problem.

materials A tennis or playground ball and a watch or clock with a second hand.

process Tell students that they are going to have to solve a problem. You want to see how long it will take the entire class to pass the ball around to every person in the class. As each person touches the ball, he or she must say, "zoom." The only rules are that everyone person must touch the ball and that each person has to say "zoom" as they touch it.

The teacher then gives the ball to a student and allows the class to do the rest. Tell the students that when they are ready, you will time their attempt. After each attempt, encourage the students to improve their time. Have them keep trying until they have passed the ball throughout the group in under 1 second. Encourage them to discuss ideas and develop a solution. Let them attempt many different strategies until you run out of time and/or energy.

Discuss the process used to find a solution and who people listened to and why. Some questions that can be asked following the activity are:

- Who were the leaders? Why?
- Who seemed to be the followers?
- What types of system emerged for people's ideas to be heard and recognized?
- Who came up with the most creative ideas? Were they the leaders?
- Did leadership of the group change during the various attempts? If so, how or why?

activity 9 Time Capsule

time 30 minutes.

purpose Students will be given a chance to evaluate the important parts of their lives. They will decide how best to represent those areas of life to their descendants, how they want to be remembered, and how they can illustrate that memory.

materials The "Time Capsule" handout, a pencil, and imagination.

process Ask students what they would like to be remembered for. Have them make a list of accomplishments or qualities that they would like their descendants to remember about them.

Give each student the "Time Capsule" worksheet and explain what a time capsule is. This capsule is going to contain a collection of items that will be placed in the earth and recovered in the distant future.

Have the students pick items from their lives that will give the people in the future a good picture of who they are. Place those items in their time capsule by drawing or writing them in. Discuss the students' choices and reasons for those choices.

follow-up Have the class make a real time capsule for their class or the school. Actually bury the time capsule with great ceremony and a marker. This can be an annual event in which the whole school can participate.

activity 10 Comparisons

150

time 20–30 minutes.

purpose The students may discover that they have many things in common and yet continue to be unique in their differences.

This activity also helps students learn to use a Venn diagram, which can be a useful tool in many other activities.

materials The "Venn Diagram" handout.

process Have students get a partner. This activity works well when the two students do not really know each other.

Tell the students that they have about 5 minutes to find out all the things they have in common and the things that are different. Students place their differences in the outside circles, with one student using the upper circle and the other using the bottom circle. Their similarities will be written in the overlapping area of the circles.

hints You can help by suggesting questions or leading the class in brainstorming some possible questions kids can ask each other once they've been paired up. Topics for questions can be about physical similarities and differences, comparisons of emotions, family makeup, likes and dislikes, skills, achievements, or travel.

Have students go to the front of the class together and share the results of their interview.

activity

11 One of a Kind

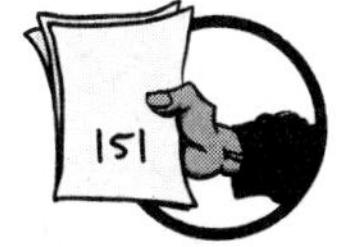

time 40 minutes.

purpose The students will realize that each person is special and unique and yet a part of all humanity.

materials A bag of roasted peanuts in the shell and enough small bowls for each small group, one larger container or bowl that will hold all the peanuts with room to spare, and the "One of a Kind" handout.

process Have students get in small groups of four or five people. Give each person the "One of a Kind" handout.

Put the peanuts in the large bowl and go around the room, allowing each student to pick the peanut they want for their own. Remind students that they are *not* to mark the peanut in any way. Tell them they will eventually get to keep their peanut but it has to be used for the activity first.

Have the students examine their peanut carefully, noticing the color and shape and any special markings or lines that are unique to the peanut. The students will then answer questions about their peanut in Part One of the handout and then draw an accurate reproduction of their peanut.

When everyone is finished drawing, have the students place their peanut in the small bowl for their group. After mixing the peanuts, have each student take a turn identifying and retrieving his or her own peanut. Ask several of the students how they were able to recognize their peanut.

Next, go to each group and have the students place their peanut in the large bowl. Ask the students if they think they could pick out their own peanut from the total group. Explain that all the peanuts are basically the same. Have students tell you the general traits of all the peanuts.

Now go to each student and have them identify and pick out his or her own peanut. If students question ownership, have them walk around the room to try to find their peanut while examining those of other students. If you have a conflict over ownership, have the students check their drawings.

Have the students answer the questions in Part Two of the handout. Then have students share how they were able to identify their peanut. Have them discuss what they learned from this activity.

Ask questions about how this activity relates to people as individuals and society as a whole.

follow-up Have students list the ways they consider themselves to be unique. You could even have students ask parents or close friends to tell them ways in which they are unique individuals. Then have the kids make a list indicating ways that they are all the same.

Use this activity preceding a lesson on prejudice or differences in cultures. This makes a good topic for an essay or journal entry.

hints If your students are like mine, the first thing they will want to do is to put the peanut into their mouths. Precede the activity by asking students to wait until after the activity to eat or mark their peanut.

If some students end up with peanuts they feel are not theirs, give them a couple of the extra peanuts at the end of the activity to make up for their separation anxiety.

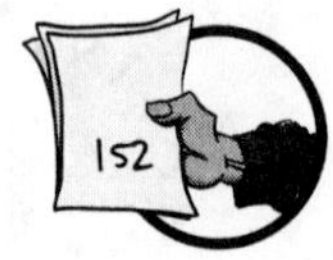

activity 12 We Have Things in Common

time 30 minutes.

purpose This activity gives students the opportunity to meet and get to form personal connections with other students. This activity can also be used as an icebreaker with new students.

materials The "Human Scavenger Hunt" handout and a pencil.

process Give each student a copy of the "Human Scavenger Hunt" handout and tell them to collect signatures from those people in the class who meet the request on the worksheet. Encourage the students to get details and additional information concerning each person they collect for their list.

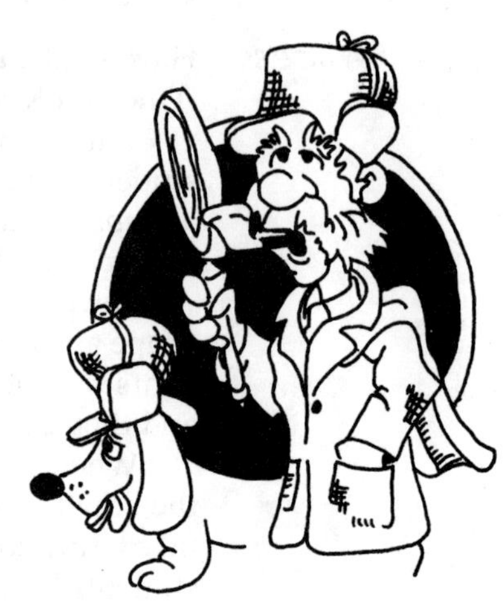

When the time period is over (usually about 10 to 15 minutes will be enough), have students sit in their seats or in a circle. Students then share their answers by taking turns with each category. Encourage them to share the details they discovered about each other. You will all get to know each other a little better during this activity; some of the interesting information that is revealed can be quite surprising.

activity 13 Life Map

time 45–55 minutes.

purpose This lesson gives the students an opportunity to look at their strengths, achievements, and goals as they record various "landmarks" in their lives.

materials Large drawing paper or poster paper, colored pencils, crayons, or markers, and the "Life Map" handout to use as an example.

process Say to the students, "You are going to make a map of your life today. Think back over the things that have happened in your life. Think about the events that have made the biggest impact on you in either a positive way or a negative way. These events have been important in shaping you into the individual and special person that you are today.

"Think also about your future. What would you like to happen in the future? How do you want to live? What special trips do you want to take? Do you want to get married? Do you have a family planned? Are you going to continue in school? How will you earn a living?"

Have students brainstorm events for the past and future. Include things like graduations, awards, jobs, marriage, children, trips, owning a certain car or house, and retirement.

After handing out materials, tell students to start from their earliest memory and record remarkable events using pictures, street signs, or symbols. Tell students to leave room between each symbol so that they can include more things as they recall them. They should make this record of their life as complete as possible, including positive and painful events. Use the "Life Map" handout as an example.

Have students identify the place on their map that shows their current age, then start developing the events they plan to have happen in the future. Refer to the list that the class brainstormed for possibilities for the future.

Remind students to be creative in their method of displaying their life maps. I have seen maps portrayed as links in a chain, burning candles with each drop of wax signifying an event, buildings under construction with each girder representing an event that supports the rest of the structure or life, and a road map with signposts along the way.

hints I allow students to talk while they are doing this assignment because they seem to share experiences and feelings about various events they are recording with others in the group. It is also a great opportunity to ask about things that are being portrayed on the maps. Students are able to share their lives with you and be recognized.

follow-up If time allows, give students the opportunity to present their Life Maps to the rest of the class. Remind students that they have the right to pass if they choose. Life Maps can also be displayed in the room.

activity 14 This Is How I See Myself

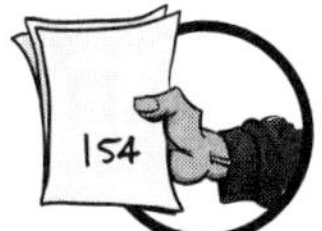

time 20–30 minutes.

purpose By allowing students a chance to focus on various characteristics and to compare those traits to their own lives, students will get a better understanding of themselves.

materials Pencils and the handout entitled "This is How I See Myself."

process Hand out the activity sheet and explain or ask for students' definitions for each of the descriptive characteristics listed on the page.

Explain that the students are to think about how each quality applies to their own lives and to their personalities.

Then give the students time to rank the characteristics on the continuum at the bottom of the page as the characteristics apply to their own personalities. The left side of the continuum is for qualities that are highly descriptive of them, and the right side of the continuum is for qualities that they feel do not apply. All the qualities and characteristics should be used on the continuum.

Ask the students for their reactions.

activity 15 You're My Kind of Person

time 20–30 minutes.

purpose This lesson provides an opportunity to acknowledge an individual's good deeds. Not only will that person's self-esteem be rewarded but the person offering the acknowledgment will also feel good because they have made a positive connection with another person. Students will learn how to receive a compliment gracefully.

materials Cut out the awards from the "You're My Kind of Person" handout. A pencil or pen will be needed. Students could even design their own rewards.

process Begin the lesson with a discussion of compliments. Guide the discussion toward the good that a supportive compliment can provide. Discuss the harm that can come from a hurtful comment, and reinforce the need for students to support each other in positive ways.

Have students then get into small groups of four or five, and give them the awards on the handout sheet. Every student should have one note for each of the members in their group.

Tell the students that each person will be given 1 minute to tell a story of a time they did something nice for another person. The teacher should time the storytelling period and allow 1 minute after each story for the members of the group to write a positive, supportive comment about the person telling the story. Each student should sign his or her name to the bottom of the award, but hold the note until the end of the activity.

After each person has told a story and all the notes are written on the awards, the students will distribute the awards they have written on to the individuals in their group. Allow time for students to read and talk to each other about the notes they receive.

follow-up Vary the individuals in the groups each time you do this activity. Have students think of different stories, or vary the topics to include:

- A time I felt really helpful
- The bravest thing I have ever done
- A time I felt really needed

hints You can do a variation of this activity by handing out paper plates to each person in class. All the students write their name on the plate. While you play music, have the students sit in a circle and pass the plates in one direction. When the music stops, each person will write a positive or complimentary comment on the plate he or she is holding. Continue the activity until there are about 10 opportunities to write compliments. Return the plates to their owners. This variation should be done only with students who know each other well and have worked together because they won't have problems thinking of something to write.

Set aside a day to thank people who have been especially helpful or pleasant. Ask students to think of people who they admire and would like to thank for being such good role models. Make cards thanking those people or thank them verbally on this day.

reminder It is important to have a discussion concerning positive and negative comments before you pass the plates so that no one receives a hurtful message when his or her plate is returned. Emphasize the good that a positive comment can have on a person's life and the harm that can come from a careless, hurtful comment. Write some examples of compliments during the discussion so that the students get a good idea of what is expected.

activity 16 Each Person's Best Point

time 40 minutes.

purpose This is one of my favorite activities. It promotes creativity, laughter, fun, cooperation, and self-esteem. This activity also increases the students' awareness of each other and of themselves as others might see them.

materials Large pieces of butcher paper or tag board and markers or crayons.

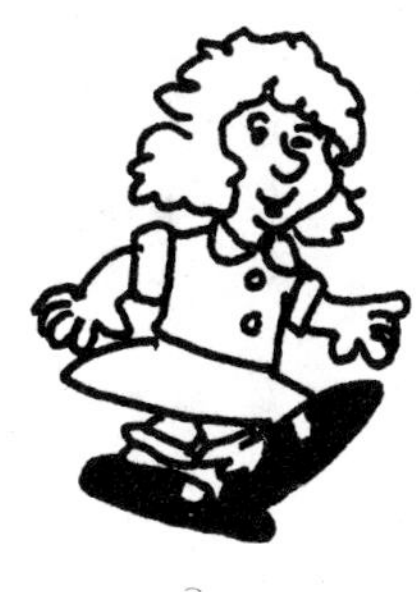

process This activity is similar to Activity 6, "Cooperative Creature," but the students will be drawing a person made up of the collective physical assets of each member of the group. In small groups of about four to six, have the students take time to look at each other closely without talking. Tell them, "You will be drawing an imaginary person. This person will be made up of the best features contributed from each member of the group. The group must discuss only the good characteristics from each person and make a list of the characteristics that will be used on their collective drawing. The person modeling the characteristic will be the person to draw that part on the imaginary person."

Allow enough time for students to share ideas and talk as they work to complete their drawing. The imaginary person should display at least two characteristics from each member of the group.

Part of the fun is sharing the drawings with the rest of the class, having each group describe the characteristic on the imaginary person and why those traits were chosen.

activity 17 Unforgettable!

time 10–45 minutes, depending on the size of the class or group.

purpose This activity allows students an opportunity to get to know each other. Each student also gets a chance to develop investigative techniques in interviewing and to see how good their imagination is in presenting or stretching the facts they receive.

materials Paper, pencil, imagination, curiosity, and a sense of humor.

process Students will act as investigative reporters while interviewing another student. Have students get a partner they do not know well.

Each member of the partnership will be given 5–7 minutes to find out all they can about the other person. The reporter will keep track of all information he or she collects about the other person and then construct a description that will make that person unforgettable to the rest of the class.

When time is up, the partners switch roles and the second person becomes the reporter.

Allow time for the partners to introduce each other to the rest of the class. Emphasize the need to make the person they are introducing unforgettable. Also remind students that this is to be a positive experience, so introductions should compliment their partner.

hint I like to use this activity at the beginning of a class with a new bunch of students. It is fun and allows everyone a chance to find out more about each other.

If time is important, have students present their partners in smaller groups. The more imaginative and creative these introductions are, the more fun and memorable the people become. You might model the activity with a student before the interviews begin to give students the idea. Take a fact and stretch it to fantastic fiction.

activity 18 It's Important to Me!

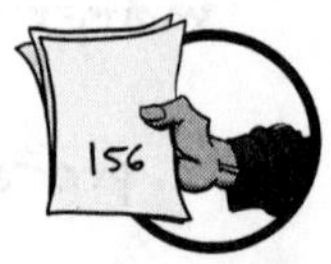

time 20–30 minutes.

purpose This activity provides students an opportunity to examine their values. They can compare their values with those of other students and develop an appreciation of the choices they make.

This activity also gives the students an opportunity to gain more self-confidence by speaking informally to the class.

materials The handout entitled "It's Important to Me!"

process Preface the activity with remarks and discussion concerning values. Are values and valuable things the same thing or different? Explain how the things you value tell us something about your values.

Begin the activity by pointing out that we all have things in our homes that are extremely important to us, and in an emergency we would save those things above all the others. Explain that they are going to experience an imaginary emergency, and they will have only a few minutes to save whatever they can from their homes.

Hand out the worksheets and give the students time to answer the questions. If you are working with students who are too young or unable to write, present the activity orally and allow each person time to think about and then share their choices with the rest of the class.

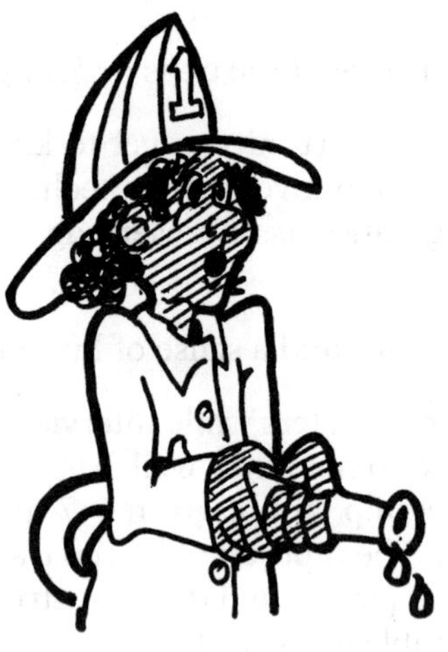

Allow time for the students to share the answers on the worksheet with the rest of the class or in small groups. Ask the students to explain why they made that choice and why it is important to them. Students should have the right to pass on sharing with the whole class.

Remind students that everyone has different values and so will choose different things that will be important to save. There is no incorrect answer and other people's values should be honored and respected. Not everyone thinks the same way, and those differences need to be acknowledged.

activity 19 This Is How I Feel

157

time 20 minutes.

purpose This activity enables individuals to recognize and acknowledge some of their feelings.

materials The handout entitled "This Is How I Feel" and a pencil or pen.

process Hand out the worksheet and ask students to seriously consider how they feel as they answer the questions on the worksheet. Ask them to go back and look at their answers when they have completed the paper.

When the papers are complete or handed in for homework, ask the students if they were surprised at themselves for some of the answers they put down and why.

activity 20 Promote Yourself

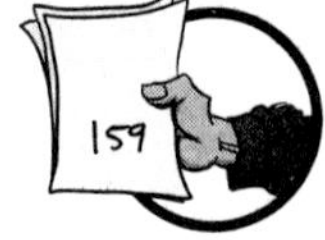

time 20 minutes.

purpose Students need to have a chance to look at their outstanding qualities and then be able to brag and be recognized for those qualities.

materials The "Promote Yourself" handout, a pencil, and a strong ego.

process Explain to students that they are going to have a chance to brag about themselves. They will make a poster, billboard, radio announcement, or commercial promoting their outstanding qualities.

Give students the handout and allow them time to create.

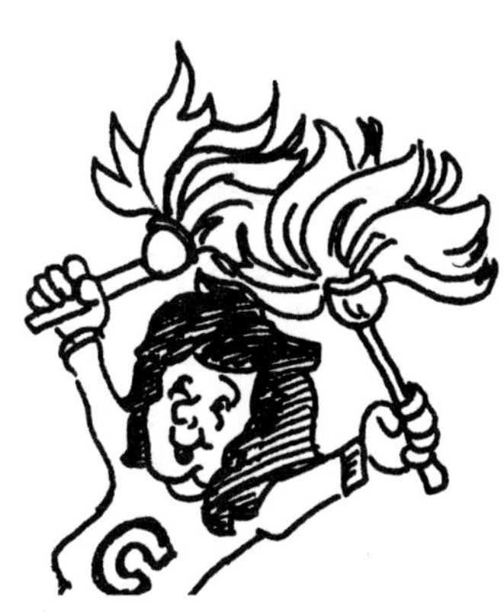

Students can then present their work to the class. Do not force students to demonstrate their work if they feel uncomfortable, but encourage them to share with the class.

You can also have students present their work in small groups. Each student in a group of four or five will be given 1–2 minutes to show and explain his or her work to the group members. This uses less class time and sometimes allows students to feel more comfortable sharing with a small group of peers.

activity 21 An Important Party

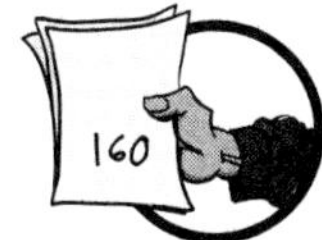

time 30 minutes.

purpose This activity gives students an opportunity to look at their values by identifying important people and influences in their lives.

materials The handouts entitled "An Important Party" and "Questions about Your Party" and a pencil.

process Preface the activity with remarks about how the people in our lives can have important influences on our behaviors and the choices we make.

Hand out the activity sheet "An Important Party."

Tell the students that they are going to host a party and that they can invite 11 other people. They are to pick any 7 people in the world they admire, but they must also pick 4 people they do not like. Include reasons why they made their choices.

After choosing the 11 people, students now have to seat these people around the table. Remind the students to seat themselves also. It is a good idea to use initials when they designate the seats, and they should not announce the people that they dislike to others in the class. They should be able to explain why the people are seated in the order chosen.

Then have students answer the questions on the second worksheet concerning their choices.

Discuss the students' reactions to the party. Students may share some of their choices of people they like and tell why they admire those people. Ask them how these choices reflect on them.

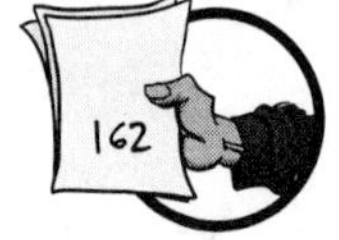

activity 22 Build a Firm Foundation

time 20–30 minutes.

purpose Placing all their strengths, dreams, and experiences in one activity can be revealing and empowering for some students. Sharing the process and the end result with other students in the class can help students get to know and appreciate one another.

materials The handout entitled "Build a Firm Foundation" and a pencil or pen.

process Hand out a copy of the worksheet to each student.

Explain that they are going to be writing or drawing in response to your instructions. They should not worry about the quality of their artistic ability. The point is that they know what is represented by their efforts.

Give the following instructions for the drawings, allowing 2 or 3 minutes for the students to complete the work:

- Space number 1 could be considered the foundation on which you base your life. In that space, indicate the person or event that has been most important in helping you develop your values. (Examples might be values such as loyalty, honesty, courage, perseverance. Remind the students that this is from their point of view and other people's thoughts should not interfere.)
- Fill the frame of your house, or space number 2, with the people or things that you use for support during difficult times in your life.
- Space number 3 is the insulation and should be filled with the people or things that protect you or make you feel secure as you go through life.
- Space number 4 is the electrical connections in your life that give you energy and a sense of excitement.
- The plumbing is space number 5. Indicate the things in your life that help you get rid of bad or hurtful experiences.
- The siding is the outward appearance of a house and is space number 6. Indicate how the world sees you or how you present yourself to others.
- Space number 7 is for the windows. What do you want to see as you look out these windows and go through life? What are your hopes and dreams for the future?
- The roof, space number 8, covers your attic, which should be filled with something big that you have always wanted to do or experience

in life. Don't limit yourself to things that are realistic—go for your wildest dreams!

- The decoration on the house is space number 9 and is what makes the house unique. What is it that makes you special and unique?
- Space number 10 is the antenna or satellite dish that brings information to your house. What do you feel very knowledgeable about?

Give students time to share their houses with others in small groups. Remind students that each person has the right to share just part of their house or to pass completely.

follow-up This can also be done as homework and made into a larger project by asking students to put this on poster paper, expressing each category with drawings, photographs, magazine cutouts, or symbolic items.

These projects, big or small, can be shared with the whole class by asking eac[illegible] house.

activity 23 H[illegible]

163

time Tw[illegible]

purpose Stu[illegible] of various birth order positio[illegible] their lives. They will also rec[illegible] order, has certain needs that mu[illegible]

materials Lar[illegible] th Order" handouts, and a pen[illegible]

process Tell[illegible] ance to "unload" their feelings[illegible] es.

DA[illegible] r ahead of time by breaking it i[illegible] eled "Only Children," the next

You may Not Like [illegible]
(what with the weight of th
But R[illegible]
Having a younger [illegible]
SCIEN[illegible]
OF
★ YOUR VERY OWN ★

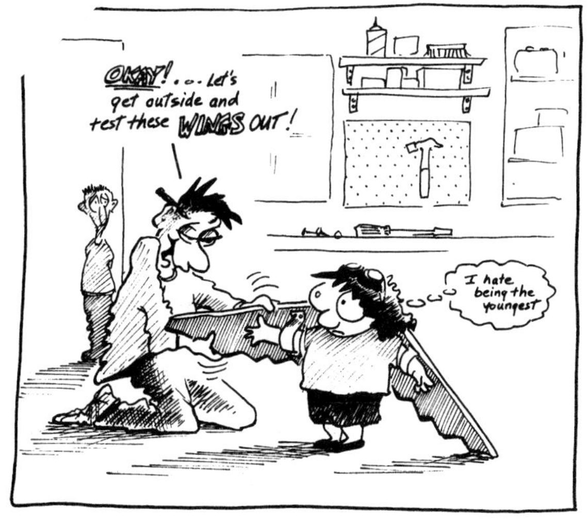

OKAY! ... Let's get outside and test these WINGS OUT!
I hate being the youngest

is labeled "First Born," the next is "Middle Children," and the last section is labeled "Youngest Children." Have a lot of chalk or markers available so that many students can be writing at the same time.

Begin class by presenting the idea that the order a person is born into their family could have an important impact on their life. Each person's birth order implies different privileges, responsibilities, and disadvantages that can affect an individual as he or she grows up. Let all students get an opportunity to tell what they like or dislike about their order of birth.

Tell the students that they will have about 5 minutes to come up to the board/butcher paper and write what they like or hate about their order of birth. Some students may fit into two or more categories because of changing dynamics within a family. They may write in the categories into which they feel they best fit.

hint I find that allowing a large group up at once is helpful because the students will talk to each other and share feelings that they may not write down. The time can be noisy, however, so be prepared and be tolerant.

Have everyone sit down again and then read the results for each category of birth order. Using the "Birth Order Factors and Personality Traits" fact sheet from the study done by *Parents* magazine, lead a discussion comparing the class results with the results of the formal study. Allow students to share personal experiences that support the findings.

DAY TWO Review the information from the study done by *Parents* magazine and remind students of their own discussion the previous day. Pass out the "Birth Order Interview" handout.

Students will use this worksheet to interview five different people about their birth order. They can take the rest of the class period to complete the interview. Directions for the paper are as follows:

- Place the name of the person to be interviewed in the large boxes that are numbered.
- Ask and record how many children there are in the interviewee's family.
- Ask and record the birth order of the interviewee using the categories suggested in the formal study: only children, first born, middle children, and youngest children.
- Place a check in the appropriate box that illustrates the interviewee's personality traits.

After completing the interview, they need to look at the answers given by the people they interviewed and think about what they know about those people personally. Then refer to the "Birth Order Factors and Personality Traits" handout and compare each interviewee with the traits proposed in the study. They should explain briefly why each person does or does not fit the characteristics of their birth order.

DAY THREE Pass out the "Meeting Needs" handout.

As a class, in small groups, or individually, determine the needs of people born in each order of birth. Use the study presented by *Parents* magazine for reference. Write the needs of each group in the appropriate space on the worksheet.

In the same work group, determine how parents can best meet those needs. Write the answers in the appropriate spaces on the worksheet.

activity

24 Goals

time 40 minutes.

purpose This activity helps establish classroom behavior practices that students will want to follow because they establish the behaviors as goals rather than as rules. Because their peers decide on acceptable behaviors, individuals will be more likely to go along with them.

materials Chalkboard and chalk or butcher paper and markers.

process Lead a class discussion on what students see as the purpose of your class and what they would like to achieve in the class. Allow time for each volunteer to speak, and emphasize the variety of answers. Goals for learning may include grades, prerequisites for college, or intellectual growth.

Students will be working in small groups consisting of four or five people and should keep in mind that they will be writing goals for the whole class. Explain that goals should be written in the present tense and there are certain steps they need to follow in making goals:

- Set a clear goal that is *very* specific in the action required. Describe only one small step at a time.
- Make sure the individual has control over achieving the goal.
- The goal should be a positive change or behavior.

Explain the purpose of a school classroom and that the goals should work toward achieving that purpose. Remind students that this is not a wish list for gum chewing and eating in class but a workable, practical set of goals for achieving the purpose of the class. An example of a good general goal would be to allow teachers to teach and students to learn in a congenial and productive atmosphere. Give students about 10 minutes to brainstorm and record goals that would work best in the classroom to establish a positive learning environment.

Give each group a large piece of butcher paper on which to display the goals that they agree will be most beneficial.

Make a large continuum on the butcher paper or blackboard. Have each group present their "best" goal and then as a class, vote on where that goal will be located on a continuum of most helpful to least helpful.

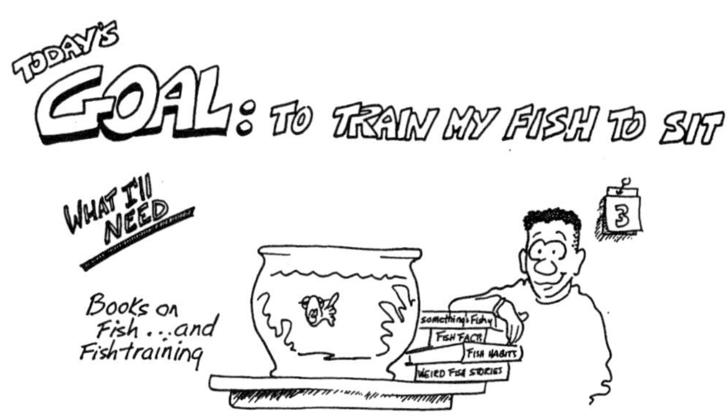
TODAY'S
GOAL: TO TRAIN MY FISH TO SIT
WHAT I'LL NEED
Books on Fish . . . and Fish training
FISH FACTS
FISH HABITS
WEIRD FISH STORIES
3

least helpful ———————— most helpful

Have students share their choices for goals until you get a good sampling. Finally, have students decide on five goals that they think will work best in the class.

As a class, decide what some of the consequences would be for each goal if there are students who choose not to work toward the goals established by the class.

hint When students complain about having to do a particular activity or assignment, ask *them* what they think the purpose of the lesson is. They will accept the assignment much better when they hear the purpose from one of their own rather than from you.

When students misbehave, call their attention to the goals set by the class and ask them if they are working toward those goals.

activity 25 Journal Topics

time 15–20 minutes per class period. This activity can be presented each day, once a week, or occasionally.

purpose The topics presented for essays will help students identify and evaluate their values and viewpoints. This activity gives studens a chance to practice their writing skills and expand their imagination.

materials All the students should have a notebook or composition book in which to keep their essays. They will also need a pen or pencil.

process Choose a topic from the list below or create a topic that would be appropriate for your students. Write the essay topic on the board and allow students time to discuss their ideas about the topic.

Have the students write a brief but thoughtful essay or poem on the topic presented. They can expand their creativity by illustrating their writings.

JOURNAL TOPICS

- How would you spend a million dollars?
- Describe a conflict you had with a member of your family.
- Write about an interesting dream you had.
- How would life be different if there were no four-wheeled vehicles?
- Write about the time you made a new friend.
- Describe an accident you had.
- Describe an interesting gift you received.
- Write about something you did that made you feel proud.
- Write a letter to your favorite character in history.
- Describe in detail your favorite meal.
- Describe the different ways you have worn your hair as you matured.
- Describe what you like most about your favorite person?
- How do you celebrate your favorite holiday?

note If you have students who are too young to write about these topics, have them discuss the topics as a class. Students get excited about having time to tell their own stories. These are also good topics to use in the "Share A Story" activity (Activity 7 in this chapter).

activity 26 I Have Responsibilities

time 10–15 minutes.

purpose All people need to recognize their own responsibility in the actions they choose.

materials The handout entitled "I Have Responsibilities" and a pen or pencil.

process Discuss the possibility that every privilege comes with a responsibility. In order to be trusted, people must prove they are trustworthy. In order to be liked, people must be friendly and kind.

Hand out the activity sheet and explain that they are to write down their responsibility resulting from each privilege listed. They may be allowed to discuss their answers with others or in small groups, because this discussion will allow them to see other points of view. Many times students will end up instructing each other in the importance of a particular responsibility.

activity 27 Important Events That Shaped My Life

time 45 minutes, or this activity could be used as a formal writing assignment and stretched out over several class periods.

purpose This activity allows students an opportunity to look at their own lives and recognize the important events that have shaped their personalities and molded them into the unique individuals they are today.

materials An imagination, a good memory, and paper and a pencil.

process Have students think about events in their lives that come to mind easily. These events might be good or bad in their estimation.

Remind the students that even terrible events leave a lasting impression on our lives and make an impact on our personalities. The students should pick the five events they feel are the most important in developing them as an individual. They should pick events that they don't mind sharing with you or with other people, because these essays may be seen by others. They will then write about those events in their lives and tell how the events have changed them.

Encourage them to write in whatever style you feel appropriate or to include pictures, awards, or snapshots that help tell their story.

hints These essays are often quite personal even though you have warned the students that other people may see them. Be careful not to share an essay with anyone else before asking the students' permission or you may jeopardize their trust in you.

warning Sometimes students will reveal information about themselves or their families that will require help or treatment by outside professionals. Make sure the students know from the beginning that you are required by law to report instances of sexual or physical abuse or behaviors that lead you to believe the students may harm themselves. If abusive situations are revealed, talk to the student and persuade him or her to allow you to share the story with a school counselor, nurse, or appropriate person at your school.

activity 28 This Is Me!

time After collecting materials from home, it may take about 30 to 45 minutes.

purpose This is a fun activity that allows students to recognize the elements of their lives and what makes them a unique individual. In sharing the posters, students recognize similarities and acknowledge differences in others.

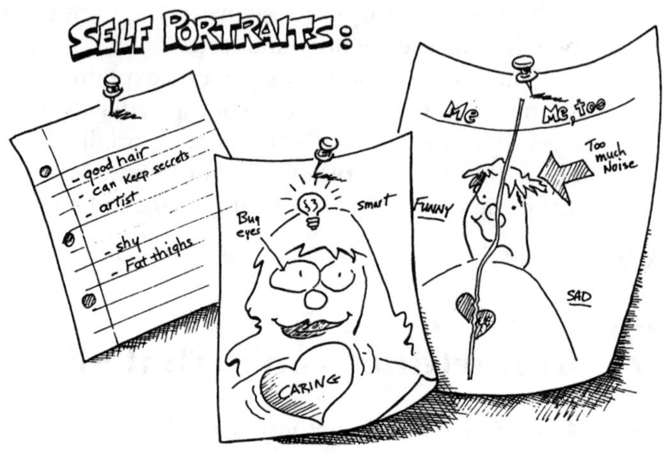

The presentation of their work will provide experience in public speaking and give students a chance to be the object of attention for a short period of time. Leaving the posters up for a while will focus attention back on each student.

materials Large poster paper or butcher paper for each student, markers, scissors, glue, and, of course, imagination and creativity. A large empty wall is helpful for displaying the end results.

process Give students time to collect pictures, awards or ribbons, class work, travel brochures, magazine pictures, and symbols of their lives. They are to collect items that will help others know more about them—what they like to do, their hopes for their future, their likes and dislikes, how they spend most of their time, and so forth.

Have students bring in their collection and give them about 30 minutes to assemble the items in a picture or display that best describes them. Emphasize that these collages will be shown to other people in the class and may be on display for parents.

Display all of the collages. Over the next few weeks, allow the first few minutes of class for presentation of the collages. Randomly choose three or four students each day to present their collages. Remind students of the importance of respecting others' work and the differences in each person's life.

hints I have found that it is a good idea for the teacher or other adults working with the students to participate in this activity along with the students. Make and present your own collage. Remember, you are a role model for kids, and they want to know more about you, too.

activity
29 My Life

time This activity may take several days using 10–15 minutes of each class.

purpose This activity will give the students a chance to review thoughts, memories, goals, aspirations, and possibilities for their future. It is a good way to get students to think about what they would like to do with their lives.

materials The "This Is My Life" handout, glue or tape, scissors, and a pen or pencil.

process Give each student the handout. Students will need to collect some of the items required. They will supply actual events and adventures from their own lives up to their current age. They can fill in goals, dreams, and predictions for their future as they work on the timeline.

Give students time each day to work on their timeline. This assignment is better if stretched over several days because it gives students a chance to form thoughtful answers.

These timelines can be displayed or presented to the class.

activity
30 Oh Look! It's Me!

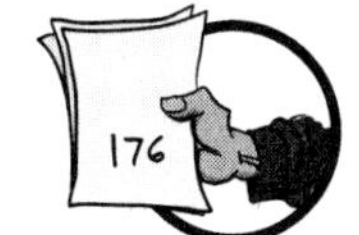

time 20 minutes.

purpose The students are given an opportunity to see how people's behavior might be affected by the opinion they have of themselves.

materials The handout entitled "Oh Look! It's Me!" and a pencil or pen.

process Tell students that they will need their imagination for this activity. They will only have about 5 minutes to write once they hear the directions.

Ask students to take a look at themselves with caring and kindness, as a friend would see them. Tell them:

> "Pretend that you can see yourself sitting in the shade against a tree. You seem to be sitting thoughtfully, kind of daydreaming. I want you to describe yourself. What do you look like? Describe in detail all the important things about your physical body that make you different and unique from everyone else. Remember to include that cute dimple, your special smile, the way your hands look, those legs that keep getting longer, the shape of your face, your latest hair style that never goes the way you want it to. Include even that little freckle that very few people know about."

When the students finish their description, give them the second page in the handout and ask them to answer the questions.

follow-up Ask students to share how they feel after completing the activity.

Collect the descriptions the students wrote and then randomly pick one to read to the class without revealing the author. See if the class can recognize the owner through their description.

WARNING: Only do this if you have told the students ahead of time that you may be sharing the descriptions with the class. The sharing sometimes leads to uneasy feelings if done without prior approval from students because these are very personal views of themselves and not really open for interpretation.

Read Virginia Satir's "My Declaration of Self-Esteem" as a conclusion to this activity. Students will leave the class with a positive impression of self even if the activity made them feel uneasy.

MY DECLARATION OF SELF-ESTEEM

I AM ME
In all the world, there is no one else exactly like me.
Everything that comes out of me is authentically mine
Because I alone chose it—I own everything about me
My body, my feelings, my mouth, my voice, all my actions,
Whether they be to others or myself—I own my fantasies,
My dreams, my hopes, my fears—I own all my triumphs and
Successes, all my failure and mistakes Because I own all of
Me, I can become intimately acquainted with me—by doing so
I can love me and be friendly with me and all my parts—I know
There are aspects about myself that puzzle me, and other
Aspects that I do not know—but as long as I am
Friendly and loving to myself, I can courageously
And hopefully look for solutions to the puzzles
And for ways to find out more about me However I
Look and sound, whatever I say and do, and whatever
I think and feel at any given moment in time is authentically
Me—If later some parts of how I looked, sounded, thought,
And felt turn out to be unfitting, I can discard that which is
Unfitting, keep the rest, and invent something new for that
Which I have discarded—I can see, hear, feel, think, say, and do
I have the tools to survive, to be close to others, to be productive,
And to make sense and order out of the world of
People and things outside of me—I own me, and therefore
I can engineer me—I am me and
I AM OKAY

—VIRGINIA SATIR

activity 31 Good Deeds and Community Service

Every job is a self-portrait of the person who did it.

—AUTHOR UNKNOWN

time Only the time you take to explain the project.

purpose This project promotes a sense of pride and well-being while providing the opportunity to be of help to others.

materials None.

process In this activity you will be enticing students to do a good deed of which they can feel proud. Pride brings a sense of satisfaction and confidence. Self-respect is earned and improves as pride in oneself increases. Give students the opportunity to gain pride in their own actions and improve their feeling of worth.

Explain to the class that a good deed is something done for somebody else without an expectation of anything in return. People often receive the behavior they give, so if someone is being kind and helpful, people may begin noticing and be kind and helpful to that person. Explain that good deeds can be expanded to include the community, schools, churches, scout troops, or friends. Find some way to help people on a regular basis.

Brainstorm a list of activities or services that meet the criteria for a community service project. This step is important in establishing boundaries for the project. Tell students that if they want to do something that is not included on the list, they need to clear it with you before using it in this project.

Have students keep track of their community service on a calendar and read over the list every once in a while. Students can try to achieve the goal of recording future service on their calendar.

Remind the students that they are helping out, expecting nothing in return. This service benefits more than the other person—it really benefits them. Their reward is a feeling of having helped, of being of some worth, and of knowing that other people appreciate them.

The highest reward for a person's toil is not what they get for it, but what they become by it.

—JOHN RUSKIN

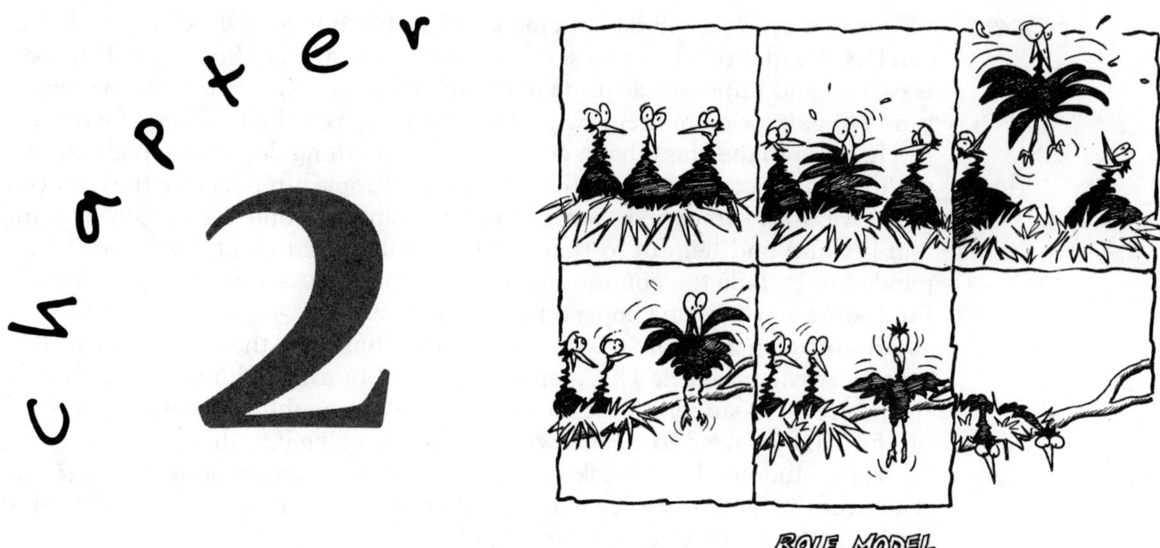

chapter 2

Relationships

Teenagers are at a developmental stage in life when relationships are very important—and complicated. Self worth is often influenced by the degree to which a person feels accepted and needed by other people.

On entering adolescence, teenagers will still listen to and depend on parents and adults for guidance, although they are probably beginning to rely more and more on role models and friends for support. Teenagers are like little birds trying to leave the nest—they are beginning to flutter their wings while watching the other birds to see how to fly.

Middle adolescence is a time of testing values and making decisions. Friends are important at this stage because of the support they offer. The group supplies the confidence needed to break the ties with parents and to begin taking on the responsibilities of being an adult. Growth occurs both physically and emotionally. All these physical and emotional changes cause a great deal of anxiety, so it is important that there is a support system made up of positive people who can share that passage through adolescence.

Oddly enough, in late adolescence teens will begin to return to the comfort and support of parents and family, but they do so as a peer. They have gained confidence and acceptance outside their family and now can accept family members and be accepted by them as an equal.

This chapter provides activities that will help teenagers develop relationships and confidence that will assist them in those early and middle adolescent years. These activities will allow students to see that they are changing and to discover what they can do to connect with others. If students can see themselves as competent and respected individuals, their opinion of themselves will grow. As they earn more self-respect, they will gain more confidence and lose that feeling of awkwardness that seems to follow and trap teenagers.

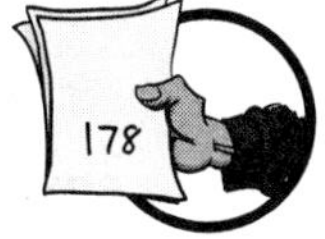

activity 1 Getting to Know You

time 20–45 minutes.

purpose Students have a chance to share ideas with each other while learning more about the people in their group. This is a good introduction or icebreaker activity.

materials The handout entitled "Getting to Know You."

process Have students introduce themselves to the group and reveal one important thing about themselves. Then have them fill out the answers on the left side of the page on the "Getting to Know You" handout.

The students then get a partner. You may want to number kids off and have even numbered students pick from the odd numbered students, or have them get in a line according to birthdays and be partners with the person to their left.

Have the students fold their paper in half so the answers do not show. Exchange papers and have the partner answer the questions on the right side of the paper.

When this is completed, allow about 3 to 5 minutes for the pairs to compare the answers on their papers and talk about the similarities and differences between their answers.

Ask the students to make a list with their partner of at least five things they have in common and five ways in which they are different.

follow-up If you have time, it is always fun to have the partners share their findings with the whole group. If time is short, have three sets of partners group together and share their findings with the small group. That way they all feel like they have shared but it does not take much time.

hints This activity may meet with some resistance at first. Most students want to get to know each other better, so with a little prodding, they will get going. It really

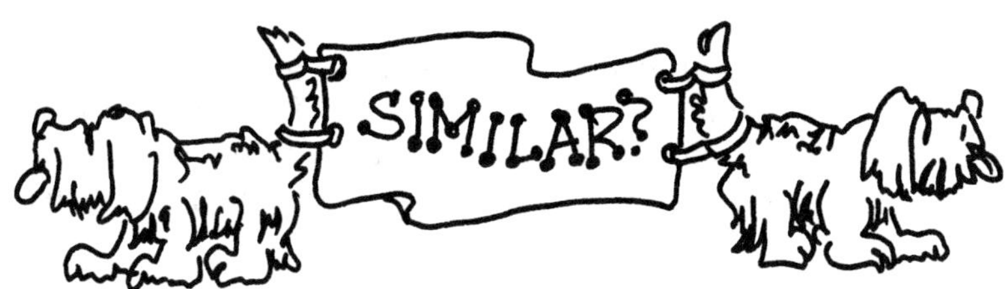

does not matter if some of the more macho kids make fun of this as they work. They are still participating, and the other students get to know exactly who they are by their behavior. Allow for variation. Sometimes the students may come up with creative ways of doing this activity.

activity 2 Ingredients for Friendship

In order to have a good friend, you must BE a good friend.

—ANONYMOUS

time 15 minutes.

purpose Students will recognize that what other students feel is important in a friendship and will evaluate their own impressions of friends and friendship.

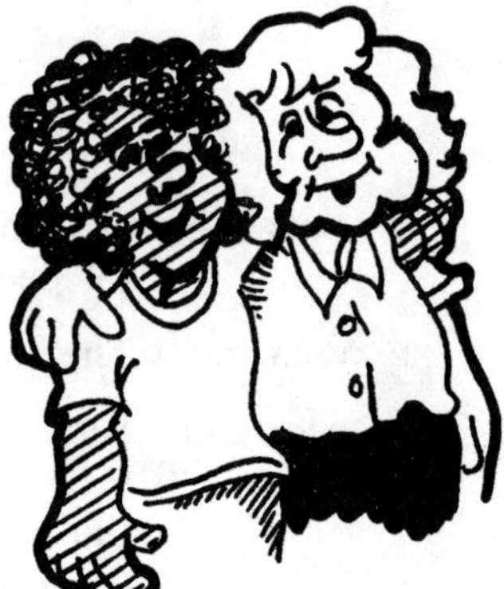

materials Large sheets of butcher paper, markers for each small work group, and blackboard and chalk.

process Students work in small groups of four to six students. Each group should be given a sheet of butcher paper and a marker to record ideas.

Ask students to think about a person in their life who has been their *best* friend. Have them think about what they really like or admire about that friend. List the things that make that person their best friend. Allow for some discussion. Suggest that the marker circulate among the group so that each person makes a contribution to the developing list.

When the list is complete, ask each group to pick two or three of the suggestions for a good friendship and write them on the blackboard. When the blackboard list is completed, ask if there is any discussion or disagreement about some of the contributions. Discuss the meaning of each of the terms and the responsibilities of each. Explain (or have students explain) what each would look like in a friendship.

The items listed below are some of the characteristics described as ingredients to friendship:

trust	confidence	honesty
dependable	understanding	loyalty
listen to you	care for you	support you
sense of humor	considerate	back you up

As students interact in class and develop friendships, remind them of the essential ingredients that go into friendships and that there are responsibilities involved in being a friend. Help students make friends by giving them many opportunities to interact, work together, and better understand each other.

activity 3 Making Friends

time 15–20 minutes.

purpose This activity offers students the opportunity to improve their skills in making friends and being a friend.

materials Large butcher paper and markers or a blackboard and chalk and the handout entitled "Most Wanted."

process Begin the activity with a reminder that there are several important ingredients to being a good friend. Being a good friend is a responsibility and takes practice. Some of the skills needed to be a good friend involve:

- the ability to develop trust, which involves keeping secrets
- empathizing with others, which involves understanding their needs and positions on various matters
- being able to communicate well with others in a nonthreatening way
- the ability to be a good listener

Have students offer their definitions for the words "trust," "empathy," "nonthreatening communication," and "good listener." Discuss the things that students can do to develop these skills. Make a heading on the blackboard or on large pieces of butcher paper for each of the skills that build friendships. Have students as a class or in small groups brainstorm ways they can demonstrate skill in each of the four areas.

Students can do the worksheet provided as reinforcement for this activity.

activity 4 My Circle of Support

time 30 minutes.

purpose This activity helps students recognize the influence they have on other people in their lives and the great influence those people have on them. Students will understand there is a responsibility that comes with this relationship.

materials The "Circle of Support" handout.

process Explain that many times the prominent people in our lives are great influences on our decisions. We also have an influence on those people.

If friends are all getting good grades, there will be pressure to get good grades to remain in the group. If friends are failing, then there is also a lot of pressure to fail to remain an accepted part of the group. The people who are prominent in our lives help shape our decisions, and therefore it is important who sits in our circle of support.

Give students the handout and explain that this activity will help them determine their circle of support. They should place the names or initials of their important people under each of the characters in the "Circle of Support" handout. Explain that they can be people in their family, friends, teachers, clergy, counselors, and other important individuals who help shape their decisions. Remind students that these supporters may be anyone who influences them or who they influence. Even role models and idols whom they have never met but admire influence their decisions.

Have the students place indicators next to the people in their circle of support as follows:

- Put a **star** next to any of those people they could go to in a time of need and know that they would help.
- **Circle** any of those people they wish they could go to for help. They may be inaccessible now because of distance or the development of their relationship.
- Place an **X** over anyone they wish they could kick out of their circle of support. They are either influenced too much by this person or are influencing this person too much. Allow students to acknowledge this need to recognize individuals who may be harmful in their lives.

Give an example of a recent important decision you made and illustrate how your own circle of support guided you in your decision. Remind students that you may rely on these people directly or indirectly.

Have students think of a decision they have made that took a great deal of thought. Use students' examples to help them see who they are relying on for support in making that decision. Help them think of the people who might have influenced them. Remind students that influence is often a two-way street.

Have students answer the questions at the bottom of the worksheet.

follow-up Have students in the group pick a recent incident that happened at school and explain how the individuals involved might have been influenced by people in their lives to act the way they did. Who might be in the circle of support for each of the participants to cause them to act the way they did?

hints I find there is often a need to discuss the person or people who were kicked off the circle of support. Students need reassurance that it is normal to have some negative influences in their lives and it is how they choose to deal with those relationships that is important. Have students brainstorm ways they can escape the influence of people in their lives who are harming them. If these people are members of the immediate family, the students might have to live with that person but they need to protect and insulate themselves in some way. They might spend time listening to music, writing a note to that person explaining their feelings and then rip it up, punch their pillow, join sports to get rid of physical frustration, or talk to friends—anything to make them feel better. If the student is a bad influence on someone, he or she might need to evaluate the relationship and try to improve his or her interactions with that person.

Leave students with the message that none of us get through life by ourselves. We all need other people for love and support. The people in their circle of support depend on the students just as the students depend on them. Our actions reflect on the people around us.

Remind students to go to the people in their circle of support when they need help, want to share their proud moments, or ask for help in carrying their burdens.

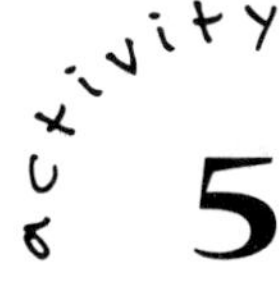

5 Making Friends

time This is a two-day lesson requiring about 20 minutes each day.

purpose This activity will give students some hints on how to build a friendship.

materials The handouts entitled "Friends" and "Talk to a Parent or Grandparent" for every student.

process Ask students to list the elements of a good and lasting friendship. Write the ideas on the board or on butcher paper.

DAY ONE Tell students there are basic skills to being a good friend. A person must work at friendship in order to make the relationship last. Have students tell you the skills needed to keep and be a good friend. List those ideas on the board.

One of the elements of being a good friend is keeping secrets. You may choose to use the role-play provided to demonstrate how easily people betray a confidence. You might want to use the role-play to open discussion concerning methods of keeping secrets.

Use the "Friends" handout and have the students think about a person whom they consider a good friend. Write that person's name in the top circle and then draw lines radiating outward to words that would describe this person or the friendship.

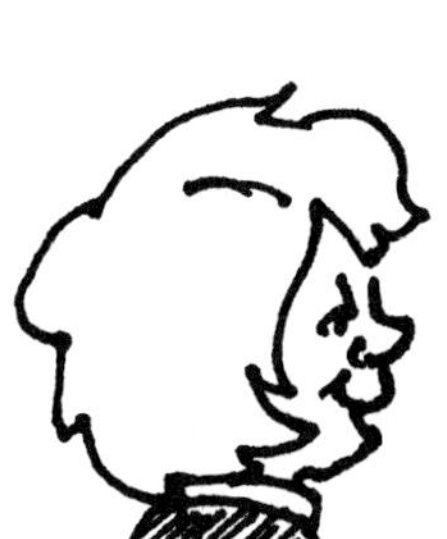

Students place their own names in the bottom circle and draw lines radiating outward to words that other people might use to describe them.

Next, tell the students that they are going to investigate friendship by interviewing people close to them. They will take the interview handout and ask a grandparent or a parent about close friends they have had through the years. If a parent or grandparent is not available, the student may interview another close and trusted adult.

DAY TWO When the interviews have been completed, ask students for their opinions and observations about friendship from the point of view of the people interviewed.

Some possible questions for discussion are:

- Why have the people you interviewed remained with their friends for so long?
- What were the important elements that made the friendship last?
- How are the people you interviewed influenced by their friends? Give some examples.
- Does friendship change as you get older? If so, how?
- Do the people you interviewed and their friends seem alike? Do they have similar characteristics? List the characteristics.

- Were you surprised by any of the answers people gave you or by any revelations as you were interviewing?
- What did you learn about friendships from these interviews?

ROLE-PLAY: CONFIDENCES

One night at a school dance, Maria told Gracy, her best friend, that she really liked Omar a lot. This was a secret. Maria didn't want anyone else to know.

The next morning Gracy and Estella had the following conversation:

Estella: I saw you with Maria telling secrets at the dance last night. What did Maria say? Come on, you can tell me. I can keep a secret.

Gracy: Estella, I can't tell you. Maria wants me to keep it a secret. I promised not to tell anyone.

Estella: Come on. Tell me—please. I won't tell anyone. I promise.

Gracy: Okay, if you really promise not to tell anyone else. Maria told me that she really likes Omar, but she doesn't want him to know. Please don't tell anyone. She will hate me if she finds out I told you.

Estella later told another friend, and that friend told someone else. Eventually Omar found out. What could Gracy have done?

activity 6 Friendships versus Values

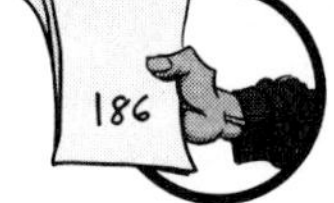

time This activity may cover two class periods.

purpose There are times when people's values may be in conflict with something friends ask them to do. This activity will help the students recognize those conflicts and learn how to deal with them.

materials You will need a blackboard or large butcher paper and the "Friendships versus Values" handout.

process **DAY ONE** Have students picture their best friend in their mind. Have them think of all the qualities that make that friendship different than a regular friendship. Ask students to share these qualities with the class as you list them on the board. (Some examples: helpful, loyal, caring, generous, supportive, playful, fun-loving, etc.)

Make another list of things that friends might ask of them. Try to elicit a wide range of ideas, from sharing lipstick to copying answers while taking a test. Ask the class to tell what qualities of friendship from the first list are required to fulfill the favors in the second list.

Ask students to select the favors that friends might ask of them that would cause problems. Giving answers during a test or borrowing a friend's new sweater might cause conflicts. Copy the list the students create.

DAY TWO Post the list of those favors that cause a conflict between friends. Discuss briefly why these favors make the students feel uncomfortable and how asking a favor like that affects the friendship.

Give students the "Friendships versus Values" handout and have them complete the worksheet on their own while thinking about a particular friend.

Students should discuss the following issues:

- What are your limits when it comes to friendship? What will you *not* agree to do for a friend? Why?

- Why will you do a favor for one friend and not do the same favor for another friend? (Like loaning money or clothing, helping with homework, or accepting advice about clothing?)
- Why do you feel more comfortable with some friends than with others?
- How can you keep your personal values and help out your friend?

follow-up Students get into small groups and rate the qualities they listed for friendship from most important to least important. Have a spokesperson from the group share their list with the rest of the class and explain why they agreed on that particular order. Compare the lists from the various small groups. Are certain qualities of friendship universally accepted as being the most important?

activity 7 Peer Pressures

188

time 15 minutes.

purpose This activity will help students recognize some of the positive and negative pressures and influences placed on them by peers.

materials A blackboard or large piece of butcher paper and markers if the activity is done as a group. Use the "Peer Pressures" handout if the activity is done individually.

process Have students define the terms *peer* and *pressure*. Explain that pressure can be quite obvious, such as when someone begs them to drink a beer. But pressure can be subtly imposed, for example, by hanging out with friends who are constantly drinking beer, even though they are not asking you to drink with them.

Students should brainstorm a list of both good and bad pressures that peers impose. Allow for some discussion because some pressure can be good or bad depending on who receives the pressure and how it is imposed. The whole point is to allow students to recognize pressures and evaluate them.

follow-up Allow students to share ways in which they have been pressured, both positively and negatively, by friends. How are they influenced by the media? The teen idols they revere?

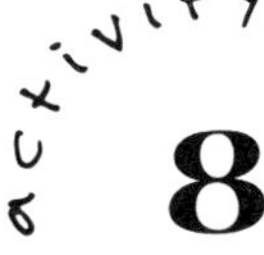

8 Peer Groups

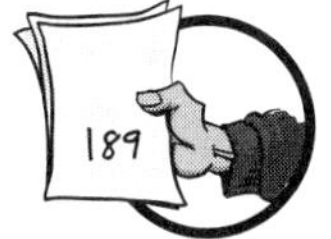

time 15–20 minutes (this is a good homework assignment).

purpose Students will recognize and acknowledge that different peer groups have different values and that the groups they choose to hang out with may influence their own behavior.

materials Handout entitled "Peer Groups" and good observation skills.

process Explain that the groups we join and the friends we have influence our values and our behavior. People are often labeled and stereotyped according to the friends they choose. Maybe this is why parents are so upset with some of the peer groups their children choose to hang out with.

Have students brainstorm all the different peer groups in their school. These groups may vary in name from region to region, but in my area of California we can identify many groupings of kids: stoners (druggies), preppies,

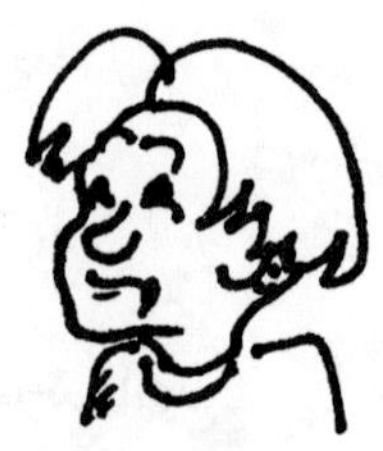

jocks, skaters (skateboarders), bladers (into roller blades), school boys/girls, nerds, geeks, gangsters, taggers (graffiti artists), cowboys/girls.

Have students discuss the characteristics of each group without becoming too negative. Remember that there are some conflicts and clashes between groups so kids might get defensive or offensive. Discuss the reasons for the conflicts between groups. Why would the jocks be antagonistic to the gangsters? Ask what images the groups project and what needs are being met by the people in those groups. Explain that we are not challenging the various groups, merely acknowledging their values and interests.

Give students the handout entitled "Peer Groups" and have them think about any one of the groups in their school. Tell students that they do not have to be in that group to report on it. They will then answer the questions about that group.

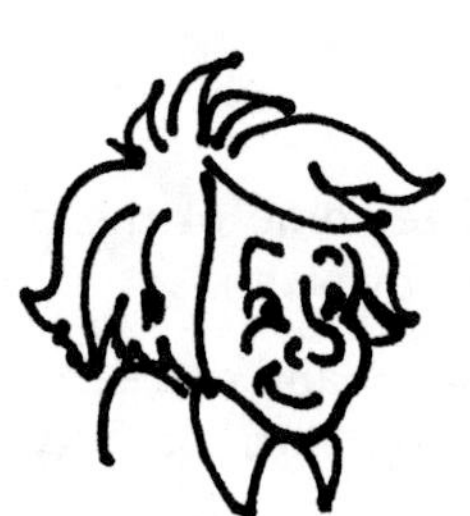

You might have students do this activity in small groups in which they can discuss the groups and the values they hold with other students in the class. A better understanding of the groups often occurs when students discuss this among themselves.

In closing, remind students that the groups we choose to join fill some of our needs and are a reflection of our personality and values. Students should think about the image portrayed by the groups they hang out with. Is this the image they choose for themselves?

follow-up When students bring their papers back after observing the peer group, have a discussion about the various groups. Put peer group headings on the board and make a list of the characteristics the students found. There may be some discussion as some of the students in that peer group disagree.

hints Be careful that students don't start labeling kids in the class. This happens at times and can be quite a surprise for some kids who think of themselves in a different way than the way they are labeled.

Keep the discussion general. List some of the groups represented in the class without naming anyone. Remember that the purpose of this activity is to acknowledge differences and create tolerance among groups. Try to show that each group has positive influences and that each group may compete with others because of conflicts in values. Remind students that it is perfectly natural for kids their age to hang out in groups. They gain confidence and support from their group as they challenge the obstacles to becoming an adult.

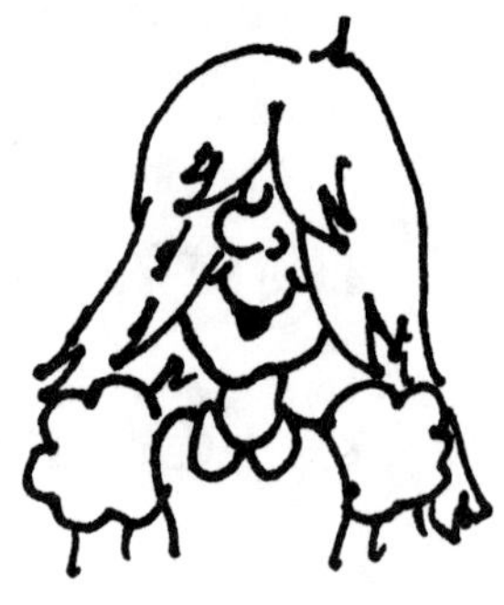

9 Role Model

190

time 20 minutes.

purpose This activity will allow students to acknowledge people they have chosen to be their role models and to examine the reasons these people are important to them.

materials The handouts entitled "My Role Model" and "Boaster Poster."

process Ask students to think about a person who has had a very positive influence in their lives. This should be someone they would like to emulate and who helps guide them even though they may not be physically present.

Unfortunately, there may be students who cannot think of a positive role model in their lives. Tell them they can use sports heroes, movie stars, or even fictitious characters whom they admire. If all else fails, ask the students to make up a hero from their imagination whom they could choose as a role model.

Make a list on the board of the positive traits these heroes and role models possess. Ask the students what they admire most about their heroes and why they chose that person. Then have the students answer the questions on the "My Role Model" worksheet, keeping their role model in mind.

After the worksheet is completed, discuss the reasons why the person they chose is important to them. Point out that many of us imitate people and behavior we admire.

We may have different role models for different areas of our lives, and we pick those people for various reasons. Sometimes we choose role models based on the way we would like to appear to others or the way we think other people want us to be rather than the way we really are. Ask students to become aware of the role models they choose and to consider whether these models help or hinder their development. Is the behavior they are emulating in keeping with the impression they are trying to make?

Ask students to consider some of the celebrities and heroes they admire but their parents detest. See if they can understand why their parents are reluctant to embrace this character as their child's role model.

follow-up Use the handout entitled "Boaster Poster" as homework for the students to make a poster or collage demonstrating the things they admire about their role model. Have students share their posters with other students in a small group activity or with the whole class.

activity 10 My Favorite Relative

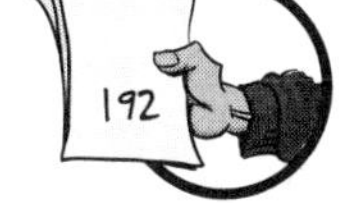

time 30 minutes.

purpose This activity will offer an opportunity for the student to build a connection with a family member. Hopefully, the lines of communication can be strengthened and the student will identify more with this person.

materials The two questionnaire handouts entitled "Questions *for* Teens" and "Questions *from* Teens" and some time outside of class for the interview.

process Ask students to interview a family member or relative they admire and respect, using the interview sheet provided. Some students may have to pick a guardian or counselor to interview but the main idea is to build a connection between the student and an adult guide. Use the questions provided and tell students that they will be answering questions as well as asking them. Explain that the information they gather is for their benefit and that questions may be excluded if they are offensive or inappropriate to their situation.

NOTE: In some states, it is against the Education Code to require students to collect or share information about their families.

When the questionnaires have been completed, ask students to share general impressions of their interview with the class. Did they learn something new about the family member? What surprised or interested them?

Have a class discussion on the following ideas:

- Do you think your family knows all the important information about you? What would you like them to know that they may not? How would you tell them?
- Do you think you know all the important information about your family member? Do you think that he or she would like you to know more? How would you find out?
- What can you do to open the lines of communication in your family and learn more about each other?
- What questions could be added to the questionnaires by you or your parents to improve the experience?

follow-up Students can make a scrapbook or collage that includes pictures of themselves and their families or relatives. Have the students write about each of the pictures, revealing the story behind the picture.

Students can share their scrapbooks in small groups or with the class. This is also a wonderful project to display to parents or to put in portfolios. This project can also lead to family history searches or a family tree research project.

hints This activity can be sensitive because some students may not be living with their family. Even the thought of their family may be painful to them for some reason. You need to have a basic understanding of the students being presented with this assignment and decide if all the students will benefit from this assignment.

If you have some reservations about including this project, individually ask the students in question who they would like to interview instead of a relative.

Do not collect the papers from this activity. If you are grading, just use the information shared in class, or walk around and see that the papers are complete. I often don't even have the students write down the answers in the interview. If you need verification, ask students to provide a signed note from the adult they interviewed with comments about the assignment. In most cases, the parents and other significant adults in the students' life really appreciate and enjoy this assignment. I have been told many times that it was one of the most enjoyable conversations they have had with the teenager and that other members of the family joined the discussion.

Sometimes the activities that are the greatest risk provide the most beneficial results!

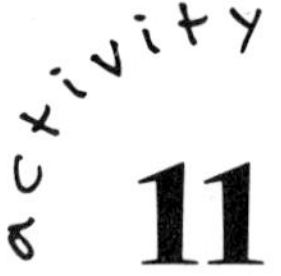

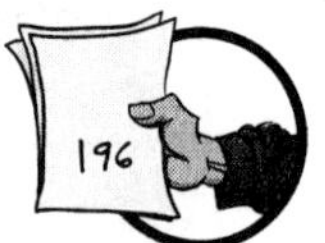

11 What Friends Think

time This activity is best done as homework, so the time taken would be just for presentation and explanation—about 5 minutes.

purpose Carefully done, this activity reinforces and even builds confidence and pride. The students are given the opportunity to see themselves through the eyes of someone who cares about them.

materials The "What Friends Think" handout.

process This activity can be sensitive and needs to be carefully considered before it is assigned. Make sure you know that all the students have someone, preferably an adult, who can share this activity with them in a caring and sincere manner.

Explain that this activity is to be shared with a person who loves and supports the student. He or she will ask this person to answer the questions on the left side of the page and then fold the paper so the student cannot see the answers. The student then answers the questions on the right side of the page. When finished, the student can compare and discuss the answers with the person helping with this activity.

hints This might be a good activity for the teacher to do with a student. Students often cherish teachers' opinions, especially when the opinions are supportive and positive.

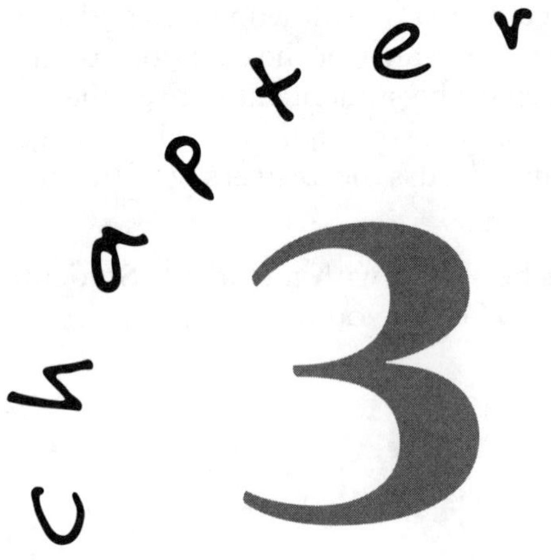

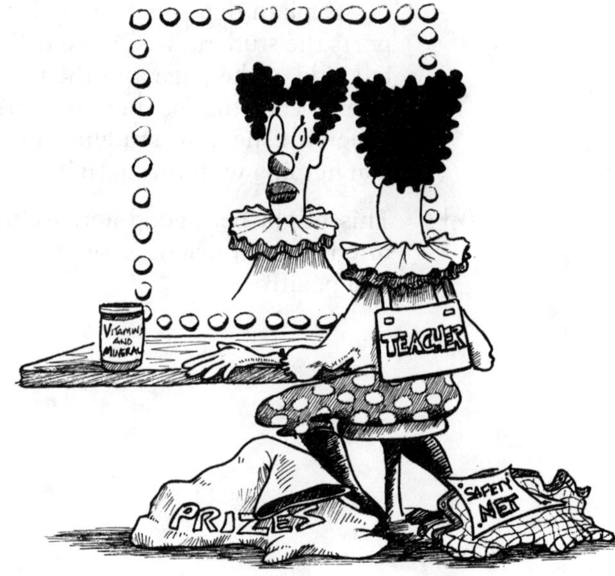

FIVE MINUTES TO CURTAIN...

Preparing for the Future

It is important that teenagers look to the future. Many students live only in the present and rarely think past the next weekend. Students need to look ahead and realize that actions they take now will have consequences in the future. These consequences can either help build a positive future or be a detriment to success.

Setting goals, and a desire to reach them, is a driving force that enables students to take control of their future. A goal becomes a focal point for teens and helps them make better choices. Success builds the confidence they need to attempt larger, more complex goals. Teenagers who are committed to a challenge have direction and a focus in life.

Goals should be based on a person's interests, abilities, and values. Many students need help discovering their strengths. The activities in Chapters 1 and 2 help students understand their strengths and values so they can set goals that are appropriate for their abilities and interests. Chapter 3 offers activities to help students learn skills that will enable them to build a positive future.

Many of the activities and skills presented in this chapter will seem familiar. Some will be easy to learn; others may take practice. All of these skills need to be practiced in order for the individual to feel comfortable using them.

Learning new skills can be exciting and helpful, but it takes patience. Tell students to take small steps in learning and using new skills. Recognize their successes and let them reward themselves. Students should learn from their mistakes, not focus on failure, and work on improving their skills. They should rely on the people who care about them for support and guidance.

This chapter is about setting goals and learning to make decisions, and it presents activities that give the students a point of focus for the future.

activity

1 Lessons from Mistakes

The greatest mistake a person can make is to be afraid of making one.

—ELBERT HUBBARD

time 10 minutes.

purpose This activity will help students understand they don't need to dwell on mistakes or failures. Instead, they can take the lesson that comes with the mistake and grow from it.

materials Two small pieces of paper and a pencil for each student and an empty wastebasket.

process Tell the students to think of a failure they have had or mistake they have made. Tell them you realize that bringing up a painful memory may make them feel bad, but that it is necessary and the end result will be worth it. Have the students write down the failure or mistake on one of the pieces of paper. They can write in code or in pictures if they don't want anyone to see what they record. They can even hide the paper until the end of the activity. No one else is going to see this paper unless they show it to someone.

Ask students to think about what they learned from that failure. Tell them all failures carry lessons that they can learn from. Ask them to write down the lesson they learned from their failure on the second piece of paper.

Tell the students to fold up the paper with the lesson they learned on it and put it in their pocket. Then have them wad up the paper with the failure on it into a little ball. On the count of three, let them throw their failure at you.

Cover your eyes with your hands and duck your head. This will only take a few seconds and the kids love it. Remind them that they only get one shot!

Once the excitement dies down, tell the students that you accept the burden of their failure—they are allowed to get rid of that failure. They are to keep the lesson they learned.

Make the point that failures are basically painful lessons that students can learn from. Tell them not to dwell on the pain or embarrassment, but to take the lesson as a gift and move on.

hints This is a very memorable activity and should be done right at the end of the class period. Refer to it in following lessons to make sure they got the point of the lesson instead of remembering that they got to throw paper at the teacher.

You will have a lot of little papers to pick up after this lesson. I have kids leaving class as I begin to pick up the papers. I have never had to do this by myself—always several students stay to help. This gives them a chance to help and gives you a chance to thank them for their thoughtfulness. They leave class feeling great and you get help cleaning up the mess.

activity

2 Who Will I Be . . . ?

The future belongs to those who believe in the beauty of their dreams.

—ELEANOR ROOSEVELT

time 45 minutes, or it can be expanded into a three-period activity.

purpose Students will identify long-range goals and discover the steps they need to take to accomplish their goals.

materials The handout entitled "Age 30."

process Tell students they will be taking a time travel trip. They will be traveling to the future, to when they are 30 years old. Take them ahead in time slowly.

Ask the students to imagine their lives at age thirty. Guide their thinking by asking them the following questions:

- What do you look like? Are you holding your age well? Are you tired or energetic? Overweight or thin? How are you wearing your hair? Do you work out or are you a couch potato?
- How are you dressed? Are you high-fashion and stylish or relaxed and comfortable? Where do you shop for your clothes? How much do you pay?
- Where do you live? Do you live in the city? A suburb? The country? Do you have a house, a condominium, or an apartment? What does your furniture look like? What type of electronics do you have?
- What kind of vehicles do you have? Car? Boat? Plane?
- Are you married? Do you have children? How many?
- Do you travel? Where do you go? Do you take your family? Do you go camping or stay in hotels?
- Do you have any pets or animals?

Explain that in order to achieve the goal they have set for themselves, they must have work that will pay for their lifestyle. Some kids may have to adjust their lifestyle to the earning ability of a chosen career.

Remind students they cannot rely on winning the lottery, marrying a millionaire, or inheriting a lot of money. They have to achieve their future themselves.

Give students the handout entitled "Age 30" and have them answer the questions. I tell students who have chosen careers as professional athletes that they should be thinking about a second career by age 30. Point out that only a few athletes earn phenomenal salaries, so most athletes rely on another income as they age.

When they have finished the worksheet, take one student's goal and go backwards from age 30, pointing out all the necessary steps to successfully achieve that career. For example, to become an attorney, they had to pass the bar and pay off education loans; finish law school; be successful in college to get into a good school of law; be successful and well-rounded in high school in order to get accepted by a good college; work on study habits and learn good skills during high school.

If there is time, in small groups have students share their ideas and steps for success. The other kids in the group will be a lot more blunt than you in pointing out discrepancies.

hints Although asking teenagers to think 15 years in the future seems impossible when they can't even plan for next week, it is important that you use age 30 as

DOWN AT THE WHO-WILL-I-BE CAFÉ

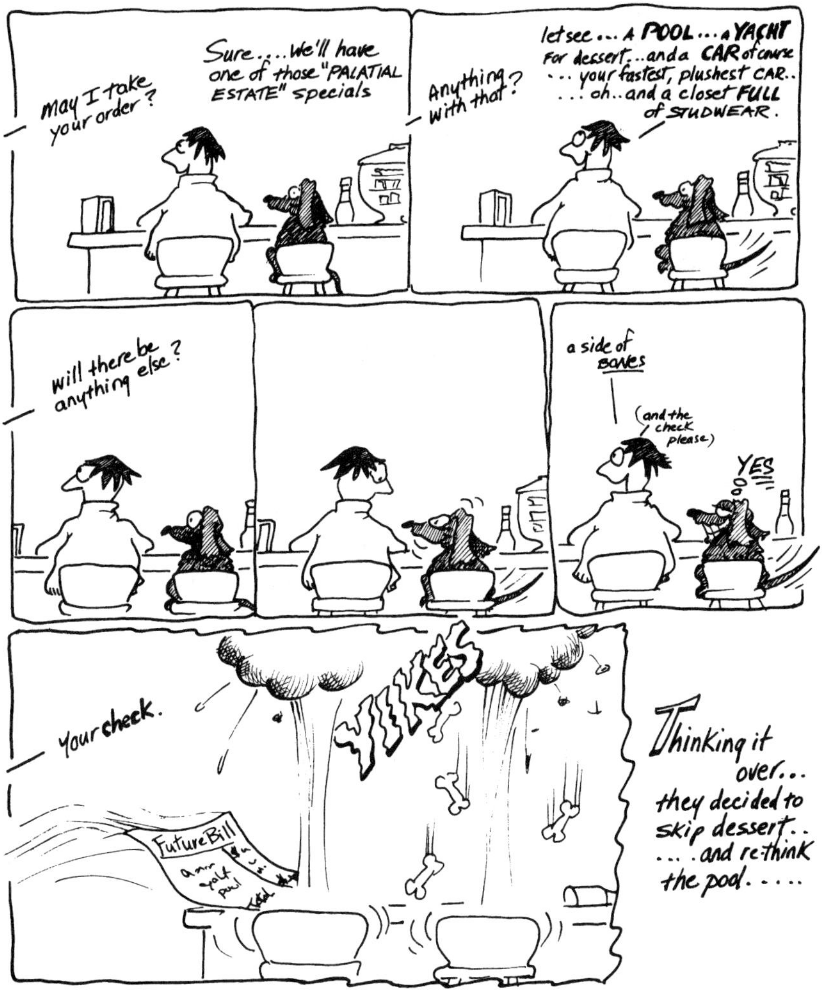
May I take your order?
Sure.... We'll have one of those "PALATIAL ESTATE" specials
Anything with that?
let see... A POOL... A YACHT For dessert...and a CAR of course ... your fastest, plushest CAR.. ...oh..and a closet FULL of STUDWEAR.
will there be anything else?
a side of BONES
(and the check please)
YES
Your check.
YIKES
FutureBill
Thinking it over... they decided to skip dessert.. ....and re-think the pool.....

a marker. If students are planning on careers in law or medicine, this is when they will be finishing their education and starting a practice. Those students planning a career in athletics will be coming to the end of that career and starting another one. This helps those who only focus on sports think beyond that career to a more reliable one.

Don't be concerned if many students choose careers that you feel are unrealistic. Hopefully, this activity will help them realize that fact for themselves. It is the process of discovering the steps they must take to achieve a goal that is important.

Remind students that their plans for the future might change—and probably will. The most important thing is that they have some goal to aim at, even though it may change as their interests change. This goal will give them direction and guide their efforts as they mature.

follow-up Another activity that can be incorporated at this point is to have students illustrate their future. Give them drawing paper and have them illustrate just how they want to live at age 30. This will also help them visualize their ideas.

activity

3 A Typical Day

time 25 minutes.

purpose This activity will help students see how they spend their time during a typical day. It often surprises people to see their day pictured and to realize how little time they have for things that are important to them.

materials The "A Typical Day" handout and colored pencils or crayons.

process Have the class brainstorm a list of ways they spend their time during a typical day. Put this list on the blackboard for reference. Tell the kids to map out a typical day using the clock-chart on the handout.

When everyone has finished charting, have the students color in their chart in the following way:

- Color the time devoted to school and schoolwork orange
- Color the time spent doing chores or working red
- Color the time spent sleeping yellow
- Color the time spent eating green
- Color the time spent doing the things they like to do for themselves blue

Have the students answer the questions at the bottom of the worksheet. Students can then share with the class or small groups any revelations they might have.

follow-up Have students complete another clock-chart. This time have them map out their day in a way that their time could be better spent to achieve goals.

hints As with many of the activities in this book, there may be quite a bit of talking and comparing clock-charts as the students work. This is a good thing. Allow students to share their days and to compare. Kids need to see how their lives compare with others.

activity

4 Setting Goals

199

Don't wait for your ship to come in; swim out to it.

—ANONYMOUS

time Three 45-minute class periods.

purpose This lesson will present guidelines and allow students to practice skills for setting goals.

materials The four handouts entitled "Be Specific," "My Goals," "Solutions to Problems," and "Alternative Solutions" and a blackboard.

process **DAY ONE** Lead a class discussion on the importance of setting goals.

Goals help people focus on particular issues or activities. Because the goal is often written, they will be reminded that the issue still needs to be addressed and will continue their efforts to accomplish that goal. Once the goal has been successfully accomplished, the person can feel a sense of satisfaction. This promotes confidence and the challenge to attack more complicated and difficult issues.

Explain the guidelines for setting goals. Each of the following guidelines should be kept in mind when writing goals.

- First **understand yourself.** Know your values, your strengths, and your interests.
- Goals should be written clearly with a **specific task** in mind. A goal should tell you exactly what you want and should be measurable.
- Goals should be **positive.** Stress things you will accomplish rather than things you will not do. Goals should improve you or society.
- Goals should be **realistic.** Listen to yourself and decide what you are willing to work for, then check to see if that goal is within realistic limits for you. Limits can be physical, social, emotional—but they are only obstacles, which often can be overcome with determination and hard work.
- You should have some **control over the outcome** of your goal. There is a big difference between a goal and a wish. You must actively seek your goal and be able to influence the outcome.
- Goals should **challenge you.** You must put effort into successfully completing a goal.

Students will practice writing short-term goals using the handouts entitled "Be Specific" and "My Goals." Advise them to break their goals into small parts. Tell them it is much easier to accomplish a task by taking small steps rather than a giant leap. If a student's goal is to get "straight A's" in school, he or she first must get an "A" in each class. To do that, he or she must set goals of handing in each assignment, studying for tests, and listening and participating in class.

Give some examples of well-written, accessible goals. Ask for volunteers to share some of their goals with the class and advise them on ways to improve the writing so it meets the guidelines offered.

hints A good daily practice is to have students set a goal for the day. Check the goals written for the previous day. Allow students to share their success. Check the goals for those students who are not successful. Help them follow the guidelines for writing goals.

DAY TWO Explain that there are always obstacles to overcome in attaining goals. The challenge in setting goals is to identify the obstacles and determine solutions to these obstacles so the goal can be obtained.

Present some examples of goals to the class or ask students to volunteer with their own goals. Have the class identify the obstacles that must be overcome and then suggest possible solutions.

Students can work in small groups to complete the "Solutions to Problems" worksheet. Ask the students to present their work to the class.

DAY THREE Suggest to the class that there are many solutions to overcoming a single obstacle. Often, individuals become obsessed with a particular solution and forget to look around for alternative solutions that might be successful.

Use an example situation. Have the class indicate the goal to be achieved. Determine the obstacle and then ask for suggestions to solve the problem. Think of the consequences of each of the choices and indicate the advantages and disadvantages of each.

Students can work in small groups of three to five students. Hand out the worksheet entitled "Alternative Solutions." Have the students work together to complete the worksheet.

hints I have had some of my classes make up situations based on their own lives and use those for the worksheets. The activity then becomes more real and relevant. If you do this, have the students write real-life situations on the second day of the activity.

Tell students the situations will be used in class and not to include real names. Have them turn in their ideas so you can preview or edit them if necessary.

follow-up Have students make and keep calendars of their goals. Have students record daily, weekly, and monthly goals. If students list several goals at a time, have them prioritize the goals. Remind students that short-term goals often lead to long-term success. Always have students refer to their goal calendars and record their successes as they are achieved.

Suggest that students use sticky notes to post their daily goals on a mirror at home so they are reminded of their goal for the day.

Remind students not to dwell on goals that have not been achieved. They can analyze their actions and choose alternative solutions, rewrite the goal, or discard the goal as it becomes obsolete. Start each day fresh with an optimistic outlook and the energy to accept the challenges presented.

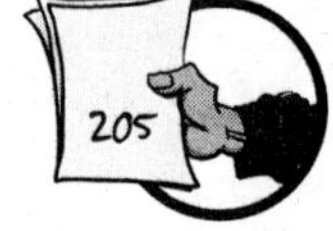

activity 5 Long-Term Goals

time 30 minutes.

purpose This activity will help students realize the steps they must take to achieve long-term goals.

materials The handout entitled "Long-Term Goals."

process Review the steps and guidelines for writing goals. See Activity 4 in this chapter.

Have the students complete the worksheet. Ask for volunteers to share their work with the class. Offer advice and suggestions. Remind the students that there may be several alternatives to overcome obstacles in achieving their goals.

activity 6 No More Rules

time 45 minutes.

purpose This activity helps students view the classroom environment and their behavior in a positive, goal-oriented manner.

materials Blackboard and chalk or large butcher paper and markers.

process Lead a discussion concerning the need for rules. I usually start by asking students to visualize a society (e.g., a school community) that has no rules. Brainstorm what that society would look like and how people would act. List their ideas on the board.

Compare the society with no rules to one in which rules are appreciated and followed. Ask why rules are necessary. Rules supply guidelines that help society:

- function more efficiently
- ensure the rights of the individuals in that society
- provide equal opportunity within the society
- promote safety and well-being

Ask students to define the words *rule* and *goal*. Ask for ways in which these terms differ. Record the students' ideas.

Explain that while rules are guidelines, a goal is more of a destination or target that a person wants to achieve. People seem to have more positive feelings about working toward a goal than being limited by a rule.

Propose eliminating rules in class and replacing them with goals. Structure the ideas as goals that everyone could work for to promote a good learning environment.

Students can then brainstorm and record the goals for the class. Use general suggestions and goals that would help all students make the most of their class, such as providing an environment in which the teacher is able to teach and the students are able to learn, respecting all the people in the class, and being prepared for class.

Guide the students in selecting several goals they think are important for the class. Discuss the obstacles that might hinder achieving the selected goals and have students suggest ways the goals can be met. Have students write personal plans for working toward the class goals.

hints This activity is especially good for reminding students of behaviors that hinder learning. You can approach the students by asking them if their behavior is helping reach the goals agreed on by the class. Then have them offer suggestions on different approaches to reach those goals. I sometimes ask the entire class to make suggestions that might help students achieve the class goals more successfully.

Students usually want to be successful in achieving goals they have helped establish, although they may rebel against rules that are imposed on them. Behaving in a successful, appropriate manner becomes something they want to do rather than something they have to do. Remember to acknowledge their achievement periodically.

activity 7 Risks and Choices

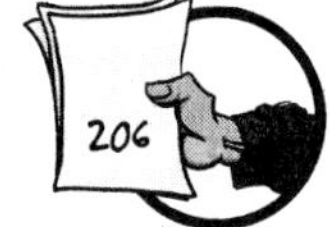

time 20 minutes.

purpose This activity will help students identify and evaluate risks and encourage them to make better choices in pursuing positive risks.

materials The poem "The Dilemma" and the handout entitled "Taking Risks."

process Read to the class the poem "The Dilemma."

THE DILEMMA

To laugh is to risk appearing a fool.
To weep is to risk appearing sentimental.
To reach out for another is to risk involvement.
To expose your feelings is to risk rejection.
To place your dreams before the crowd is to risk ridicule.
To love is to risk not being loved in return.
To go forward in the face of overwhelming odds is to risk failure.
But risks must be taken because the greatest hazard in life is to risk nothing.

The person who risks nothing does nothing, has nothing, is nothing. He may avoid suffering and sorrow, but he cannot learn, feel, change, grow or love. Only a person who risks is free.

—AUTHOR UNKNOWN

Poem reprinted with permission. Crisp Publications, Inc., 1200 Hamilton Court, Menlo Park, CA 94025; 800-442-7477 or 415-323-6100.

Discuss the meaning of the poem. Explain that most of the decisions made in life involve some degree of risk. Even not doing anything may involve some risk. Consequences will occur no matter what, so it is up to the students to weigh the consequences of decisions before they happen so the risk can be reduced.

Tell the students a risk is like taking a chance. There may be unforeseeable or frightening outcomes or even an element of danger involved. They need to evaluate the risks and the consequences as much as possible *before* they act in order to minimize the danger.

Put students in small groups of three or four and give them the "Taking Risks" handout. Have them work together on the handout. Allow time for discussion within each group. They will record their ideas on the handout provided.

At the end of the activity, remind students that everyone has fears and faces risks every day. It is important to challenge ourselves by stepping beyond our zone of comfort and evaluating the risks we take in order to create powerful, fulfilling lives.

hints It is important to remind students that there are some risks not worth taking because they endanger their health, safety, reputation, or friendships. Students need to evaluate the risks they are taking and determine whether the price they may have to pay is worth it.

activity 8 S.T.A.R. Decisions

208

time 45 minutes.

purpose This activity enables students to learn and practice a system for making dependable decisions.

materials The "S.T.A.R. Decisions" handout.

process Ask students to tell you the difference between a good and a bad decision. Basically, a good decision is one you do not regret making and a bad decision is one you later regret.

Tell students they will be learning a method for making decisions that will help them make more good decisions. Learning decision-making skills will increase their chances of making better decisions, which can provide more freedom and control in their life.

Describe the S.T.A.R. method of making decisions. The summary of the S.T.A.R. method of making decisions is as follows. The first letter of each step in the process spells the word STAR:

S — stop
T — think
A — act
R — re-act, review, or reevaluate

Use an example that would be real for your students, such as whether students should wear uniforms at school or if they should be allowed to chew gum at school. Take them through the process as a class.

First you **STOP.** You are giving yourself space to think without being pressured. Get away from the pressure your best friend is putting on you and take time to listen to your own thoughts.

THINK. Use the following list to write down all the positive, negative, and interesting facts (facts that are neither good nor bad but should be considered) about the decision you have to make.

Positive	Negative	Interesting
1.	1.	1.
2.	2.	2.
3.	3.	3.
4.	4.	4.
5.	5.	5.
↓	↓	↓

Think about how you *feel* about each item in the columns after exhausting all your ideas for each column. Circle the items that are of extreme importance to you.

The next step is to **ACT.** Make your decision based on the reasons you listed. Pay extra attention to the items you circled because they are important to you. Consider what the consequences of your decision will be. How will you feel if you decide according to the items that are most important?

The last step is to **RE-ACT** (or **review,** or **reevaluate**). After you have made your decision, look back at how things are turning out. Should you continue with the choice you made or change your mind?

hint I often use the example of whether a young teenager should be sexually active. This is very effective in gaining the students' attention. By this point in my class, I have a rapport with the students, and we are preparing for the unit on human sexuality.

This question is one that students rarely take the time to think through, so using class time forces kids to face the issue. This also gives you a chance to demonstrate mature behavior while discussing sensitive issues. Students will be a bit embarrassed and shocked at first, but if the teacher can talk about the subject without faltering, so will the students.

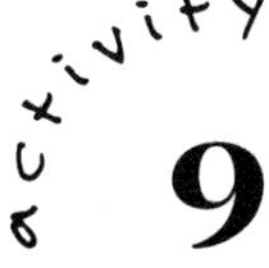

9 What Would You Do?

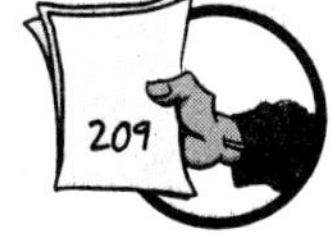

time 45 minutes.

purpose To allow students to practice making decisions using the situations provided and receive reinforcement from peers.

materials The handout entitled "What Would You Do?" for each group.

process Have students get in groups of four or five students. Tell them to work together to solve the problems posed on the worksheet using the S.T.A.R. method of making decisions. Refer to Activity 8, "S.T.A.R. Decisions," in this chapter.

The students should write down their answers, revealing each step they made in the thought process to arrive at the final decision. If time allows, have each group present its work to the class on one of the topics. Discuss the merits of their ideas.

activity

10 My Choices Have Consequences

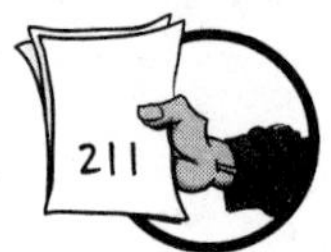

time 45 minutes.

purpose Students will become more aware of the consequences that result from the choices they make.

materials The handout entitled "My Choices Have Consequences" for each group.

process Have students get in groups of three to five students. Tell students that all the choices people make result in both good and bad consequences. It is important to think ahead and anticipate those consequences so they can make better choices and avoid unfortunate results.

Use an example situation to illustrate how to complete the worksheet. Put the responses on the board so all the students can see them. I often use an example of a really hungry student stuck in class, who has to wait an hour for lunch. What can the student do? Ask the class for suggestions and write their answers on the board. Allow for creative solutions without commenting. The resulting consequences will demonstrate whether they are good choices.

Explain that each of the choices listed will result in good and bad consequences. Ask the students to list consequences for each of the choices they offered. Below are some examples:

1. Eating during class
- ⇨ not hungry anymore
- ⇨ no lunch left for lunch time
- ⇨ may get in trouble

2. Going to the nurse to get a snack
- ⇨ not hungry anymore
- ⇨ bother the nurse without being sick
- ⇨ miss out on class

Give each group the handout and tell them to work as a group to make choices about the problems presented and to list good and bad consequences for each choice.

activity

11 Lifeboat

214

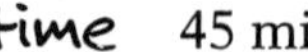

time 45 minutes.

purpose This activity allows students to practice making decisions in a group setting.

materials One "Lifeboat" handout for each small group.

process Students brainstorm socially acceptable ways to come to agreement when people in a group are totally deadlocked in disagreement. Some examples: vote, draw straws, flip a coin, or roll dice. Remind students that it is important to pick the method of solving disagreements *before* they come to an impasse.

Put students in groups of four or five. Tell them to choose a method for solving disagreements as soon as they get into their groups. Then explain that they will be making life and death decisions! People's lives will depend on them. Read or have the students read the problem to be solved and the descriptions of the characters involved. The students will have 10 minutes to make their decisions. A person from each group will report to the class about the choices they made and the reasons for those choices.

List the names of the characters in the story on the board with a brief description of the character's statement. This could be done before the students come into class. As each group reports, record its choices on the board. After each group has reported, allow time for argument and discussion between groups.

important Before students leave class, tell them that there are no right or wrong answers in this activity. It is merely an exercise in thinking and making decisions. The choices made are based on their values, and values differ just like people do.

hints I always take the opposite argument to the one being presented and force students to justify their choices. If a group seems deadlocked in disagreement, have them tell you ways they could solve the problem in a socially acceptable manner.

activity 12 Take My Advice

216

time 30 minutes.

purpose The situations presented in this activity allow students to practice making decisions.

materials The "Take My Advice" handout for each student.

process Tell students they will be working on their own today to give advice to a friend. They will be given a worksheet with various problems listed, and they will use the decision-making process to arrive at answers to the problems.

Remind students to review the steps to making good decisions. They should be thinking about setting goals, taking small steps in changing behavior, and learning lessons from making mistakes. Refer to Activity 8, "S.T.A.R. Decisions," and Activity 10, "My Choices Have Consequences," in this chapter.

activity 13 Commitment to Change

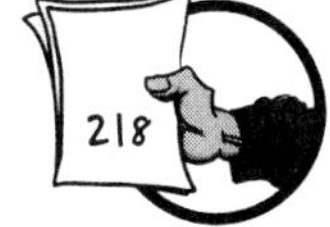

time 30 minutes.

purpose To help students understand the steps involved in changing behavior.

materials Large piece of butcher paper and markers for each small group and the "Commitment to Change" handout for each student.

process Begin the discussion by comparing the process of changing someone's behavior to going on a trip. First you decide where you want to go. Then you gather maps and information on routes to get there, pack, and make arrangements for accommodations. Finally, you get started on your trip. As you travel, you check maps and road signs to make sure you are on the right path.

The process of making changes in life is a lot like planning a trip—take it one step at a time.

Use an example for comparison, such as the fear of taking tests in school. Because of this fear, the student avoids tests by staying home. Low grades affect the student's total grade point average. Have the students help by offering steps for change.

- *Identify the problem behavior.* You are afraid of taking tests.
- *Identify the behavior you want instead.* You want to face tests unafraid, with confidence.
- *Gather information and ask advice.* Think of the worst things that could happen and the best things that could happen. Focus on the good as you gather information on what to do.

  Worst things that could happen:
  - you might forget everything
  - you will look foolish for not knowing the information
  - you will disappoint yourself, your friends, and your family

  Best things that could happen:
  - you do well on the test and overcome your fear
  - your parents and friends will feel proud of you
  - your grades will improve and you will gain confidence

  Then get advice from successful students on taking tests:
  - they study every night for a week before the test
  - they make flash cards for review
  - they study with friends and quiz each other

- *Choose a plan of action.* Develop a plan outlining specific ways to overcome your fear.
  - set up a place and time to study at home
  - get help from a friend
  - study diligently every night for a week before the test
- *Evaluate your progress.* As you get closer to the day of the test, quiz yourself on the material. Study the difficult information.
- *Reward yourself as you successfully complete each portion of your plan.* Remember that your goal is to feel more confident going into the test. Reward yourself in ways that will not impede your progress. Stick to your plan and revise it as necessary.

After that long explanation, students will be ready to do something! Have students pick a behavior they want to change and follow the steps in devising a plan to change that behavior. Have them answer the questions on the handout.

Remind students to be their own cheerleader in working for change. Look for support from every direction. Get friends and family members to help during difficult times.

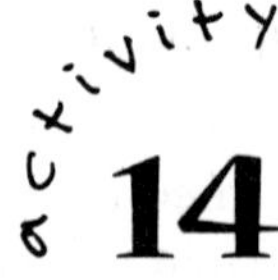

14 This Is the Way I See It . . .

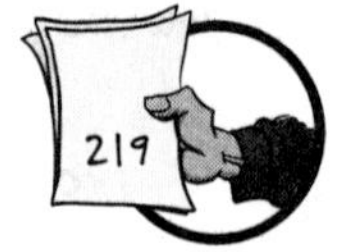

time 30 minutes.

purpose This activity will give students the opportunity to see that people interpret events differently based on their values, experiences, and beliefs. How people interpret an event makes a difference in the choices they make.

materials The handout entitled "This Is the Way I See It . . ." for each student.

process Explain to the class that decisions are based on the way people interpret certain events. People react differently to an event because they perceive or interpret the event differently. Perception of an event is a very personal experience that is based on the experiences the person has had. A person's actions will seem correct to that person even though others may disagree with the choice.

Have the students complete the worksheet entitled "This Is the Way I See It . . ." Ask the students to share their reactions and answers in class. Acknowledge the differences in interpretations and explain that there are no right or wrong answers.

activity 15 Making Mistakes

222

time 30 minutes.

purpose This activity will help students look at mistakes from a positive viewpoint by accepting the lessons learned from mistakes and moving on.

materials The handout entitled "Making Mistakes" for each student.

process Lead a class discussion concerning mistakes and the reactions people have to them. Propose the idea that people can decide how to react to a problem. Remind students that they have a choice in the attitude they display. Keep going back to the premise that all events are learning experiences. Tell students to take the time to look at their choice, decide how they feel about it and what they learned from it, and move on.

Inform the students you realize that sounds easy. There will be times when they get discouraged or think they are complete fools. The students still need to think about the messages they are sending themselves. There are several judgments people make about themselves that can lead to negative thoughts and actions. If people tell themselves something long enough, they begin to believe it.

List on the board the types of negative thinking people fall prey to.

- focusing only on their faults
- believing everything will work out without any effort from them
- imposing too many "shoulds"
- jumping to conclusions by making a judgment before having all the information available
- exaggerating the importance of an event
- expecting perfection from themselves every time.

Have students write down a negative thought they find themselves having a lot. Have them indicate the message the thought sends to them, then replace the negative thought with a positive one.

Situation	Negative Thought	Message	Positive Thought
Bad hair day	"I really look ugly today."	"I don't look good enough to be around people."	"This is my chance to try a new hairstyle."

Have the students brainstorm situations to use on their worksheets. Hand out the worksheets and give students time to complete the assignment.

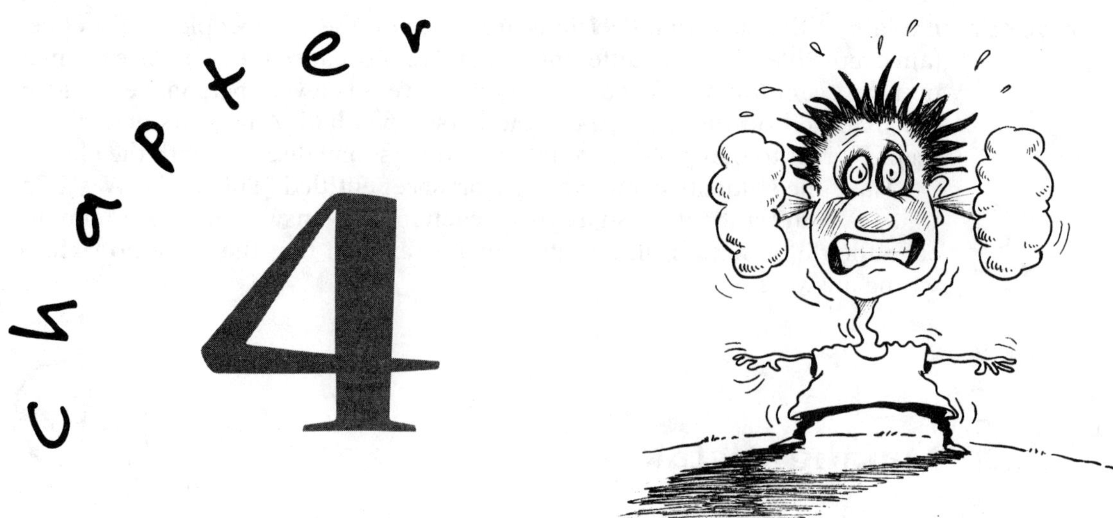

Chapter 4

Dealing with Stress

Stress is the effect any situation or event has on the body and mind. Stress that is not relieved causes uncomfortable reactions in people. Physical reactions such as a headache, stomachache, asthma, heart problems, or muscle spasms are often caused by repressed feelings. Many real medical problems are caused by stress.

Stress can lead people to cover up feelings by taking on habits that are dangerous. Smoking, drinking, or taking drugs are all ways of masking feelings and relieving stress. Stressful situations can overwhelm individuals to the point of feeling out of control.

Life has become more complex, and with this complexity comes the pressure to make choices, to accept responsibility for decisions, and to cope within socially acceptable limits. Young people today face demanding situations at a much younger age than did people in previous generations. It is essential that teenagers learn to deal with stress and feel free to explore their options in an open, caring environment.

Students need to explore their feelings and gain experience using effective tools to cope with the stressful environments they encounter daily. Learning to set goals and make choices are part of coping with stress. Students also need to learn to recognize stress in their lives and actually channel that energy into productive behaviors.

This chapter will help teenagers identify possible stress-filled situations and learn how to deal with unavoidable stress.

activity

1 Identifying Stress

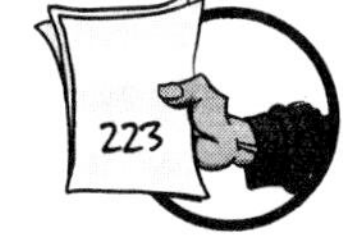

time 45 minutes.

purpose This activity will help students determine their stress level.

materials The "Identifying Stress" handout for each student.

process Tell students they are going to evaluate their level of stress. Ask them to fill out the worksheet entitled "Identifying Stress."

When students are finished, discuss what the different stress levels indicate. Talk about where students might receive help if they are upset about their score. Remind students that they will be learning about ways to deal with stress in the next few days and that stress can actually be helpful once it is identified.

activity

2 Identify Your Feelings

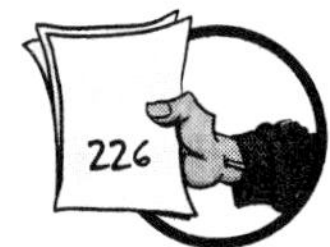

time 15 minutes.

purpose Students identify feelings that have been caused by stressful situations.

materials The handout entitled "Identify Your Feelings" for each student.

process Hand out the worksheet and have the students read over the list of feelings. Tell them to choose the feelings that best express the reactions they might have to the situations on the worksheet.

When completed, the students can compare their reactions with other students in a small group. Have a class discussion concerning the different ways people react to various situations. Reinforce the premise that there is no correct feeling for any particular situation. Everyone reacts based on their own feelings, perceptions, and past experiences.

The choices people make can affect their attitude and behaviors. Constantly choosing to complain and whine can make a person depressed and angry. However, if they choose to accept problems as a challenge, they may have a more positive, pleasant attitude.

activity 3 Reactions to Stress

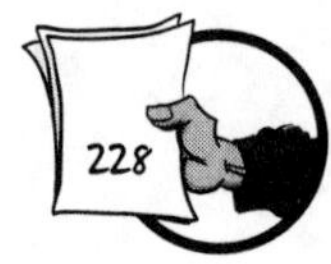

time 45 minutes.

purpose This activity helps students discover healthy ways to cope with the stress they experience.

materials The handout entitled "Reactions to Stress" for each student.

process Students brainstorm the most frequent causes of stress in their lives. Write their answers on the board so everyone can see. Have students consider the causes of stress and compare those answers to their own experiences. You can offer some ideas from an adult perspective to show students that many stressors remain the same.

Discuss some general suggestions for coping with stress. (See Activity 5, "Coping with Stress," in this chapter.)

Have students get into small groups of three or four students and focus on one of the stressful situations the class listed. Have them suggest and discuss ways to cope with the situation in a healthy way. Each group can share its ideas with the class.

Use the "Reactions to Stress" worksheet as a focal point for discussion of which reactions to stress might be considered healthy and which might be considered detrimental to a positive well-being.

hint Use a continuum on the board to place the reactions to stress from most healthy to least healthy. Remember that rating the reactions to stress is arbitrary and can change from day to day.

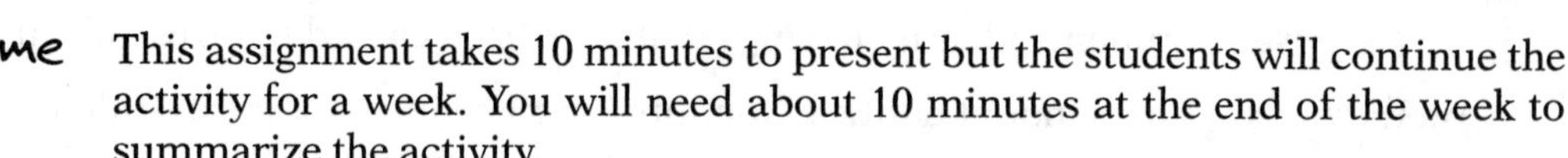

activity 4 Stress Calendar

time This assignment takes 10 minutes to present but the students will continue the activity for a week. You will need about 10 minutes at the end of the week to summarize the activity.

purpose This activity gives students an opportunity to identify stressors and to keep a continuous record of the incidents.

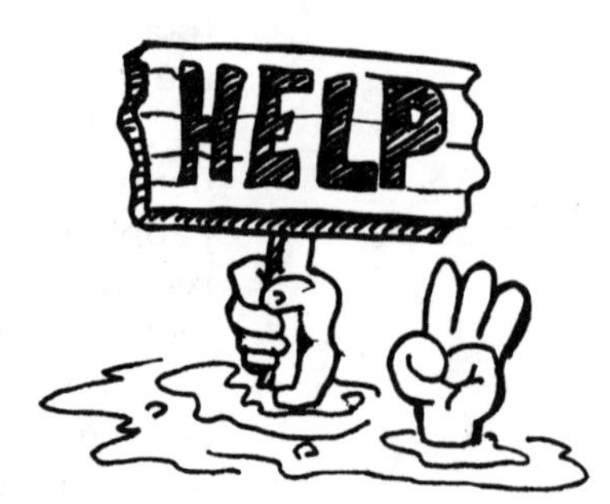

materials The "Stress Calendar" and "Stress Calendar Conclusions" handouts for each student.

process Give students the "Stress Calendar" handout and ask them to record stressful situations they experience during the week. Ask them to be sure to write down how they felt. Have students look at any patterns that may develop in their charts.

At the end of the week, take some class time to have the students look back over their behaviors and stressful situations for the week. Have them look for any connections between stress and the time of day, the activity, or people they were with, or any other things that may trigger stress for them. Have the students write a conclusion about their own stress triggers on the "Stress Calendar Conclusions" handout.

From *Building a Positive Self-Concept: 113 Activities for Adolescents* by Marjorie Jacobs, Blossom Turk, and Elizabeth Horn.

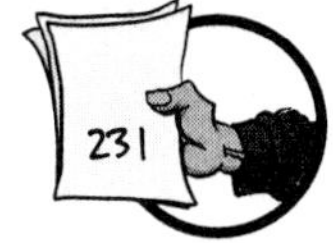

activity 5 Coping with Stress

time 10 minutes for presentation; 5 minutes each day if you use this in class as an attention break or stress reliever or 45 minutes if you present and then have students try each stress reliever.

purpose These exercises and suggestions give students a plan for learning to cope with stress and encourage students to develop their own plan.

materials The handout entitled "Coping with Stress" for each student.

process Make up packets of the "Coping with Stress" handout and give them to each student. Explain the exercises and activities to the class and suggest that they incorporate some of them into their lives when dealing with stress. If time permits, take a few minutes at the beginning or end of class to practice one of the methods of dealing with stress.

hints When I first started using these activities, many students complained, "This is not a physical education class and we shouldn't have to do exercises in a classroom." Ask the students to indulge you by trying it. You will find that the students soon look forward to the activities and will often suggest that they be continued even after the unit on stress is over. Many students even asked to do some of these activities in other classes or before a test.

follow-up Have students prepare a joke they can share with the class for practicing the laughter method for relieving stress. Remind students that the jokes should be material that can be shared in school and should not hurt anyone's feelings. Give some examples of acceptable jokes before having students prepare their own.

Make the exercises fun. Laugh a lot and relax with the students. You will find that you look forward to the activities, too—you have a bit of stress in your job!

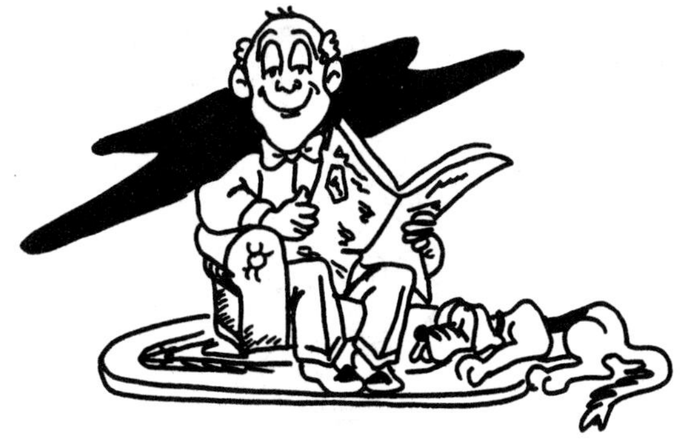

activity 6 How Do You Cope?

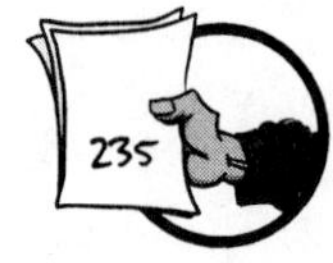

time 15 minutes.

purpose This interview activity helps students see how adults cope with stress and build lines of communication between students and adults.

materials The "How Do You Cope?" handout for each student.

process Give each student the handout. Explain that adults as well as teenagers experience stress in many ways. Students will interview three adults whom they feel handle stress well. Students can interview teachers, parents, coaches, or club leaders.

hints You will keep your friendships with other teachers by telling students to ask a teacher at the beginning of a class. That teacher can write his or her answer on the board for all of your students to copy.

activity 7 Take That!

236

time 45 minutes.

purpose This activity gives students a chance to compare their typical reactions to stress with those of other students in the class. Students will be able to identify responsible reactions to frustrating situations.

materials The handout entitled "Take That!" for each group.

process Students work in groups of three or four. Give each group the worksheet. Tell the students to read each of the situations on the worksheet and to discuss their reactions as if they had experienced the trauma.

Have students identify the initial problem for each situation. They should then brainstorm ways of solving the problem and list those ideas on the worksheet. Circle the ideas for coping that the students think would be the most positive and healthy.

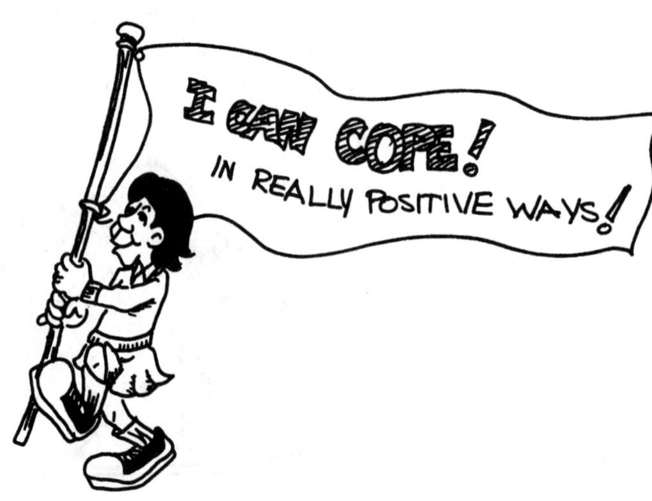

activity

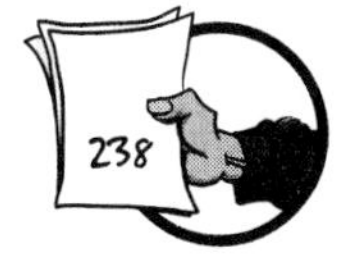

8 This Hurts Me

time 30 minutes.

purpose Students identify hurtful situations in life. Reevaluating the situation may diffuse the pain of the experience.

materials The handout entitled "This Hurts Me" for each student.

process Tell students that all people experience hurtful times in their lives. Give an example of a painful situation in your own life that you feel comfortable sharing with the class.

Tell students they are going to express one of their most painful moments on the worksheet. Ask them to draw a picture that represents that painful experience. The students should record the way they felt when the ordeal occurred and how they feel about it now. Have them notice if their feelings have intensified or receded. How would they have changed their reaction? Have them consider the amount of control they had and what they learned from the experience.

Remind students that this is a very personal paper and that no one else will see their paper unless they want to share it with someone.

Have students put this exercise in their journal, if they have one. It can be kept with a notebook or in a binder. They should look at their paper and check their feelings to see if they have changed as they gain distance and perspective on the incident.

hints Because you shared a painful situation in your life, many students may volunteer their own examples. Warn the students before you allow them to share that these experiences are very personal and should be respected by each person in the class.

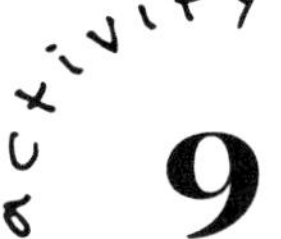

9 Good Choices and Changes

time 45 minutes.

purpose Students will identify upsetting situations, describe their feelings, and make choices to resolve problems in a constructive manner.

materials The handout entitled "Good Choices and Changes" for each student.

process Explain that the experiences people have may affect their feelings. Many of the things we live with cannot be controlled, such as age, ethnic background, and family income. There are, however, situations that you can control.

Discuss various uncomfortable or unpleasant situations that teenagers experience and list them on the board. Have students indicate whether or not they can control each of the things listed.

Take one of the situations the students agree they can control and use it as an example. Have the students describe the feelings stemming from that experience. Change the reactions to the situation and describe how feelings might be changed. Identify barriers to achieving the change and then discuss how those barriers can be resolved.

Suggest to students that becoming obsessed with situations that cannot be controlled may cause unnecessary stress. The first thing people need to do when trying to deal with stressful situations is to evaluate whether they can control the outcome. It they can't, let it go. Choose your battles.

Have students complete the worksheet in the same way.

activity 10 Emergency Plan

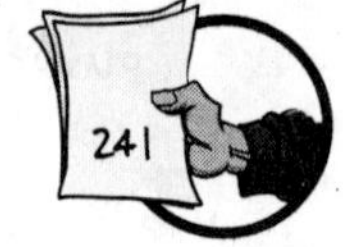

time 15–45 minutes, depending on the method of presentation.

purpose This activity gives students a plan to use and resources to contact in case of emergency situations.

materials The "Emergency Plan" handout for each student.

process Discuss civil defense emergency plans that cover circumstances of fire, earthquake, flood, severe snow, war, and so forth. Explain that these plans are developed before the emergency occurs so that people can be prepared and act rationally in a time of chaos.

Have students fill out the "Emergency Plan" resource guide using their own resources and phone numbers for community resource groups that you list on the board. Students can also investigate phone numbers for those resources in telephone books available in the classroom. If students work in groups, each group could have access to a phone book and check each other for accuracy on phone numbers.

When the students have completed their "Emergency Plan," explain how to contact the support services. Discuss the importance of trying all methods to solve problems before resorting to these community resources.

activity 11 Power Packed!

time 45 minutes.

purpose This activity gives students a chance to discover new words and use a dictionary while demonstrating positive self-esteem.

materials Each student will need drawing paper and markers, colored pencils, or crayons and access to a dictionary.

process We tend to act out what we believe about ourselves. The more we hear something, the more we believe it. Students reinforce their positive beliefs by making a poster showing themselves in their most powerful attitude. They look up words in the dictionary that describe them at their best and surround the powerful picture of themselves with these words. The words should be positive, give them a sense of power, and show them at their best.

follow-up Have students share these posters with the rest of the class. The students can applaud each poster, which enhances the student's feeling of power and accomplishment.

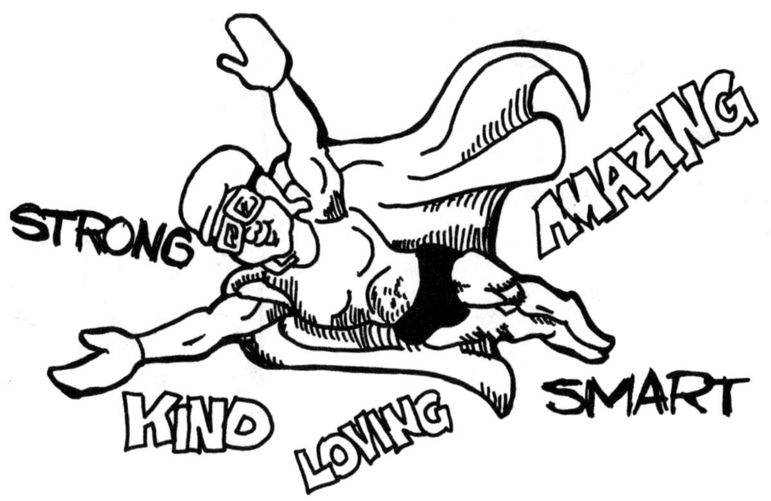

hints You may have a noisy room while the students create these posters. Allow them to help each other and talk about their choices. It might be necessary for you to check spelling and to be supportive when students pick words that may be questionable.

These posters are great for decorating the room and for reminding students that they have terrific qualities.

This is a good exercise with which to end the unit about coping with stress. It leaves students with a sense of power. Self-confidence and a positive attitude are important in creating powerful individuals who can take charge of stressful situations and become stronger with each confrontation.

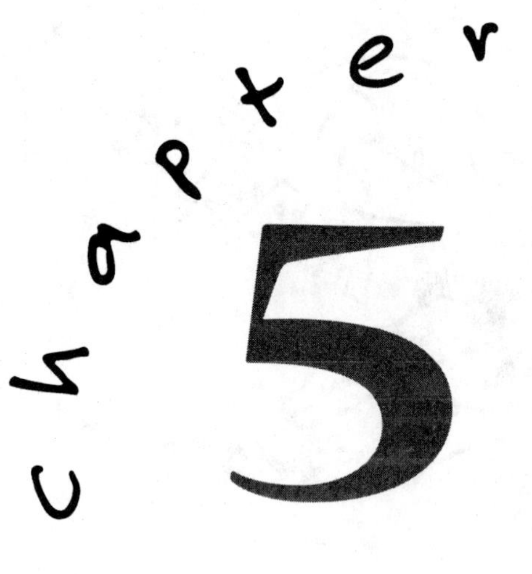

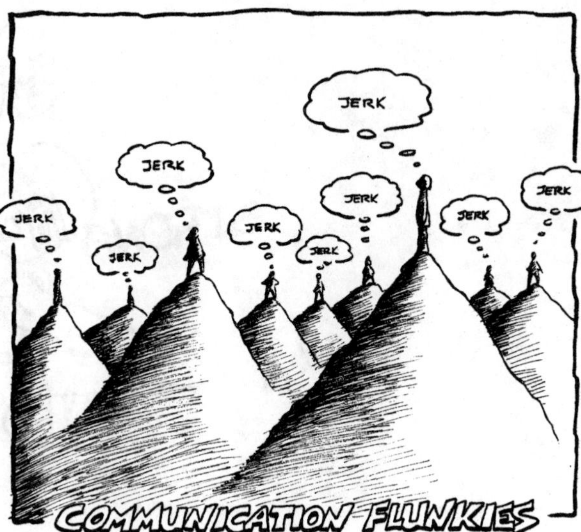

Communication

Communication is something at which most teenagers feel they excel—look at all those hours spent on the phone. If teenagers are so good at communication, then why do they so often feel misunderstood?

Communication is basically an exchange of thoughts, feelings, and emotions. There are many forms of communication—some are written, verbal, and nonverbal. Communication takes place all the time, both consciously and unconsciously. Communication affects relationships and is a link to other people.

People can control their image through their style of communication. The old "Golden Rule" applies to communication—treat other people the way you would like to be treated. Take the time to think about how you would like to be treated and then treat other people in that manner. They will reciprocate, probably in the same way.

There are some skills people can learn in order to be more effective communicators. This chapter presents activities that help students recognize various attitudes they may be assuming and help them become familiar with different forms of communication. Students are given an opportunity to practice different methods of communication that improve their ability to be understood successfully.

activity **1**

Body Language

time 20 minutes.

purpose This activity helps students realize and appreciate the importance of body language in delivering a message.

materials The handout entitled "Body Language" for each student.

process Explain that nonverbal communication is called *body language*. Many people use a form of body language by *signing* or talking with hand gestures. However, everyone uses body language every day. Explain that attitudes and emotions are clearly conveyed by posture, gestures, blushing, facial expression, and clothing.

Give each student the "Body Language" handout and have the students complete the worksheet. Help students recognize the commonly used forms of body language.

activity **2**

Sending and Receiving

time 45 minutes.

purpose This activity helps students identify the basic components of communication and learn effective communication skills.

materials Blackboard and chalk or an overhead projector and the handouts entitled "Sending Clear Messages" and "Am I Clear?"

process Present the two basic parts of communication—listening or *receiving*, and speaking or *sending*. Ask the students to give an example of each from their own experience.

Communication is an exchange of thoughts, feelings, and emotions that can take place in a variety of ways. Communication can be verbal, written, and nonverbal (sign language or body language). Information is sent consciously and unconsciously regardless of the method of communication.

The way we communicate can influence our lives in many ways. Relationships can be made and lost. Business deals are affected. The way we are perceived by others is built on our ability to communicate effectively. Information and education are built on effective communication.

There are two basic parts to communication: sending and receiving. If you want to be an effective communicator, you need to learn to send clear messages and be a good listener.

Some of the methods for **sending** clear messages are as follows:

- Repeat the message.
- Use gestures or body language to clarify and define your message. Make sure your body language agrees with your verbal language.
- Use "I" messages that include your own experiences and feelings to personalize your message.
- Organize your thoughts and be clear in your delivery of the message.
- Develop a friendly rapport with listeners so they will believe you and want to listen.

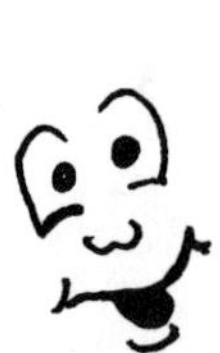
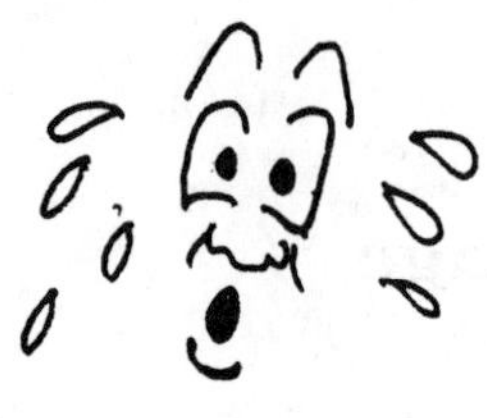
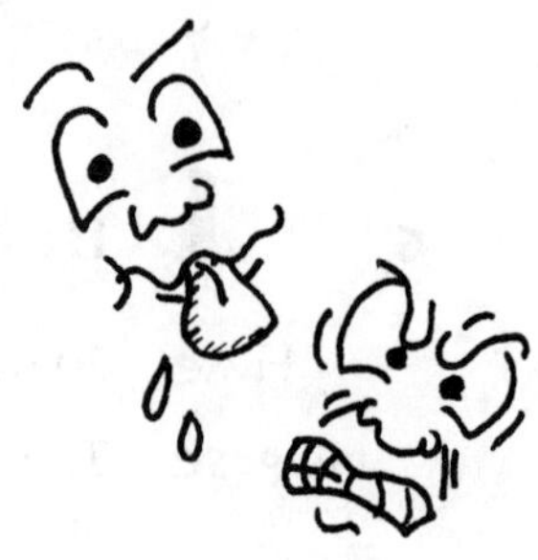

Some of the ways you can improve your methods of **receiving** messages are:

- Hear the message that is being sent by experiencing the feelings of the other person. Put aside judgment and criticism—listen.
- Look at the person sending the message and give him or her your full attention.
- Use gestures or body language to clarify and define your message. Make sure your body language agrees with your verbal language.
- Ask questions to assure that you have heard correctly.
- Repeat the important parts of the message.
- Be aware of body language—yours and theirs.
- Don't interrupt.

Emphasize the importance of body language in communicating with people. It has been said that 80 percent of all we know is learned through eyesight. Many times the way a person behaves speaks much louder than what they say because other people rely heavily on vision for learning. Use an example of contradictory messages—for instance, telling your date that kissing is as far as you want to go but being very sensual in your actions by gently caressing the other person's ear. What message is really being sent? Ask students to give you some examples of contradictory messages from their own experiences.

Have students practice sending clear messages. Students can work with a partner or in small groups of three or four. Give them the "Sending Clear Messages" handout that has students role-play different situations and try to be clearly understood. Only the person doing the role-play should read the situation so the listeners don't have any clues as to the message being sent. Have students take turns role-playing and listening.

Have the partner or the other members of their group tell the message that was actually received. The students can then compare to see if the message they received was the one intended.

Another way of using the handout is to cut out each of the situations and call on a student to role-play the response for the entire class. Then the audience can respond by explaining what they understood the message to be.

follow-up

Have students do the "Am I Clear?" handout as homework or during extra time available in class. Topics should be routine activities that people take for granted —making a peanut butter and jelly sandwich, for instance. It is really fun to bring in a jar of peanut butter, jelly, a loaf of bread, a knife, and a plate. Have students follow the directions exactly as given on how to make a sandwich. Don't volunteer any steps. I always give the successfully completed sandwich to the student who provides the clearest directions.

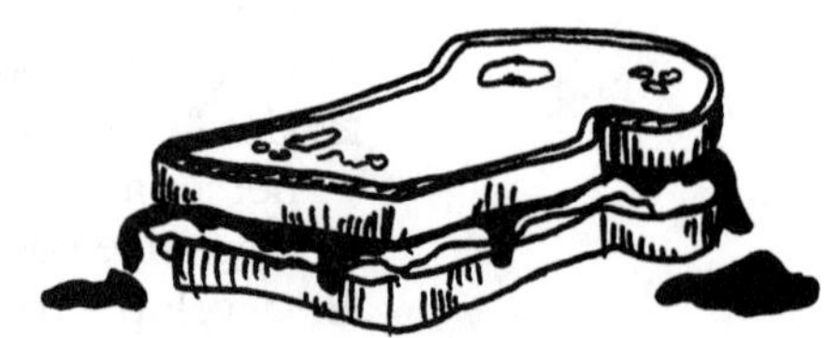

activity 3 Explain a Puzzle

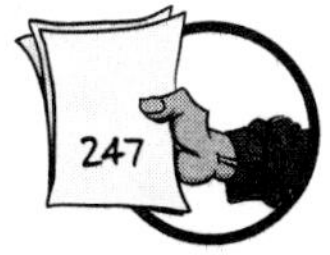

time 10 minutes.

purpose This activity gives students experience in public speaking and helps them clearly organize their thoughts.

materials Copy the shapes from the "Explain a Puzzle" handout and paste them on three-by-five cards. Make additional cards if you need more- or less-complicated shapes. Each student will need a piece of paper to write on.

process Ask for a volunteer from the class. Choose a confident, assertive student. Give the student a card that has one of the copied shapes on it. Tell him or her to hold this card with *both* hands and not to let anyone in the audience see it.

Tell the volunteer to give directions to the class—without using hand gestures or making any other body movements—for drawing the shape. The students follow the directions to the best of their ability. Only allow three questions from the audience for clarification.

When the volunteer is finished giving the directions, have him or her show the class the shape. Walk around to see how many students were able to replicate the shape. It is interesting to see just how close some students got to the actual shape being described.

hint The frustration level may get high. This is a fun activity, however, and is a good way to begin class each day during the unit on communication. Allow two or three students a day to deliver the directions.

activity 4 Clear Directions

time 10 minutes.

purpose This activity gives students experience in public speaking and helps them organize their thoughts to produce clear directions.

materials You will need blindfolds for half the students in the class. Prepare three-by-five cards ahead of time, naming landmarks in the room or objects to which students can be directed.

process Explain that people who can organize their thoughts well and can speak clearly have a better chance of being understood. Tell students they are going to practice giving clear, well-organized directions.

Each student will pick a partner. One person will be blindfolded and will receive directions. The other person will be giving directions to a specific object in the room (or outside if it's a nice day).

Have the person giving directions pick a three-by-five card with a landmark from the room posted on it. That student then has to direct the blindfolded partner to that landmark using as few directions as possible. Tell students they *cannot* say that their partner is "getting hot or cold."

Reverse roles and test the partner's ability to give clear, well-organized directions.

hints This activity can become loud. Tell students they are to move slowly and with caution in order to avoid injury. If there are many students participating at the same time, there might be some confusion. See what works best for you.

This is a terrific activity to take outside on a warm day to break the monotony of being in the classroom.

activity

5 Trust Me

time 20 minutes.

purpose This activity helps students appreciate the importance of body language.

materials Blindfolds for each student in the class.

process Explain to the students that listening is a large part of communication, but noticing the speaker's body language often reveals the true meaning of their message.

Have students get into groups of four or five people. Give each student a blindfold and decide on a topic to discuss. Use a topic you decide on or choose from the following possibilities:

- explain how to tie your shoe
- explain how to brush your teeth
- give directions to your house from the school
- give directions from this room to the cafeteria or office
- describe the interior of your room at home or this classroom

Each student will have 1 minute to speak without being interrupted by the other members of the group. Time each interval and rotate turns so each member of the group gets a chance to speak.

Discuss reactions to this activity as a class. How well were they able to follow the meaning of the speaker? What difficulties did they encounter? How does this exercise compare to speaking on the phone? What are the advantages and disadvantages of not being able to see the person speaking?

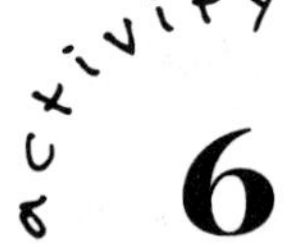

6 Listening Skills

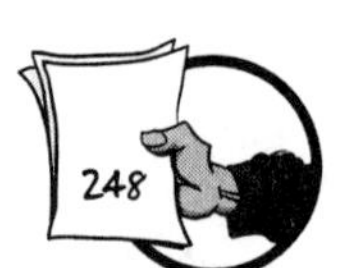

time 20 minutes.

purpose The students practice effective communication and become better listeners.

materials The "Listening Skills" handout for each student.

process Review the skills necessary to be a good listener as presented in Activity 2 in this chapter.

Students work in groups of three. Each student will answer Part One of the worksheet.

Pick a topic for conversation and then have one person begin by speaking about the topic for 1 minute. The second student is the listener and should be demonstrating all the skills attributed to good listening. The third person in the group is the observer and watches the person listening to see whether they demonstrate good listening skills. At the end of the minute, the observer will answer the questions about the listener on Part Two of the worksheet.

Repeat the activity, rotating positions until each member of the group has been speaker, listener, and observer.

follow-up At the end of the activity, ask the students to point out the people they felt were exceptional listeners and tell their reasons for choosing those people. Kids love to hear praise from their peers. It is somehow more valid coming from another student than from a teacher.

activity 7 Recognizing Attitudes

249

time 45 minutes.

purpose Students will identify attitudes and their effects on communication.

materials The "Recognizing Attitudes" handout for each student.

process Explain to the students that the attitudes they display when communicating are important in eliciting a response.

Three general choices can be made when communicating:

- *Non-Assertive or Passive.* Passive behavior places responsibility for making decisions on the other person. This behavior is weak because it allows others the advantage. It could also mean not taking any action at all in a situation that warrants a response.
- *Assertive.* This is a nonthreatening method of communication and is a direct way to express feelings and thoughts. After communicating, both people leave with a feeling of being treated honestly and fairly.
- *Aggressive.* This method of response imposes your own way, often at the expense of other people's rights. It might embarrass or humiliate someone or create hard feelings. A person who behaves aggressively assumes little responsibility for the consequences of their actions.

Each method of behavior is valid when used at an appropriate time. Tell students to think before they act and make sure their behavior reflects the appropriate attitude for the situation. There are times when they need to communicate in an aggressive or passive manner. Assertive behavior is the most desirable attitude in the majority of communication situations because it is clear and nonthreatening.

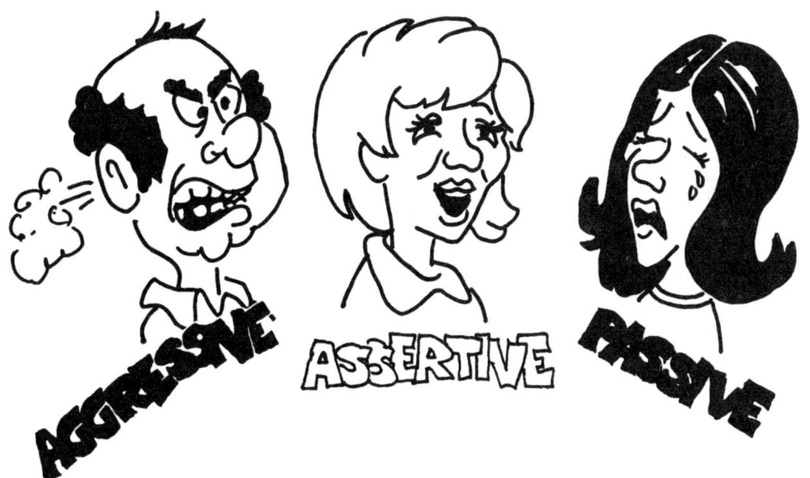

Teenagers often find themselves in a position with adults in which they don't really have control. Assertive behavior can be helpful in attaining their communication goals while keeping them out of trouble.

Give each student the handout entitled "Recognizing Attitudes." Tell the students to work on the assignment by themselves, but they can get help from people around them or in their small groups.

answers The following is a list of the possible answers to the handout questions with explanations. Sometimes the answer may vary depending on the delivery of the person sending the message. A variation of this activity is to have students role-play situations in class and have the class respond by naming the type of attitude.

1. The first response is aggressive—you are being rude without regard for your brother. The second response is passive—you made him guess at your feelings and needs. The third response is assertive—you expressed your desires in a polite manner.
2. The first response is assertive—you expressed your feelings and protected your friend in a polite manner. The second response is passive—you did not protect your judgments about loyalty to your friend. The third response is aggressive—the others know how you feel but you embarrassed them and put them down while doing it.
3. The first response is aggressive—angry behavior will elicit an angry and defensive response from the clerk. The second response is passive—you are not solving the problem. The third response is assertive—you are giving the person a chance to correct their mistake without making them feel bad.
4. The first response is passive—allowing them in front of you makes your turn seem less important. The second response is assertive—you took care of your needs in a polite manner and allowed the person the opportunity to get in line behind you and correct his or her behavior. The third response is aggressive—pushing someone and yelling only makes him or her want to push and yell back.
5. The first response is aggressive—you are demonstrating a lack of responsibility for your actions and your angry behavior will only provoke anger in your parents. The second response is passive—you have not addressed the problem. The third response is assertive—you are accepting your responsibility and addressing the problem of being grounded in a mature and polite manner. (You still might have to accept their punishment, however.)
6. The first response is assertive—you have been direct in your preference. The second response is passive—you are forcing the other person to choose for you when he or she wanted your opinion. The third response is aggressive—you have expressed your preference but in a way that puts down any further discussion.

activity

8 Practicing Assertive Behavior

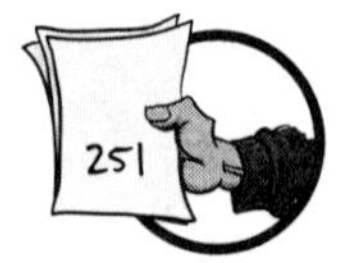

time 30 minutes.

purpose This activity gives students the chance to practice using assertive behavior.

materials The handout entitled "Practicing Assertive Behavior" for each student.

AT THE PARTY...

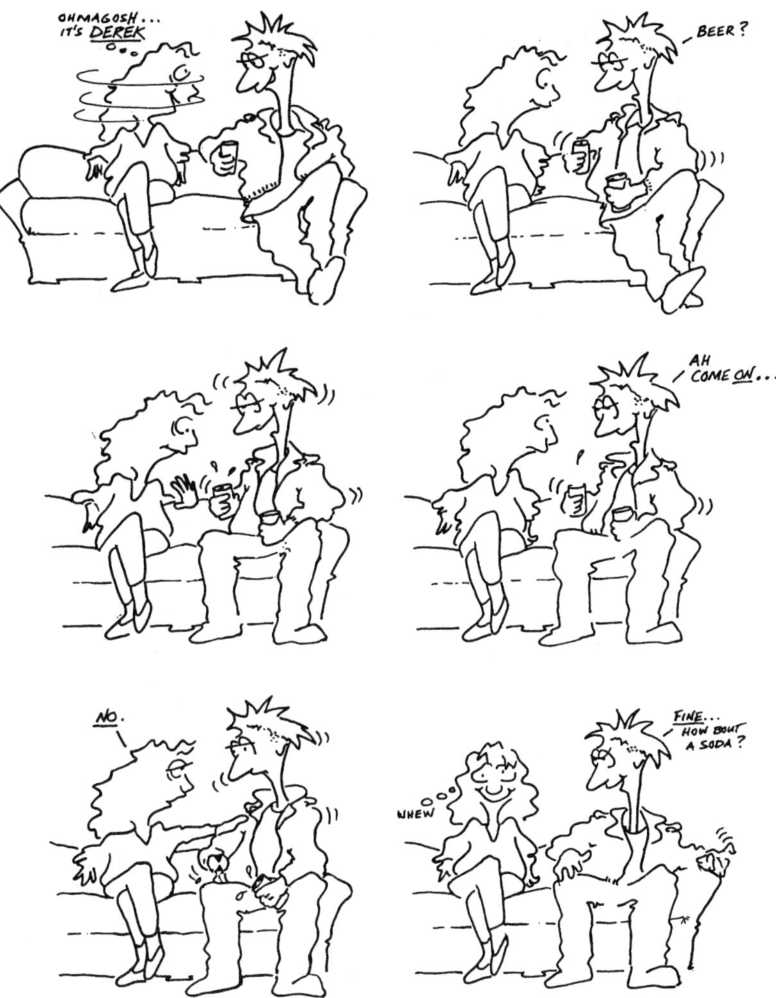
OHMAGOSH...
IT'S DEREK
BEER?
AH
COME ON...
NO.
WHEW
FINE...
HOW BOUT
A SODA?

process Remind students that they need to practice using assertive behavior—it doesn't just occur naturally. Review the tenets of assertive behavior. Have students ask themselves the following questions:

- Are you presenting a clear message?
- What would your response be if someone said this to you?
- How would you feel if someone said this to you?
- Is this an assertive statement—honest and direct, yet respectful of the other person's rights and feelings?
- Am I accepting responsibility for my choices?

Hand out the worksheets and have students write their own assertive responses to the situations.When the worksheets are complete, ask students to act out their responses for the class. The class can evaluate each response for assertiveness.

activity

9 Friendly Refusals

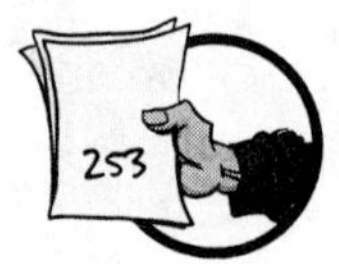

time 45 minutes.

purpose Students learn the steps to making an effective friendly refusal and practice refusing a request made by a friend.

materials The "Friendly Refusals" handout for each student.

process Make the following presentation concerning friendly refusals.

It is fairly easy to refuse a request from someone you do not know or care about. You can say "no" and leave or be rude and not worry because you will never see that person again. It is much more difficult to refuse a request from a friend. You want to realize your own needs but also want to remain friends. What can you do?

Effective friendly refusals do many of the following:

- Include the word "no" in the refusal. Most people need to hear "no" to really understand that your response is a refusal.
- Repeat the refusal using several variations.
- Give a reason for the refusal—explain the problem.
- Provide an alternative. Including your friend in a future activity shows your willingness to be with him or her.
- Walk away or change the subject to end the discussion. They can choose to go with you or they can do whatever they were going to do in the first place. You can't change their behavior, but you can stick up for yourself.

Present an example, such as a situation in which a friend walks up to you at lunch during school and wants you to leave school with him or her for the afternoon. You don't want to for various reasons. Your response could be:

> "No. I don't want to cut school because I am falling behind in science and I need to be in class to understand the material. Besides, if you get caught you will be sent to the office and your parents will be called, which could mean big trouble. Let's go shoot some hoops now and then after school we can go to my house for a while."
>
> Turn and walk to the basketball court.

Have the students practice refusals by writing a friendly refusal for each of the situations presented on the handout. When they finish, have the students exchange papers with a person sitting near them and evaluate each other's refusals. They can also act out their refusal with a partner.

activity

10 Refusal Role-Play

255

time Two 45-minute class periods.

purpose This activity allows students to practice writing and delivering a friendly refusal.

materials The "Ineffective Refusal Role-Play," "Effective Refusal Role-Play," and "Refusal Role-Play: Friendly Refusal" handouts for each small group.

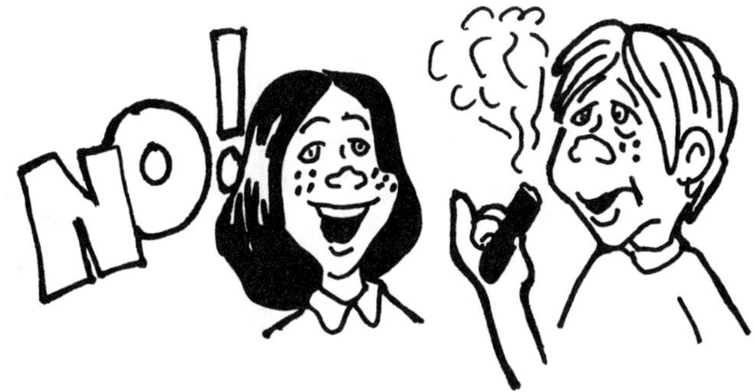

process **DAY ONE** Review the steps to a friendly refusal as explained in Activity 9, "Friendly Refusals," in this chapter.

Ask for a male and a female volunteer to present a role-play of a friendly refusal. Suggest that the class listen to the refusal and evaluate its effectiveness.

Have the students act out the ineffective refusal first. The class can evaluate the refusal.

Ask for two more volunteers—male and female. Have them act out the effective refusal. Have the class evaluate the refusal. List ways in which this refusal is better than the ineffective refusal.

Have students sit in groups of three to four students and write a script using an effective friendly refusal.

DAY TWO Have each group present their skit to the class. The audience will evaluate the effectiveness of the refusal.

Have the steps to a friendly refusal written on the board and check off each step if the audience agrees that the step has been used in the refusal skit. Suggest that the refusal could be more effective if all the steps are included during this practice. Having the class evaluate the refusals allows for more practice for the entire class and gives them a sense of participation.

hints Some of the refusal topics may be inappropriate for class, so take time on the first day to preview each group's work and offer suggestions. The one thing I find the students have a difficult time remembering is that this is to be a *friendly* refusal. Emphasize friendliness as one of the criteria to be met when evaluating the skits.

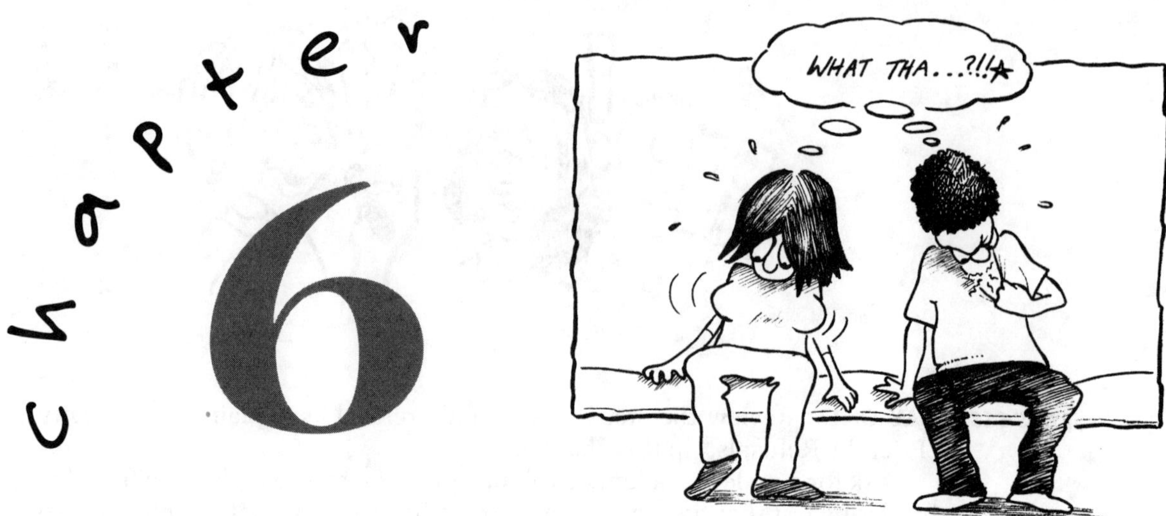

Human Growth and Development

This chapter contains lessons that may cause the most concern among parents and yet be the most interesting to teens. I cannot stress enough the importance of full disclosure to parents of the nature of these lessons. Include parents in discussions of materials presented. Send letters home explaining the proposed topics of discussion. Hold parent information evenings in which you present the nature of the materials used so that parents can relieve their anxieties by asking questions. Create homework assignments that require students to involve adult (parental) participation. This keeps the parents informed and opens lines of communication between students and adults.

Parental permission is necessary and essential in maintaining a class on human growth and development that includes family life education. Develop a letter of permission that meets the legal requirements in your state. The letter should inform the parents of the content of the class and when the student will be participating. A date for previewing materials or for meeting the teacher and asking questions should be included.

I have found that the majority of parents support the need for teenagers to be fully informed on issues of human growth and development. Parents' biggest concerns are about the teaching of morals or values in the classroom. I have satisfied their concern by assuring them that I merely present the facts of human growth and development. Students rely on the values and morals learned at home to make decisions and judgments. The teacher guides students to discover their own values. These values, based on their family background, are often strengthened as students become involved in discussions in which they are sharing their ideas with other students.

I have found the best tools to have at your disposal are a firm belief that this information is essential to healthy development; training in teaching this information; a philosophy with which you feel secure; and a supportive administration that has faith in your ability to be tactful and discreet. Develop these tools fully. Take workshops and classes to strengthen skills in teaching this material. Keep your administration informed and volunteer to present to parents while including your administrators as backup. Be well prepared in every meeting, class, and conference.

Keep in mind that adolescents are confused by the changes they are experiencing. They need to have some references they can look to for reinforcement. You may be an important link in helping your students mature into healthy, responsible adults.

Present the information in a clear, factual, straightforward manner. Reassure students that the material may embarrass them—as it may embarrass you at times. But that is a natural reaction to material that is considered taboo by much of our society. Allow students to express their discomfort. You can demonstrate appropriate reactions to the embarrassment by modeling ways to react maturely. Remember that the students are learning behaviors as well as information. Guide the students in learning appropriate behavioral choices as you would guide them in correcting mistakes on a worksheet. Allow for growth.

Individual students may confront you with questions about what is normal and if they are within those bounds of normalcy. I try to help them understand that many people worry about being normal. I can provide facts about what they can expect as they mature. I often refer them to significant adults in their lives who can help them with moral or values clarification.

This chapter offers a lot of background information that supplements the activities. Information about the basic physiology of the male and female reproductive systems is included, along with brief comments and responses to questions that teenagers often ask. I have found that lecturing in modest doses, reinforced with activities, promotes learning the necessary facts and building attitudes of respect and responsibility.

The objective of this chapter is to help students learn the facts of human growth and development. They will experience personal growth and maturity as they improve their ability to interact successfully with others. While in a safe, protected, and controlled environment, the students will also gain skill in making decisions that enable them to reach life goals.

activity 1 Classroom Guidelines

time 15 minutes.

purpose This activity helps students understand the guidelines that are necessary to learn sensitive information.

materials Blackboard and chalk and a prepared poster reminding students of mature, responsible behaviors. Each student will need a composition notebook for keeping a personal journal.

process Tell students that this is the first day of lessons concerning human growth and development. Explain that many people feel uncomfortable when talking about these topics. Discuss the reasons people might feel uncomfortable talking about sex. List some of the students' ideas on the board.

Explain that it is normal to feel uncomfortable or embarrassed because of all the reasons listed. In order to make the students feel more comfortable and at ease in the classroom, suggest that some guidelines are necessary.

The following is a list of guidelines that may establish a comfortable atmosphere.

- *All questions are valid and will be addressed.* Assure students that no question is stupid or dumb. Provide a question box so students can avoid embarrassment by asking questions anonymously.
- *Students are to assume their most mature and respectful attitudes.* Ask students to use scientific or medical terminology in class rather than slang terms.
- *Be respectful of each person in the class.* Students are at various levels of physical and emotional maturity. Everyone is in transition, so allow for differences with tolerance and patience.
- *A rule of confidentiality applies to the class.* Respect the students' confidentiality but explain that there may be times when you encourage them to talk to counselors or parents.

Pass out composition notebooks to each student. Students will keep a journal of the information and the lessons covered in this unit. They should make entries in their journal each day. Students should record the guidelines for behavior in their notebook.

Set up the journal using the following categories:

- *Lesson or topic for the day.*
- *Brief description of the lesson.* This could include notes taken in class, pictures and diagrams, synopsis of the discussion, or any other method of recording the information presented in class.
- *New vocabulary.* Record new terms and the meanings of those terms.
- *What I learned.* The students tell what they gained from the class discussion or activity.
- *How the information affects me.* The students draw a relationship between the topic of discussion and their own lives.
- *Questions I have.* List any unanswered questions.

activity 2 Differences between Boys and Girls

time 45 minutes.

purpose This activity allows students to become comfortable while developing an understanding of the feelings and differences in the opposite sex. This activity promotes critical thinking skills.

materials Two large sheets of butcher paper and markers. One sheet should be titled "Advantages of being a girl" and the other titled "Advantages of being a boy."

process Remind students that they should demonstrate a high level of maturity during this activity. They should also remember to use scientific or medical terms when writing on the butcher paper.

Have the boys sit on one side of the room and the girls sit on the other side. Give both groups a sheet of butcher paper and four markers. Give them about 10 minutes to make a list of the advantages of being their gender. They will be showing their poster to the other group at the end of the 10 minutes. Have them record ideas in a positive manner and refer to body parts only *once* on their chart.

Monitor the students as they record their ideas to ensure a respectful presentation. Because this is the first activity in the unit, many students will test the limits of acceptable behavior. I find that this is a great time to model mature behavior and make constructive criticism. It is important to allow students the opportunity to learn from mistakes rather than discipline a breach in behavior. Point out each breach in appropriate behavior tenderly. You are trying to develop an atmosphere of comfort and safety, and you can only do that by understanding and allowing for change.

Post the two completed lists and read them aloud. Lead a class discussion allowing students to question or object to various ideas presented on the lists. Students should be able to explain why they disagree and be able to support their theories.

activity 3 Puberty

time 45 minutes.

purpose Students learn to recognize and better understand the changes taking place in their bodies during adolescence.

materials Lots of energy, good humor, and patience.

process Lead a class discussion about puberty.

Puberty is a stage in development when a person's body changes from a child's body into that of an adult. It is an exciting time during which you experience physical, social, and emotional changes that will prepare you for being an adult.

The most obvious changes occur physically. You grow taller and your body takes on adult characteristics. Some emotional changes occur as well. You begin to reject your parents' guidelines and accept those values that your friends consider important. You may identify strongly with friends—even to the exclusion of family.

You want to rely on yourself but lack the confidence and experience of an adult, so you depend on your friends for support and confidence. You may also feel lost and alone. You may feel confused because you alternate between wanting to be nurtured and comforted like a child and changing into a wild, hormonal beast locked in conflict with adults.

Your body is changing. Secondary sex characteristics develop, indicating that you are changing from a child to an adult.

Everyone grows and develops according to a pattern that is right for them. Girls tend to start puberty about two or three years earlier than boys. For girls, this process might start as early as age 8 or as late as age 16—or older. Boys begin puberty as early as 10 years old or as late as age 18. These changes occur according to nature's own clock.

The following list includes some secondary sex characteristics.

- The female's body shape or contour will change. Hips will become rounder and wider and breasts grow and become fuller. These changes prepare the body for childbearing.
- Girls begin to menstruate. Menstruation is discussed in Activity 8 later in this chapter.
- The vulva, which is the outside of the female genital organs, changes. The tissues become fleshier and the vaginal opening becomes larger.
- Male sex organs begin to grow larger. The testicles grow at a rapid rate and the scrotum begins to hang lower. The penis doesn't usually begin to grow until there is a noticeable change in the size of the testicles.
- Males experience more erections and may start having nocturnal emissions, commonly called "wet dreams."
- The voice changes in both boys and girls. As the voice box, or larynx, grows, the vocal cords get longer. The voice will take on a deeper, more resonant tone. This change is especially dramatic in boys. Sometimes the larynx will grow in a manner that causes the voice to "crack" and seem out of control.
- Hair grows in the pubic or genital area and under the arms. Hair on the legs becomes heavier and more coarse. Males develop facial hair.
- Pimples develop in most adolescents as the oil glands in the skin become more active. Pimples may occur on the face, neck, shoulders, or chest, where there are more oil glands than in other parts of the body. Pimples are oil glands that become clogged and fill with a whitish pus. There is no cure for pimples, but keeping hair clean and away from the neck and face may help. Washing prevents the pores in the skin from clogging and allows those pores to remain open.
- Increased sweating or perspiration will occur as the sweat glands become more active. Perspiration under the arms, on hands and feet, or around the genital area may increase. This perspiration may have an odor. Bathe regularly and wear clean clothes. A good deodorant may become necessary.

These changes occur at different rates from person to person. Talk to an adult or doctor if you are worried about the rate at which you are developing.

All the changes that take place are controlled by *hormones*. These are substances produced by many different glands in the body. Some hormones control body changes directly while others control the production of still more hormones. The pituitary gland, which is located in the brain, is thought to produce the hormone that starts the whole process.

Hormones produced in the pituitary gland travel through the bloodstream to the reproductive glands located in the genital region. The reproductive glands produce their own hormones that control the changes that occur in your body during puberty.

journal entry Have students record the required information in their journals. Lead the students through the journal topics, reviewing the information on puberty, secondary sex characteristics, and hormones. Students can draw a human body and indicate the areas where secondary sex characteristics will occur.

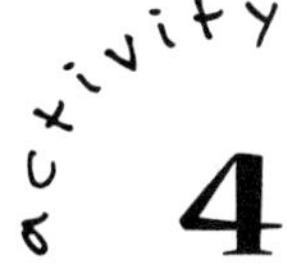

4 Am I Normal?

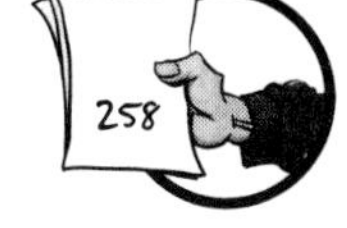

time 15-minute explanation.

purpose This activity opens lines of communication between the teenager and a significant adult.

materials The "Am I Normal" handout for each student.

process Ask students to define the word *normal.* Then have students brainstorm what being normal means to them. Point out that there may be many ideas of what is normal.

Give each student a copy of the handout. Tell them to interview a significant adult in their life. They can talk to a parent, grandparent, counselor, adult friend, or teacher. Have them ask the adult the interview questions on the handout. Remind students that the adult should have the right to pass on answering a question.

Students should not write down the answers to the questions but merely talk about the questions with the adult. The adult will sign the worksheet in the space provided, confirming that the interview has taken place.

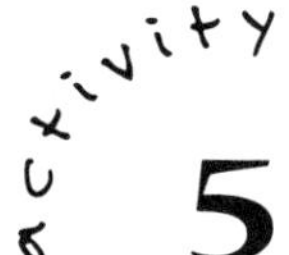

5 Everything You Want to Know—And More

time 45 minutes.

purpose Students gain knowledge and appreciation about topics that concern them during adolescence.

materials Students will need their journal notebook and access to three-by-five cards. You also need to prepare a question box. The box is a place in which students can put questions on cards if they are too embarrassed to ask the questions in class.

process Tell students to list the things on the card that they have questions about as you lecture and to place the card in the question box. You can draw cards out of the box at a later time and give a brief explanation of each topic or term.

Below is a list of topics that concern teenagers:

- *Loss of virginity.* The membrane that partly closes the vaginal opening is called the *hymen.* This membrane will break during the first time a girl has intercourse, if it is still intact. Girls today are very active and many times the hymen is stretched or broken during normal childhood activities, so there may not be any bleeding during intercourse. The girl is still a virgin if she has not had sex, even if the hymen is broken.

- *Menstruation.* It is okay for a girl to swim or take a bath while she is having her period. It is even possible to have sex at this time, although it may be messy. The possibility of becoming pregnant still exists.
- *Breasts.* During puberty, a girl's breasts will begin to grow, sometimes by developing a hard lump under the nipple. The lump should go away eventually. Breasts come in all sizes and shapes. Some girls' breasts may start to grow at an early age, others may start to grow later. It is not unusual for one breast to become larger than the other breast. As boys begin puberty, their breasts will sometimes become full and seem as if they are going to develop. This is usually a reaction to the onslaught of hormones and may last for a while and then return to what is considered "normal."
- *Penis.* As a boy begins puberty, his penis and testicles grow. The penis will grow to a length determined by the genetic plan he inherited from his parents. The sac containing the testicles, called the *scrotum,* will lengthen and allow the testicles to hang further from the body. Sometimes only one testicle will drop while the other remains closer to the body. Erections occur, causing the penis to swell and stiffen. Erections can happen in sexual situations or from ordinary circumstances.
- *Dreams.* It's normal for girls and boys to begin having dreams concerning sexual fantasies. These dreams can cause physical reactions. A boy may experience a "wet dream," in which his penis becomes erect and ejaculation occurs. Girls may experience physical stimulation as the vagina becomes moist with lubricating fluid.
- *Emotional changes.* It is normal for adolescents to feel huge shifts in emotions. A fight for independence from their parents is normal. There may be times when adolescents feel both dependent and independent at the same time. It is also common to feel isolated—as though no one else feels the same way. Most teenagers would be surprised to know how many of their friends feel the same way.
- *Growth.* Boys and girls grow at a rapid rate during adolescence. Their feet and hands begin to grow first and the rest of the body is not far behind. It takes time for their minds to adjust to the changes in body size, so they may be clumsy and awkward for a while. This passes eventually. They may also feel tired more often because growth demands a lot of energy.
- *Heterosexuality and homosexuality.* Studies have been done that show that a person's sexual orientation may be established long before adolescence. Some people believe that sexual orientation is determined before birth. As adolescents undergo the physical changes that alter the shape and size of their body, they also go through stages in emotional relationships. It is common to develop close ties to members of the same sex during childhood and adolescence. These close relationships occur regardless of a person's final sexual orientation.
- *Love and/or sex.* Love and sex do not necessarily go together. Someone can feel sexual excitement for a person and not love them. Also, a person can love someone but not feel sexually aroused. Frequently, sex is a compelling force in a loving relationship, but there are many ways to show someone love without having sex.
- *Masturbation.* The word *masturbation* describes the action of a person stimulating his or her own genitals to a point of sexual excitement. There

are many rumors about masturbation—the person will go blind or crazy or grow hair on the palms of his or her hands, for instance. These rumors are not true. Many people have strong religious or moral beliefs regarding masturbation and feel that it is wrong. It is rarely physically harmful but may cause feelings of guilt if someone is brought up in an environment in which masturbation is believed to be wrong.

- *Body odor.* As boys and girls progress through adolescence, their bodies produce more hormones and more perspiration. Their sweat often carries a strong odor. It is important to practice good personal hygiene by bathing regularly and using deodorant.
- *Complexion.* Hormones make adolescents perspire more and also make the skin produce more oils. If the oils are left to clog pores and hair follicles, and inflammation develops that results in pimples. The best treatment for pimples is to wash regularly and keep the area free from makeup. Teenagers should get proper nutrition and go to a doctor if the problem is severe.

hints Always advise students to talk to their parents if they are concerned about something happening in their bodies. You, as the teacher, can also be a resource.

journal entry Allow time for students to make the journal entry for the day. You may need to write some of the topics of discussion on the board for reference.

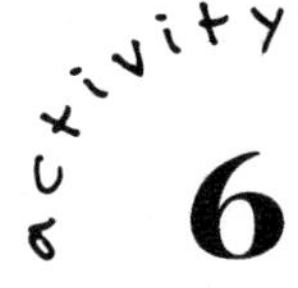

6 Male Reproductive System

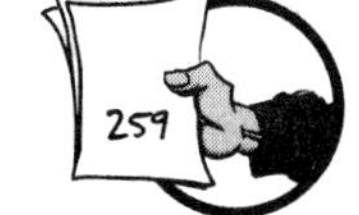

time 45 minutes for the discussion and 15–20 minutes for the activity.

purpose Students learn to describe the path the sperm follow during ejaculation. They will also gain an appreciation and understanding of the male reproductive system.

materials The diagram of the male reproductive system and the "See What You Have Learned" handouts and colored pencils.

process Lead a discussion on the male reproductive system.

The reproductive cell produced by the male is called the *sperm.* It is the smallest cell in the human body. More than 1,000 sperm cells can fit on the head of a straight pin. Once the male starts producing sperm during puberty, sperm will be continuously produced for the rest of his life. As he reaches old age, sperm production will slow down.

Sperm are produced in two glands, called *testicles,* which are located in a skin-covered sac called the *scrotum.* The scrotum also contains a muscle that acts as a thermostat by raising and lowering the scrotum, thus controlling temperature in the testicles. A constant temperature of 95 degrees is necessary for the production of sperm.

Ask the students if they have ever wondered why the testicles are externally located on the body. Many of the most important organs in the body are well protected, such as the brain inside the skull and the heart and lungs protected by the ribs. The testicles, however, are located in a vulnerable position. Why? Well, sperm can only be produced at a temperature of about 95 degrees. People's body temperature is about 98 to 99 degrees, which is too warm for the production of sperm. The testicles are located outside the body to provide the cooler temperature necessary. The muscle in the scrotum pulls the testicles closer to the body for warmth in a cold environment and relaxes to allow the testicles to hang as far from the body as possible in a warm environment.

Once the sperm are produced, they travel to the *epididymus,* which is a holding area in which the sperm mature. It takes the sperm about four to six weeks to mature and travel through the extensive tubular system in the epididymus.

Once the sperm are mature, they travel into the body through a tube called the *vas deferens.* The sperm are then stored in an area of the vas deferens called the *ampulla* until they are ejaculated when the male becomes sexually excited. Sperm live for about 24 to 48 hours once they mature and are absorbed back into the body if they are not ejaculated.

The *seminal vesicles* produce a white sticky fluid called *seminal fluid.* The seminal fluid mixes with the sperm and is called *semen.* The sperm become very active in the semen, which allows them the mobility required for fertilization. The *prostate gland* also contributes some fluid to the semen and helps during ejaculation by squeezing the vas deferens and pushing the semen into the *urethra,* which is the tube that travels down the center of the *penis.*

The urethra carries the sperm through the penis. It is also the pathway for urine traveling from the bladder through the penis. When a man has an ejaculation and the sperm are forced from the vas deferens through the urethra, a tiny valve at the bottom of the bladder closes, making it impossible to pass urine at the same time.

As a man becomes sexually excited, he has an *erection.* The penis enlarges and becomes firm and rigid. The erection starts when the male becomes excited in his brain. His brain sends out chemical messengers in the bloodstream to the entire body. The messengers cause many blood vessels to close down but allows the blood vessels in the penis to open. Blood then rushes from other parts of the body to fill the millions of blood vessels in the penis, filling it much the same way as a water balloon. The more liquid that rushes into the penis, the larger and more firm the penis becomes.

An *ejaculation* occurs as the muscles around the prostate gland and the muscles in and around the penis contract. These muscle spasms force the semen into the urethra and out of the penis in several spurts of fluid. About a teaspoon of fluid is ejaculated. The action of the muscles contracting and causing the ejaculation is called an *orgasm.*

Many things can cause sexual excitement and an erection. The erection can be sudden and take just a few seconds to occur, or it may take a much longer time. Erections can happen from thinking about a girl, looking at sexy pictures, or having pants that are too tight and rub against the penis—or for no reason at all. This can be embarrassing for a boy if he is in public, but erections are natural. Not all erections end in ejaculation. If an erection does not end in an ejaculation, the penis will get soft again.

One sign that a boy has begun puberty is the ejaculation of semen. Sometimes an erection occurs as a boy sleeps and dreams. A sexually exciting dream can cause an ejaculation. This is called a "wet dream" or a *nocturnal emission.* Wet dreams are natural and a signal that the boy is becoming an adult.

After the discussion, give each student a copy of the handout and colored pencils. Allow time for students to complete the activity. Encourage students to work together. This promotes discussion and success in completing the activity.

journal entry Provide time for students to make journal entries for the day.

follow-up You could also use the unlabeled diagram to test the students' knowledge of the male reproductive system. Have the students find and label the parts of the reproductive system.

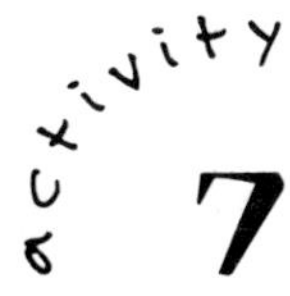

7 Female Reproductive System

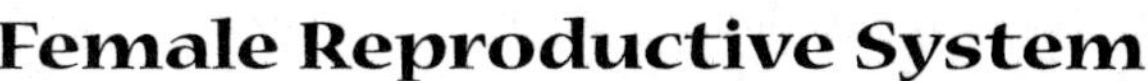

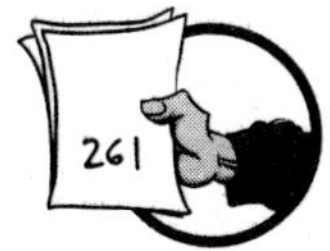

time 45 minutes for the discussion and 15–20 minutes for the activity.

purpose Students learn to describe the female reproductive system. They also gain an appreciation and understanding of the female reproductive system.

materials The diagram of the female reproductive system and the "See What You Have Learned" handouts and colored pencils.

process Lead a discussion on the female reproductive system.

The reproductive cell for the female is called the *ovum.* In contrast to the male reproductive cell, which is the smallest cell in the body, the ovum is the largest cell. It is about the size of the head of a straight pin and can be seen without a microscope.

The ovum is produced in glands called *ovaries,* located on either side of the lower abdomen. Females are born with all the ova they will ever need. However, only a small fraction of the total number of ova will be used in the woman's lifetime.

Puberty begins as the pituitary gland in the brain releases a hormone called *FSH* (follicle stimulating hormone) that travels in the bloodstream to the ovaries. The ovaries are then stimulated to begin producing ova and another hormone called *estrogen.* Estrogen then travels through the bloodstream causing many of the secondary sex changes that occur during puberty.

As estrogen levels in the body rise, the pituitary gland starts making another hormone called *LH* (lutenizing hormone) and slows down the production of FSH. The LH travels to the ovaries and causes an ovary to release a mature ovum. *Ovulation* is the process of the ovum bursting from the ovary. Ovulation occurs about once every 28 days and will usually alternate from one ovary producing an ovum one month to the other producing an ovum the following month. Sometimes, however, each ovary may produce an ovum or several ova can be released from one ovary. If two ova are later fertilized by sperm, fraternal twins will result.

While on the subject of twins, take the time to clear up some misconceptions. *Fraternal* or *nonidentical twins* are created when two ova are produced and fertilized by separate sperm. Fraternal twins can consist of a boy and a girl or two babies of the same sex but they will be no more alike than any other brother or sister. *Identical twins* are formed when one ovum is produced and fertilized by one sperm. Very early in the growth and development of the ovum, as it splits into more and more cells, it occasionally pulls apart into two separate groups of cells, which will become embryos. These twins will be of the same sex and look identical because they have the same origin—the same sperm and ovum formed both individuals. In the rare instance of *conjoined twins,* one ovum is fertilized by one sperm as with identical twins. Instead of later pulling apart completely, the groups of cells remain connected at one point. This point of connection forms the linkage between the two bodies. This linkage can be at any point and the twins may share organs or limbs. Sometimes surgery can be performed to successfully separate the twins if they are not sharing important organs.

Return to the discussion of ovulation. The ovum bursts out of the ovary during ovulation and is drawn into the *Fallopian tubes.* The Fallopian tubes have finger-like projections that pull the ovum into one of the tubes. These tubes are about the thickness of a strand of spaghetti and about four inches long. They are lined with tiny hairs called *cilia* that move back and forth and push the ovum along the tube toward the uterus.

The *uterus* is a muscular organ about the size of a clenched fist. This is the place where a baby grows and develops during pregnancy. During pregnancy, it is called the *womb.* The uterus is lined with a spongy tissue rich in blood vessels called the *endometrium.* When the ovum bursts from the ovary during ovulation, another hormone is produced from the torn tissue of the ovary. This tissue is the *corpus luteum* and produces the hormone *progesterone.* Progesterone causes the endometrium in the uterus to become even thicker and more nourishing for a fertilized ovum.

If the ovum has not been fertilized by sperm, the corpus luteum stops making progesterone and the lining begins to break down. Because the ovum will not develop and is not going to need the support and nourishment of the endometrial lining, the lining begins to loosen from the inside wall of the uterus. The lining will slowly pass from the uterus, through the *cervix,* the opening at the bottom of the uterus, and into the vagina.

The *vagina* is an opening that connects the uterus to the outside of the body. It is only about three to five inches long but can stretch to accept the penis during sexual intercourse. The vagina is sometimes partly covered by a thin flap of skin called the *hymen.* When a woman has intercourse for the first time, this tissue can tear or rupture, causing a small amount of bleeding. Some people think the hymen is important in proving a woman's virginity. Some women are born without a hymen and others may stretch or tear the hymen during a normally active life while participating in activities like horseback riding or gymnastics. When the hymen does tear during intercourse, or any other time, there may be a small amount of blood and a minimal amount of pain. The pain and bleeding may vary somewhat from person to person.

All the organs we have discussed so far have been internal. They are located inside the woman's body. The external portion of the female genital region consists of the *labia minora,* the *labia majora,* and the *clitoris.* The labia are folds of skin that help protect the opening to the vagina. The labia minora come together at the front of the body and form the clitoris. The clitoris is very sensitive to touch and becomes firm when sexually stimulated.

When the discussion is completed, give each student a copy of the handout and colored pencils. Give students time to complete the activity. Allow students to work together. This promotes discussion and success in completing the activity.

journal entry Allow time for students to make journal entries for the day.

follow-up You could also use the unlabeled diagram to test the students' knowledge of the female reproductive system. Have the students find and label those parts of the reproductive system on their diagrams.

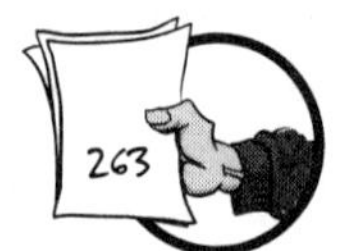

8 The Menstrual Cycle

time 45-minute presentation.

purpose The students will gain an understanding of the menstrual cycle.

materials Students will need their journal and the "Menstruation" handout.

process Lead a discussion about the menstrual cycle.

Sometime between the ages of 9 and 16, most girls begin to *menstruate.* When the ovum is not fertilized by sperm, it disintegrates after a few days. Because the *endometrium,* the thick lining in the uterus, is no longer needed, it begins to break down and slowly pass from the body. This is the process of menstruation.

It takes about 3 to 7 days for the endometrium to pass from the body. During this time, a girl will wear a sanitary pad inside her underpants or a tampon inserted into her vagina to absorb the bloody tissue. She changes the pad or tampon every few hours as it fills with blood. The amount of blood that leaves the utcrus can vary between a tablespoon to about a cup. The amount varies from woman to woman. Each woman has her own pattern, which may change at times depending on illness, travel, or emotional turmoil.

When her period is finished for that month, her body will immediately begin the task of building a new endometrium in the uterus. This prepares the body for the next month when ovulation occurs. This cycle is called the *menstrual cycle* and takes about 28 days. This cycle will continue to repeat itself every month until the woman reaches about age 45 to 55. At that time, her body will gradually stop having this cycle and she will go through *menopause.* After menopause, the woman will no longer ovulate and will no longer be able to have children. Sexual activity can remain an important part of a woman's life long after she passes through menopause.

As a girl starts having her menstrual cycle, the length of the cycle may vary from month to month as her body adjusts to this new process. It may take a couple of years to finally settle down into a regular, dependable cycle. An irregular cycle may occur again as the woman reaches the time of menopause. The body must adjust again to the cycle ending.

A young woman may be a little uncomfortable during her period. She may experience cramping pains in her lower abdomen or back. There may also be a feeling of bloating or fullness a few days before the menstrual flow actually begins. She may have a shift in emotions that can cause a few difficult days. These symptoms are often referred to as *PMS—premenstrual syndrome.* Most women experience some of these feelings at some time during their life but seem to be able to overlook the discomfort and go on with their normal activities. Severe discomfort caused by menstruation could be a signal that something is wrong. A woman should always listen to her body and go to the doctor if she has questions. If the discomfort continues, medication can be prescribed to alleviate the problem.

The following diagram illustrates the menstrual cycle. Start counting the days of the average 28-day cycle on the day that bleeding begins.

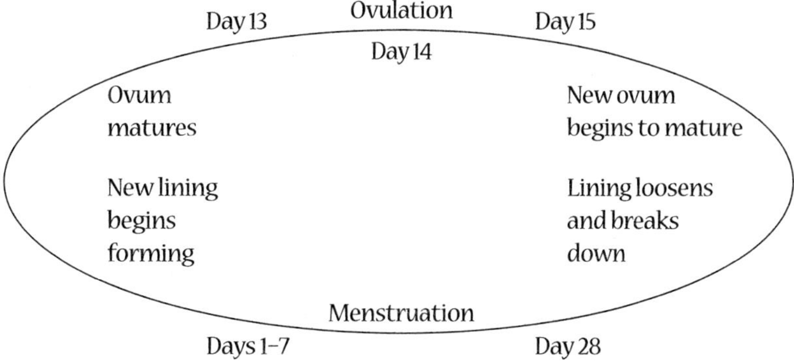

journal entry Allow time for students to write in their journals. You may need to lead the writing to emphasize and review important points.

activity 9 You Bet Your Life!

time 30 minutes.

purpose This activity graphically illustrates the risk involved in having intercourse while practicing the "natural selection" method of birth control.

material blackboard and chalk.

process Draw the diagram of the 28-day menstrual cycle on the board. Review briefly as you label each event during the cycle. (See the illustration that follows.)

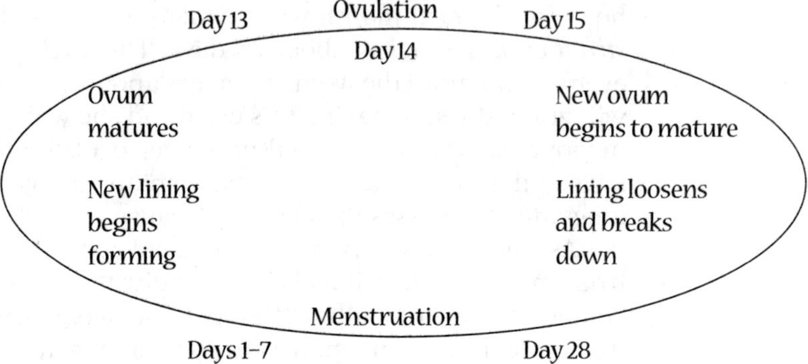

Challenge students to "Bet Their Lives." Tell them to pretend that they are on a date some Friday night and have been persuaded (against their better judgment) to have intercourse. They are not prepared with any form of birth control and so are going to hope they are in a safe time during the menstrual cycle and will avoid pregnancy. Remind students that this happens all too often with teenagers because they often feel that nothing can happen to them. It is always someone else, "that" kind of girl, who gets pregnant.

Tell students they will have one vote to guess the time during the menstrual cycle when a woman can become pregnant most easily. Ask them to raise their hands when you point to the event during the menstrual cycle in which the woman would be most fertile.

Remind the boys that this affects them, also. Fathers can be held financially responsible for their children until that child reaches the age of 18 in most states. Women will definitely be affected if they are pregnant because their lives will change, whatever they choose to do about the pregnancy. Their choices are:

- keep the baby and raise it
- have the baby and put the baby up for adoption
- have an abortion

All these choices will affect the future well-being of the mother.

Point to each event during the menstrual cycle on the diagram on the board. Record the number of votes for each guess of the time when a woman will be most fertile. Remind students that if they know the time of the month when a woman is most fertile, they should avoid having sex at that time if they don't want a pregnancy to occur.

Record all the votes. Build up the suspense by describing the life the students will lead if they have made an incorrect choice.

Ask students to think about having to go home this afternoon and tell their parents that they are pregnant or have just gotten a girl pregnant. Ask them to visualize their parents' response.

Finally, refer to the votes and the menstruation chart. Point to ovulation as the time when a woman is most able to become pregnant. Remind students that even if they were correct in their vote, pregnancy might still occur because every woman is different and may ovulate at a different time during the cycle. Women are also affected by emotional and physical changes during their cycle that can vary the normal time of ovulation. Tell students that there is *no* time during the cycle that is completely dependable and that having sexual intercourse is risking pregnancy.

Remind students that sperm live for 24 to 48 hours. If a woman has intercourse on day 12 or 13 of her cycle, she may risk pregnancy because the sperm might still be viable enough to cause conception to occur. The ovum lives for 3 to 5 days. Engaging in intercourse on day 15, 16, 17, or even day 18 might result in pregnancy.

Trying to avoid pregnancy by avoiding intercourse around the time of ovulation is called the natural selection method of birth control and is not very effective.

activity 10 Reasons for Abstinence

time 45 minutes.

purpose Students will acknowledge and be aware of reasons for choosing abstinence at their age.

materials A sheet of large butcher paper and markers for each group.

process Establish small groups of four or five students. Give each group a large piece of butcher paper and a marker.

Ask students to define the word *abstinence.* Write the ideas on the board that best describe the term. Tell students they will have 10 minutes to list reasons for teenagers to remain abstinent. They will be sharing their lists with the rest of the class.

At the end of 10 minutes, each group will display its list. Each group chooses a spokesperson who will offer two of the group's reasons for abstinence. Give all the groups a chance to share and keep going around the room until all the ideas have been presented.

Allow time for discussion.

activity 11 Recognize Affection

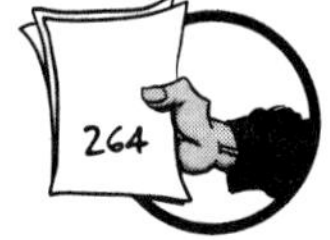

time 15 minutes.

purpose Students are reminded that there are many ways to show affection without having sexual intercourse.

materials The handout entitled "Recognize Affection" for each student.

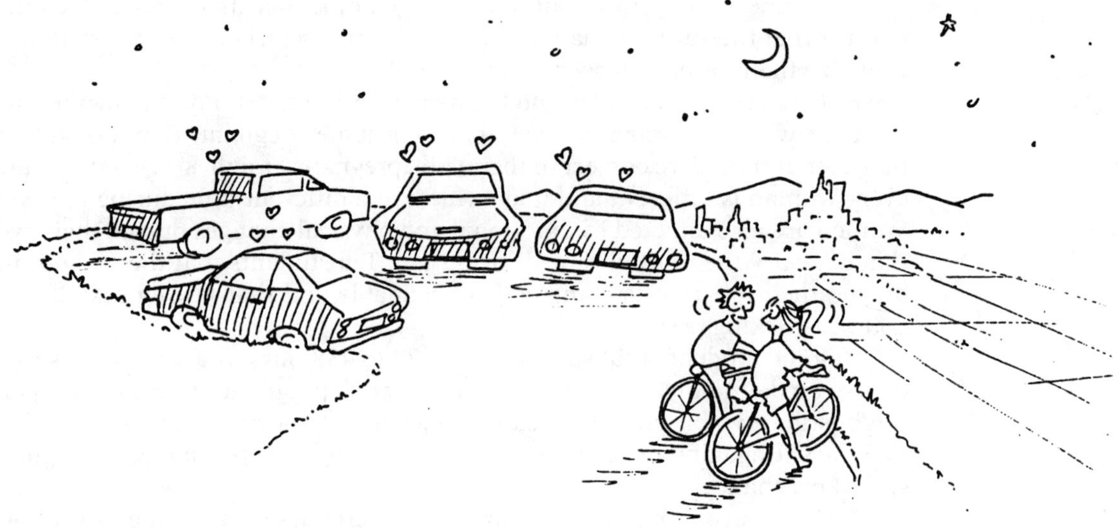

process Offer a personal story about a date you thought was especially romantic. Make up a story if you are shy! Or describe your favorite romantic scene from a movie.

Ask students to volunteer some examples of romantic moments they have seen in the movies or on television. Have them explain what made that moment romantic. Point out that the romantic moments probably did not include intercourse although they may have led to intercourse later.

Give each student a copy of the handout entitled "Recognize Affection" and tell them to answer the questions on the paper. They will also be categorizing their romantic suggestions on a continuum. The ideas should be placed on the continuum according to their rating.

hints Tell students you realize these papers are very personal and that they will not be shared with other students in the class.

Be aware that some parents may disapprove of this activity. I have found that parents need to understand that the purpose of this activity is to show students there are many ways of demonstrating affection without resorting to sexual intercourse. Many parents feel that their children are too young to even be thinking about these things. Some parents disapprove because of religious practices that frown on displays of affection. However, don't skip this assignment out of fear. This activity is effective in illustrating to students the various ways to show affection without the need for sexual intercourse.

activity 12 Pregnancy

265

time 45 minutes.

purpose Students become aware of the stages of fetal development during pregnancy. They develop an appreciation of the miracle of birth.

materials Students will need their journals. It is helpful to have a large chart or pictures illustrating the stages of pregnancy. The "Fetal Development during Pregnancy" and "Fetal Development" handouts can be given out to each student for reference, but try to have more detailed charts available.

process Lead a discussion about pregnancy and fetal development.

Pregnancy occurs when the ovum from a woman is fertilized by the sperm from a man. Students often ask questions about exactly how this happens.

Women and men share an act called sexual intercourse. This is an intimate act and usually happens when two people want to be especially close. Sexual intercourse can be a wonderful experience when it is shared between two responsible people who love each other.

The man becomes sexually excited and has an erection that causes the penis to become firm and rigid. Once erect, the penis can slide easily into the vagina of a woman. The vagina is able to stretch to receive the penis.

The genital area on men and women is filled with many nerve endings that can be stimulated in ways that are pleasurable. These feelings will travel to the brain and cause the whole body to be stimulated. As that feeling increases, it may result in an orgasm. In a man, an orgasm causes the sperm to be ejaculated from the penis into the vagina. The sperm must then travel through the uterus and into the Fallopian tubes to the ovum.

The sperm scatter as they are ejaculated and only a small percentage of the total amount will make it to the ovum. The sperm that don't get to the ovum will gradually leave the body by draining out the vagina or by being absorbed. Sometimes millions of sperm are ejaculated at one time. Of the sperm that do get to the ovum, only one may penetrate the outer chemical coating and fertilize the ovum. Fertilization does not occur every time an ovum and sperm are present, but it could.

When one sperm penetrates the outer coating of the ovum, a chemical reaction takes place that repels the other sperm, allowing only that one to enter the ovum. The process of the sperm entering the ovum is called *conception*. The sperm and ovum each have chromosomes that carry the map or code for the baby that will develop. The sperm carries half of the traits and the ovum carries the other half. When the two chromosomes combine, the traits that are dominant or stronger will prevail. These traits are inherited from the mother and the father, each supplying half the traits necessary to make a new human being.

The fertilized ovum begins to grow and divide into more and more cells as it makes its way to the uterus and settles into the thick, spongy lining that was prepared for just this reason. The developing ovum is now called an *embryo*.

By the end of the second week of pregnancy, the cells in the embryo begin to specialize into nerve, bone, muscle, and other specialized tissues. The embryo is about the size of a grain of sand at this point.

When the embryo is about 6 weeks old, it will begin to move, and the testes or ovaries will begin to form. At the end of the first 3 months of pregnancy, which is called the *first trimester*, the embryo will be about 3 inches long from head to toe. All organs will be functioning and there will be coordinated movement such as thumb sucking and grasping.

In the *second trimester*, or the fourth, fifth, and sixth months of pregnancy, the baby continues to grow and develop. By the end of the fifth month, the baby's heartbeat can be heard. The baby is about 8 to 12 inches long and weighs about 8 ounces—one-half pound.

The *third* or *last trimester* is the time of most rapid growth. The baby, or *fetus*, has a good chance of survival if it happens to be born by the end of the seventh month of pregnancy. A *premature birth* is one that occurs before the full 9 months of pregnancy are finished. The baby will be about 15 inches long and weigh about 3 pounds by the end of the seventh month of pregnancy.

By the end of the ninth and final month of pregnancy, the normal, healthy baby will be about 20 inches in length and weigh about 7 or 8 pounds. All the organs will be mature and functioning.

The developing baby is actually a little like an astronaut while inside the mother. It is in a protected environment and is attached to a source of oxygen and nutrition. The baby floats in a liquid called *amniotic liquid* that is held inside the amniotic sac. This fluid is the "water" that comes out when a mother is nearing childbirth and her "waters break." The fluid protects the baby from outside injury.

The baby is attached to a *placenta* by the *umbilical cord.* The placenta filters the baby's blood, processes nutrition, and provides oxygen for the baby. The umbilical cord connects the placenta to the belly of the baby and acts as the baby's lifeline. When the baby is born, the placenta is called the *afterbirth* and is delivered after the baby is born. The umbilical cord is cut, and the place where it attached to the baby forms the navel or belly button.

journal entry Provide time for the students to write in their journals.

activity 13 Childbirth

269

time 45 minutes.

purpose Students learn about the process of childbirth.

materials The "Stages of Labor" handout and the students' journals. It is helpful to have a large chart or pictures illustrating childbirth.

process Lead a discussion about the process of childbirth.

When a baby is ready to be born, the mother will experience muscular contractions in her abdomen or lower back. This is called *labor.* The muscular wall of the uterus contracts to push the baby into position to be born. The contractions begin slowly and feel like mild cramping, then increase in intensity and frequency as labor progresses. Labor may be over quickly or last a long time, depending on the woman and the pregnancy. A doctor may be called on to help if labor continues for too long.

At some point during labor, the amniotic sac will break from the pressure of the contractions. The liquid inside will flow from the vagina. This is when the woman's "water breaks." A doctor may have to break the sac just before delivery of the baby if the sac does not break naturally.

The cervix, which is the lower part of the uterus and the opening into the vagina, will begin to *dilate.* The cervix opens as the baby pushes downward toward the opening. At this point, the baby is usually in a position with the head pointing toward the cervix. Some babies are born either feet first or in a different position that can make birth more difficult. As the contractions get stronger, the baby is forced through the cervix into the vagina, which is called the *birth canal* during childbirth.

The baby's head will appear outside the woman's body. This is called *crowning.* Shortly after that the shoulders and body will follow. The umbilical cord is cut and the baby is cleaned, weighed, and evaluated, and then presented to the mother.

After the baby is born, the mother will experience more contractions, and the *afterbirth,* or placenta, will be delivered. The whole process of childbirth, from the first contractions to the delivery of the afterbirth, usually takes about 10 to 14 hours. Of course, many women tell stories of labor that took a much longer or much shorter time. Some women think childbirth is very painful while others think the birth process is not too bad. Most women tend to overlook the pain they had when they see their baby and experience the delight in the new life they brought into the world.

If difficulties arise during labor or birth, a *C-Section,* or *Caesarean delivery,* might be required. In this case, the doctor will prepare the mother for surgery and make an incision in the abdomen. The baby can then be easily lifted from the mother. This is an easy way for a baby to be born because the child is not forced through a small opening. It is not as easy for the mother to recover from. It may take longer to get back on her feet.

Use pictures or charts to illustrate the stages of birth. There are some good books and charts available through teacher resource supply stores and bookstores. Give students the "Stages of Labor" handout and have them identify the appropriate illustrations. Students can use the illustrations for taking notes during the presentation.

journal entry Provide time for students to write in their journals.

activity 14 Birth Control

time Two 45-minute periods.

purpose The students will learn about various methods of birth control and recognize the failure rate for each. Those students who are sexually active become informed about the methods of birth control.

materials Several sample boxes of different brands of latex condoms and one latex condom for each class.

process **DAY ONE** Lead a discussion about the various methods of birth control.

Becoming sexually active is an extremely important decision that needs to be made after much thought and deliberation. It is not something to enter into lightly. You need to think about the consequences of sexual activity and be prepared to accept the grown-up responsibilities that sexual activity brings with it. You must be prepared to accept the role of parent even if you are not planning to have a child. Using birth control can help prevent pregnancy but is not foolproof. The only thing that will ensure you against pregnancy is to abstain from sexual intercourse.

The subject of birth control is a sensitive topic because there are so many religious and philosophical issues concerning its use. If you are thinking of becoming sexually active or planning on using some method of birth control, speak to an adult who can counsel and guide you.

Most contraceptive forms of birth control work by preventing the sperm from fertilizing the ovum, by preventing ovulation, or by preventing a fertilized ovum from growing in the uterus. The following list describes various forms of contraceptives:

- *Spermacides.* These are usually in the form of foams or jellies that are supposed to stop the sperm from reaching the ovum. They are not especially effective when used alone but can be used with other types of contraceptives to increase the rate of prevention. Most spermacides can be purchased over the counter in pharmacies and supermarkets. The directions for each type may vary, so read the instructions that accompany the package. Spermacides are 80–90 percent effective, but are much less effective if used improperly.

- *Diaphragm.* This is a dome-shaped cap made of soft rubber that is filled with spermicide and then placed over the cervix. Sperm are ejaculated into the vagina but are blocked by the diaphragm as they try to make their way into the uterus. This device can only be obtained by prescription from a doctor because it must fit the cervix. It is reusable and can be left in the body for extended periods of time. The diaphragm is 80–95 percent effective, depending on proper use.
- *The Pill.* The birth control pill is made of female hormones and is meant to be taken every day according to a schedule. While you are taking the pill, you will be held at a certain point in the menstrual cycle so that you do not ovulate. Forgetting to take the pill for even one day can result in pregnancy if you are sexually active at that time. The pill must be obtained by a doctor's prescription and needs to be monitored for effectiveness. When used correctly, the pill can be 99 percent effective. If the woman is careless in using the pill, the rate of effectiveness can be as low as 60 percent.
- *Norplant Implants.* The implant works the same way as the birth control pill does but removes the chance for human error. The implants are small plastic tubes containing hormones that are slowly released into the bloodstream after being inserted under the skin in the upper arm. This is a surgical procedure that must be done by a doctor. The Norplant Implant is 99 percent effective.
- *Condoms.* These are the only contraceptives that are used by the male. A condom is a thin tube of latex, a form of rubber, that is unrolled over the length of the erect penis to keep the semen from entering the vagina. It should only be used once and then thrown away. Condoms are often taken for granted as an easy method of birth control. You must read the instructions for using condoms so that you apply the condom in the correct way to provide maximum protection. Condoms are readily available in supermarkets, pharmacies, and many other places. There is no age requirement to purchase condoms. If used properly and correctly, the condom can be 90 percent effective. Improper use can lower the rate of effectiveness to 65 percent. Using a combination of condoms and spermicide correctly can increase the rate of protection.
- *Natural Selection* or *Rhythm Method.* This method requires keeping a record of the changes in the menstrual cycle to pinpoint the day of ovulation. You must avoid having intercourse around the time of ovulation. It is not a very effective method because predicting ovulation is uncertain and avoiding intercourse during the time of ovulation is difficult.
- *Withdrawal.* Withdrawal is not really a method of birth control, although it is commonly accepted as a choice. During intercourse, the male withdraws the penis from the vagina before ejaculation occurs. Withdrawal relies primarily on the male realizing he is nearing orgasm and then trusting he will withdraw at the point when intercourse is the most exciting. It is rarely effective.

There are certainly more methods of birth control, such as vasectomy and tubal ligation, which are permanent methods of preventing pregnancy. I presented only the most common types and the methods that a teenager would be most likely to consider.

hint Be sure to emphasize the importance of seeking responsible adult advice when making a decision about becoming sexually active or in choosing a form of birth control.

journal entry Allow time for students to make entries in their journals.

DAY TWO This is the presentation on condoms. It is important that students be aware that latex condoms are the *only* method of birth control that provides protection against pregnancy *and* against sexually transmitted diseases.

Start the discussion by listing the three types of condoms available: novelty condoms, sheepskin condoms, and latex condoms.

- *Novelty condoms.* These are condoms that often provide little or no protection to the person using them. They are offered merely for amusement and are only available in specialty shops or in adult stores catering to people above the legal age.
- *Sheepskin condoms.* These are good quality condoms that offer protection against pregnancy. They will not protect people from the AIDS virus, however. Because these condoms are made from animal tissue, they have pores. Even though the pores are small enough to prevent sperm from passing through, the AIDS virus is much smaller than sperm cells and can easily pass through the openings and cause infection.
- *Latex condoms.* These condoms offer protection against pregnancy *and* sexually transmitted diseases, including AIDS. Because they are a type of rubber, they have no pores that allow any transmission of fluids. Latex condoms are relatively inexpensive and readily available.

Present the various brands of latex condoms available by holding up the boxes. Many students are surprised at the variety of manufacturers. Emphasize the importance of reading the label on the box to ensure the condoms are going to protect against pregnancy and sexually transmitted diseases.

CARE OF CONDOMS Condoms are weakened by heat and friction. Keeping a latex condom in a wallet in a back pocket for a long time is risky. Body heat and the friction caused by normal movement during the day will affect the condoms' reliability. It is safer to keep condoms in the box and put one in a wallet prior to needing it. If a condom is kept in a wallet for a long time, exchange it after about three weeks and throw the old one away.

Women can carry condoms in a purse as long as the condom is protected from sharp objects by a carrying case. Remind students that even though women do not wear the condom, they are protecting themselves by ensuring the reliability of the condom. They are protecting themselves and their partners.

Take a latex condom out of the wrapper and show it to the class. Demonstrate the difference between a lubricated and an unlubricated condom. Explain that if additional lubrication needs to be applied, only water-based lubricants should be used with latex condoms. Using vaseline or baby oil may destroy the latex condom because they are petroleum-based products and may react with the latex.

Point out the "reservoir tip" that catches the fluid from ejaculation. Demonstrate the application of the condom using two fingers for a model. Remind students that they would be putting the condom on the penis—not fingers.

hints I recommend using fingers instead of vegetables or fruit because of the humor that may develop around those objects at lunch. Also, use two of your *own* fingers rather than asking for a student volunteer. This reduces the possibility of embarrassment and teasing.

Explain that the condom is put on at the time of the erection. The condom is unrolled to the base of the penis. After climaxing, the condom should be held at the base of the penis while the penis is withdrawn from the vagina. The condom is then rolled about half way down the penis and taken off, with care taken not to spill the liquid inside. The condom is then tied and thrown away.

You can illustrate the strength and reliability of the condom by stretching the condom over a closed fist. This will graphically illustrate that the condom will fit most men and that it is a strong product. Condoms are 90–95 percent effective with proper care and use.

To end the demonstration, I walk around the class and allow students to feel the lubricated and unlubricated condoms while I am holding them.

journal entry Allow time for students to make entries in their journal.

warning Make sure you have the consent and support of the administration and the parents in your community before presenting this material.

activity 15 Teen Parents

time 45 minutes for the presentation and about 20 minutes for follow-up the next day.

purpose This presentation allows students to make a direct connection with real teenagers who have gotten pregnant and are struggling to make their lives successful. This activity demonstrates the difficulties in being a teenage mother.

materials You will need to contact a teen parent class or find another resource for reaching teen mothers willing to speak to your students about the difficulties of being a teen mother.

process Contact about four or five teen mothers and/or fathers. Make sure they understand that the goal of the presentation is to have your students realize the difficulties in being a teenage mother or father. Interview the young parents to make sure the story they are going to present carries the message you have as an objective.

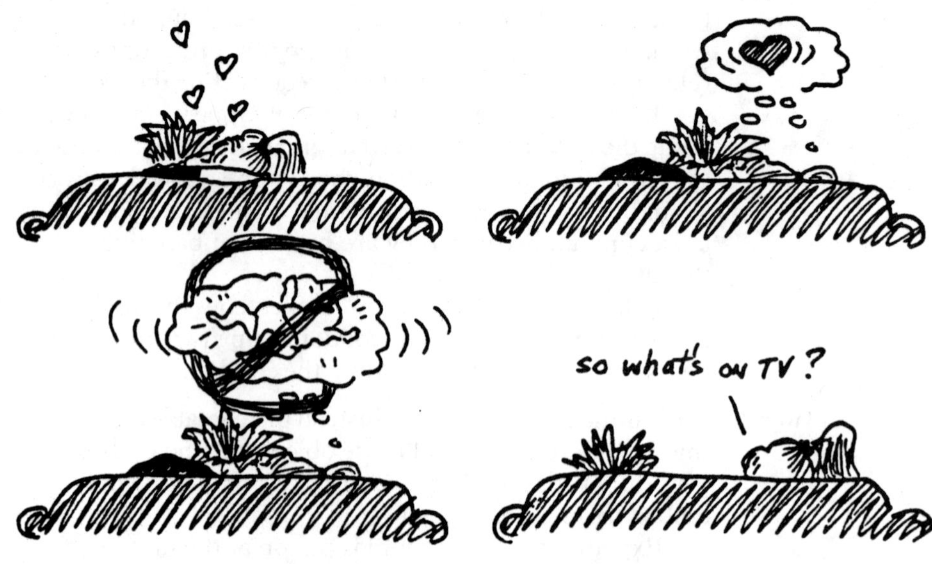

On the day of the presentation, have the teen parents sit at tables in the front of the class. Remind students that they can ask questions but are to be polite and respectful.

During the day following the presentation by the teen parents, provide time for discussion and questions the students may have for you.

I have found this activity one of the most powerful ways to reach students with the message that teen pregnancy is difficult. Students invariably comment on the impact made by the teen mothers.

hints I have the students write thank you notes to the teen mothers. I ask the students to explain what they learned from the presentation. After reading each note to ensure a respectful comment, I send the notes to the teen mothers.

The following is a list of sample questions for a teen parent panel.

1. What is your age and the age of the father?
   a. How old were you when you got pregnant?
2. How did you feel when you found out you were pregnant?
   a. How did you tell your parents? How did they react to the news?
   b. How did you tell the father and how did he react to the news?
   c. Have you experienced any changes in the way friends, family, or your partner relate to you now?
3. What did you consider as your options after discovering the pregnancy?
   a. What are the difficulties you encountered with each of the choices?
4. Describe the emotional and physical changes that take place during pregnancy.
   a. Did you have any special cravings while pregnant?
   b. What are some of the difficulties you encountered during pregnancy?
   c. How have your parents helped you during pregnancy?
5. Did you plan to get pregnant or was it an accident?
   a. Were you using any type of birth control?
   b. Had you discussed the possibility of pregnancy with your partner before becoming sexually active?
6. Are you and your partner still together?
   a. How does your partner help with the responsibilities of pregnancy and parenting?
7. How has the baby changed your life?
   a. How have your plans for the future changed?
   b. Describe a typical day while caring for a baby.
8. What are some of the most difficult decisions that you have had to make because of this experience?
9. What new pressures do you feel now that you are pregnant or a parent?
10. How is your life different from a typical teenager's?
    a. What do you miss most about being a typical teenager?
    b. Describe your social life as a teen parent.
11. Were you able to talk about sex with your parents and family?
    a. Who did you talk to about sex?
    b. Where did you get information about sex?
    c. What will you do to prepare your child for dating when he or she reaches puberty?
12. Did you feel pressured to have sex?
    a. Have you discussed the possibility of pregnancy with any of your friends that you know are sexually active?

13. Describe birth.
    a. How did you know it was time to go to the hospital?
    b. How long were you in labor?
    c. What were you feeling at the time?
    d. Did your child experience any adverse effects?
14. How have your plans and goals for the future changed after becoming a parent?
    a. What are your expectations for your child?
    b. How will you reach the goals you have set for yourself and your child?
    c. How do you meet your financial responsibilities?
15. What was your worst fear when you were pregnant?
16. What are some of the sacrifices you have made as a teen parent?
17. What can a teen father do to be a good parent?
    a. What are the teen father's responsibilities?
18. Do people treat you differently in public if they know you are a young parent?
19. If you could turn back the clock, what would you have done differently?
20. What message would you like to leave with the students?
    a. How do you think we could cut down on the number of unexpected teen pregnancies?

activity 16 Responsible Choices

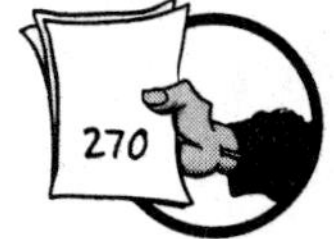

time 30 minutes.

purpose This activity provides students an opportunity to practice making responsible choices.

materials The "Responsible Choices" handout for each group.

process Students work in small groups of three or four people. Review the process for making decisions from Chapter 3, Activity 8, "S.T.A.R. Decisions."

Give each group a copy of the handout and tell them to work as a group to complete the worksheet. Encourage the students to share ideas and opinions. They should agree on the solutions after the discussion of options.

activity 17 Sexually Transmitted Diseases

time 45 minutes.

purpose Students gain knowledge about sexually transmitted diseases and available treatments.

materials The handout entitled "Sexually Transmitted Diseases" for each student.

process Lead a discussion on the common forms of sexually transmitted diseases.

One of the consequences of being sexually active is the possibility of contracting a sexually transmitted disease (STD). There are many different varieties of STDs, but all are transmitted primarily through sexual activity. Therefore, if you are not sexually active, your chances of getting or having any of these diseases will be low.

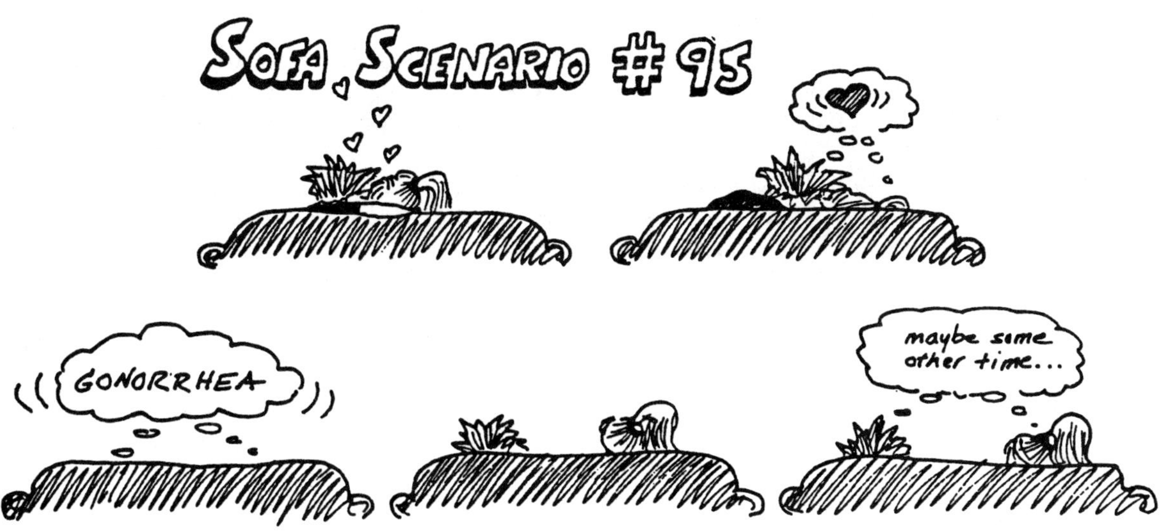

Sexually transmitted diseases used to be called venereal diseases. They can be painful and cause a lot of damage. Most STDs can be treated and cured if you recognize the signs of the disease and go to a doctor. Some STDs will clear up by themselves and some, such as AIDS, cannot be cured and can end in death. It is important to be able to recognize the signs and symptoms of all these diseases and to get treated.

Many people feel embarrassed when they think they have a sexually transmitted disease and often do not go to a doctor or clinic for help. If left untreated, the disease can cause serious damage and can be spread to more people. Most STDs are easily treated by using high doses of antibiotics.

The most common signs and symptoms of sexually transmitted diseases are listed below. If you are sexually active and you develop any of these symptoms, go to a doctor for treatment.

Women	Men
✔ An unusual discharge or strong odor from the vagina ✔ Pain in the lower abdomen ✔ Burning or itching in or around the vagina ✔ Bleeding from the vagina that is not your regular period ✔ Pain deep inside the vagina when having sex	✔ A pus-like drip or discharge from the penis, usually having a strong odor

Symptoms for Both Men and Women

- ✔ Sores, bumps, or blisters near the sex organs or the mouth
- ✔ Burning or pain during urination or during a bowel movement
- ✔ Swelling in the groin or around the genital region
- ✔ Sore throat, redness, or swelling in the throat
- ✔ Fever, aches, and chills throughout the body

Most of the time you will notice several symptoms rather than just one. You can have a sexually transmitted disease without showing any symptoms. If you notice any symptoms, (1) go to a doctor or clinic and get treatment, (2) tell your sexual partner so he or she can get checked for STDs, and (3) stop having sex until you are cured of the disease.

To reduce the risk of sexually transmitted diseases, limit your sexual partners. The more partners you have, the more likely you will encounter someone with an STD. Know the background of your partner. If you are sexually active, you need to talk with your partner about past sexual encounters he or she has had with other people and whether he or she has any signs or symptoms of disease. Know the symptoms of STDs and look for signs that your partner may have one of the diseases. Have a health examination every 6 months and ask the doctor to look for signs of disease. Use a *latex* condom during sexual intercourse. The latex condom is the only form of birth control that provides some form of barrier between you and your partner. The most reliable form of protection against sexually transmitted diseases is not having sexual intercourse.

journal entry Allow time for students to write in their journals.

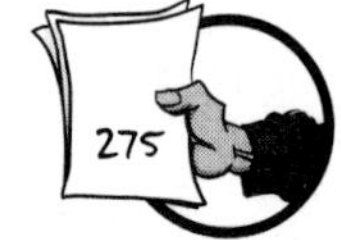

activity 18 Reporters on Sexually Transmitted Diseases

time 2 hours or at least two class periods.

purpose Students practice working together cooperatively while discovering information about sexually transmitted diseases. This activity develops leadership skills and allows students to solve problems of organization and cooperation.

materials The "Information Guide for Reporters" and "Newsflash!" handouts for each "newspaper group" and packets of resource materials for each sexually transmitted disease the students will be researching.

process **DAY ONE** Place students in work groups with enough students in each group to cover the number of topics being researched.

Place packets of information on each sexually transmitted disease to be researched around the room with a sign designating the topic.

Explain the activity. Describe how a newspaper crew functions to produce a newspaper. The staff meets and the editor assigns the stories to be reported on for the day. The reporters then disperse and gather information on their stories and verify facts. Everyone returns to the office, where they meet with the editor and report the information found during the investigation. The editor and reporters work cooperatively to organize all the incoming information into a presentable paper, and send it off to be printed. The finished paper then is available to the public.

The students in this activity work in much the same way. They will collect data and present that information in a cooperative effort.

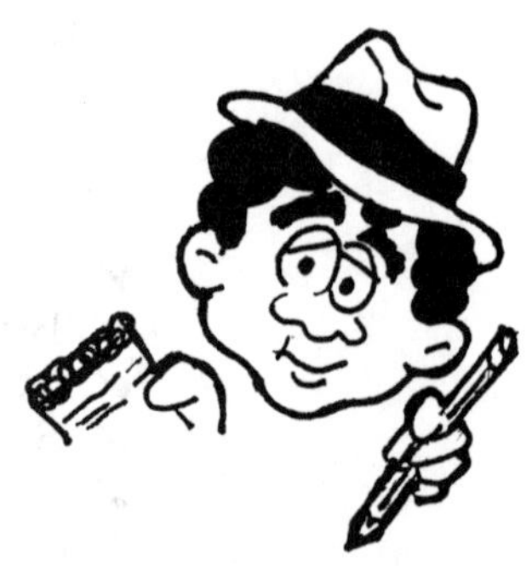

Each newspaper group will meet in an assigned area of the room that will function as their meeting place or office. They will then elect an editor. The editor will act as a reporter and will accept the additional job of coordinating the efforts of the reporters and overseeing the placement of facts gained through investigation and research. Students should pick a name for their newspaper and write that name on the handout.

Students will be assigned or choose a topic to investigate. One reporter from each newspaper will then take the "Information Guide for Reporters" handout and go to his or her topic table and gather facts for the story. They will find other reporters from other newspapers reporting on the same topic. Explain that it is acceptable to help each other discover the facts about the topic even though they are from competing newspapers. Students should have 20–30 minutes to gather information. This will take you to the end of the first hour or even overlap a bit into the second hour.

DAY TWO Remind students to meet at their office and report back to the entire staff on the topic they researched. Explain that it is important for each reporter to have correct facts and to report accurately because they are the only source of information for the other students in the group and will supply the necessary information on that topic for the finished newspaper. Allow 15 minutes for the presentations to their groups.

The editors then begin to collect the facts and help the reporters organize the information to be consolidated into the newspaper that is the final product. The editor oversees the placement of data and makes final decisions on the problems and conflicts that occur. Together, the staff collates the data into a final presentation using the "Newsflash!" handout.

When the "Newsflash!" is complete, it can be checked by the Editor-in-Chief (the teacher) for accuracy. If mistakes are evident, send the reporters back to the research areas to correct the facts until the finished product is acceptable. Then the "Newsflash!" can be turned in.

follow-up This activity can be made more challenging by having each group actually make a real newspaper on their own rather than merely answering the questions on the "Newsflash!" handout. A guide for making the newspaper might be necessary and more time would be needed for the assignment. You can incorporate the use of computers and produce a professional finished product.

Some of the finished newspapers have been used as information sheets and handed out to all students in the school or made available to parents.

hints Some students may get confused after being sent to report on their assigned topic. The teacher's main concern at this point is to make sure each topic area has the correct number of students. Circulate to the various topic areas to act as a resource and to assist in gathering important facts.

activity 19 Spreading Infectious Disease

time One 50-minute class period.

purpose This activity clearly illustrates the spread of one STD from one infected person to many others. Behaviors can be illustrated that will eliminate, minimize, or increase the risk of contracting an STD.

materials Enough three-by-five cards for all the students.

process Have enough three-by-five cards for each student in the class and mark an "X" on the back of *one* of the cards. Pass out the cards to the students.

Have the students write the numbers 1, 2, 3, and 4 on their cards. Ask them to walk around the room collecting signatures from four different students and return to their seats.

Have the students look at the back of their cards and have the student with the "X" on the back of his or her card stand. Students should check their cards to see if the "X"-infected student's name is on *line number one.* Ask those students to stand. They had *first contact* with the infected individual.

Have the students check *line two* on their cards. If the "X"-infected student's name *or* the name of any of the students standing are written on line two, those students should stand.

Have the students check *line three* on their cards. If they have the names of any of the students standing up written on line three, they should stand also.

Finally, the students check *line four* on their cards. If they have the names of any of the students standing up written on line four, they should stand. The number of students now standing represents how a sexually transmitted disease is spread from one person to another.

Have the students sit down again and ask for comments or opinions about the spread of infectious diseases.

activity 20 AIDS/HIV Puppet Show

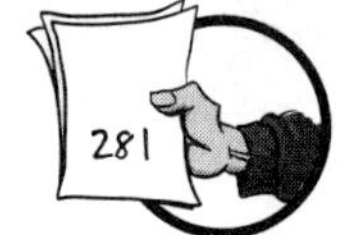

time One 50-minute class period.

purpose Students gain a good understanding of the immune system and how HIV affects the immune system in the human body.

materials Four Styrofoam cups, four tongue depressors, glue, some cardstock, and the illustrations on the "AIDS/HIV Puppet Show Puppets" handout.

process Make the puppets by following the directions on the handout.

Explain to the students that AIDS stands for Acquired Immunodeficiency Syndrome. The name explains the disease. *Acquire* means to get. *Immuno* refers to the immune system in the body. *Deficiency* means to break down or give out. And *syndrome* refers to a condition or illness. In other words, AIDS is a condition or illness that breaks down the immune system in the body. AIDS is the name of the disease.

HIV is the name of the germ or virus that causes the disease. HIV stands for Human Immunodeficiency Virus. It is a virus that attacks humans by breaking down their immune system.

AIDS is one of the most serious health problems we have ever faced. It attacks all types of people. It doesn't matter who you are—but it does matter what you do.

HIV attacks the immune system. The immune system includes white blood cells and, therefore, pervades your whole body. There are actually several types of white blood cells. Show the students the three puppets labeled T4, B, and T8. Explain that each puppet represents millions of cells and they each have specific duties to perform in fighting disease and infection.

The T4 cell is like a scout for the cavalry. The T4 cell travels throughout the body looking for infection, germs, viruses, or things that are not part of your original "equipment." When a T4 cell finds one of these, it instructs the B cell to kill the infectious agent. This cell attacks the germ, virus, or infection and kills it. This cell needs to be told when its job is complete. That is the job of the T8 cell. It is a comforting blanket that surrounds the B cell and tells it to stop killing.

Explain that so far, this system has worked perfectly in all the students' bodies because they are all alive and healthy. When a person is sick, the cells in the immune system work to overcome the infection. A fever is often a result of the war waged against infection.

HIV enters the body in two very specific ways—both of which you can avoid. The easiest way to catch AIDS is by having sex with an infected person. The virus is carried in the semen or in vaginal fluids. The virus can enter the body through the vagina, penis, rectum, or mouth. The chance of contracting AIDS increases if you have a sore, cut, or rash in any of these areas.

The second most common way of catching AIDS is by sharing drug needles and syringes with people who have the virus. When a person injects drugs, a small amount of blood remains in the needle. If the person is infected, his or her blood contains the virus. If that needle is then used by another person, they will become infected.

Some babies of mothers infected with the AIDS virus can be born with the virus because it can be transferred from the mother to the baby before or during birth.

Some people have gotten AIDS through blood transfusions. In 1985, it was recognized that HIV is carried in the blood, so now blood is tested before it is used for transfusions and blood products. Donated blood is routinely checked for the AIDS virus, and the chance of becoming infected by receiving blood or blood products is slight. You will not become infected, however, from donating blood.

So, the two most common ways a person becomes infected is by having unprotected sex with an infected person or by sharing drug needles.

Use the puppets to show that HIV enters the bloodstream and finds the T4 cells. It merges into the T4 cell and remains inactive in the T4 cell for a few months or maybe even several years. The person is now considered to be HIV positive. He or she has the virus and can infect other people but is not sick and does not demonstrate any symptoms of the disease. That person may not even realize he or she is infected.

Eventually, the virus becomes active and starts to use the proteins in the T4 cell to replicate. As it uses up the T4 cell, it sends out thousands more HIV to infect and use up other T4 cells until the individual is left with no T4 cells. With no "scouts" to warn the B cell, the immune system is unable to fight infections. The individual begins to display symptoms of AIDS and contract more and more opportunistic infections and diseases until he or she dies. A person is considered to have full-blown AIDS when his or her T4 cell count drops from 2,000 per cubic centimeter, which is normal, to below 200.

An indication of full-blown AIDS is a type of pneumonia called Pneumocystis carinii. Another common disease that affects people with AIDS is Kaposi's sarcoma. It is a form of cancer that causes purple blotches and bumps on the skin. Some of the long-term effects from AIDS can be devastating. It can affect the nervous system and damage the brain. It can cause the victim to experience loss of memory, loss of coordination, blindness, or even mental disorder.

The number of people estimated to be infected with the AIDS virus is staggering when you realize the dangers involved. The people who are infected with HIV but show no sign of the disease pose the greatest danger to those people not infected. In fact, they may not even realize that they are infected unless they receive a special blood test that indicates the presence of HIV. Even the test is not foolproof, however. Many times the presence of the virus cannot be detected until several months after infection.

No cure has been found for AIDS. There are new treatments being developed all the time. Most of the treatments involve many expensive drugs that work to block the virus from entering the T4 cell. Protease inhibitors are types of drugs that act together to prevent the virus from using the proteins within the T4 cell.

Using a combination of drugs to block the virus and then to inhibit its use of proteins has battled the virus in several ways. This is a very expensive treatment and therefore is prohibitive for many people. This treatment is also toxic and can only be used on about one-third of the people infected with HIV. So far, it is not a cure.

The way to avoid getting AIDS is to avoid any behaviors that might put you at risk. This list from *Understanding AIDS* by the U.S. Department of Health and Human Service shows the behaviors that put you at risk for catching AIDS.

- sharing drug needles and syringes
- anal sex, with or without using a condom
- vaginal or oral sex with someone who shoots drugs or engages in anal sex
- sex with someone you don't know well (a pickup or prostitute) or with someone you know has had several sex partners
- unprotected sex (without a latex condom) with an infected person

Safer behaviors include:

- practicing abstinence
- sex with one mutually faithful, uninfected partner
- not using drugs or sharing needles

Your chance of catching AIDS is minimal if you are not engaging in any of the risky behaviors. If you are sexually active, talk to your partner about his or her past sexual history. If the person has had many partners, your risk factor increases. Use a latex condom to place a barrier between you and your partner. Use a spermicide or lubricant in the tip of the condom and covering the outside to provide additional protection. Remember, however, that not having sex is the only safe sex.

AIDS is a deadly disease, but it is preventable. Gain knowledge about the disease and practice behaviors that will keep you safe.

hints After presenting the puppet show and explaining how HIV infects the immune system, ask if any of the students can think of ways that AIDS could be cured. It is amazing how perceptive students can be in presenting possible cures. Students will want to inject more T4 cells into the system, find a way to block HIV from connecting with T4, figure out ways the B cell could be "turned on" to kill HIV, and transfuse all the old blood with new. All these methods are actual treatments that are used in one form or another in treating patients with AIDS. The discussion actually becomes quite exciting.

This could even be made into an assignment. Have students suggest a method of curing or stopping AIDS and explain their logic in an essay. Students can draw charts illustrating their ideas.

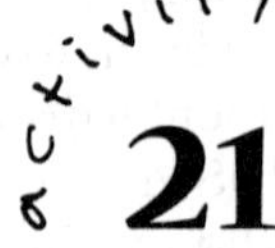

21 How Do You Feel?

time One class period if the answers are discussed in class. This is often used as a homework assignment.

purpose This activity allows students to demonstrate the knowledge they have gained about sexually transmitted diseases. Students will test their values in the safety of a classroom.

materials The handout entitled "How Do You Feel?" for each student.

process Hand out the worksheet and ask students to answer the questions. When the worksheets are complete, discuss the possible answers with the students.

answers The following are possible answers to the questions on the worksheet:

1. If you chose not to join in the blood ritual, you were smart. Be a part of the club but choose a different test of loyalty. These people are your friends but AIDS is carried in the blood and is difficult to detect. It is just too big a risk to permit an opening for the AIDS virus.
2. The fact that you share a bathroom will not harm you. As long as you don't share the drug needle or have intercourse with the person, you will be safe. The person who shoots up drugs is definitely at risk for having AIDS.
3. If you decided to go to a dance, movie, party, or someplace where it would be impossible to have sex, you made a good decision. Having sex, especially with someone who may have had many partners before you, puts you at risk for AIDS and other sexually transmitted diseases. Talk to your partner about his or her past sexual history.
4. You will not become infected from a hug or from breathing the same air. AIDS can only be transferred through blood-to-blood contact in an open wound or from transmission of sexual fluids.
5. Try to inform your friend of the risk she is taking by agreeing to sex without using a condom. She is putting herself at risk for AIDS and for sexually transmitted diseases.
6. Unless you share drug needles or have sex, she is not a danger to you. If she is open about her infection, it might be a good idea to ask the teacher to give the whole class more information about AIDS.

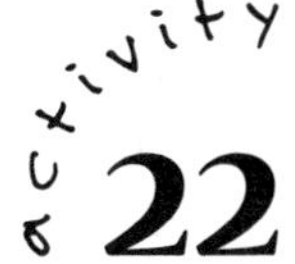

22 Test Your Knowledge of AIDS

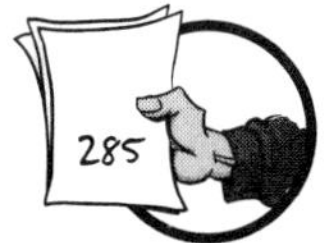

time 30 minutes.

purpose Students will demonstrate their knowledge and understanding of the information presented about AIDS and HIV.

materials The handout entitled "Test Your Knowledge of AIDS" for each student.

process Provide each student with the handout. Give the students about 10 to 15 minutes to answer the questions.

Discuss the answers with the whole class. A copy of the answers and reasoning supporting the answers is provided below.

answers

1. True. A person with AIDS can look and feel perfectly healthy. The person may not even realize that he or she is infected with the virus.
2. False. Anyone can become infected with AIDS at any age. Some babies are infected at birth if their mothers have AIDS.
3. False. You cannot catch AIDS by donating blood. The blood is taken from you, not put into you. The needles used in the procedure are used once and thrown away.
4. True. The virus attacks T4 cells, a type of white blood cell. The T4 cells are eventually eliminated, making it impossible to fight infections of all types.
5. False. There is no cure for AIDS at this time.
6. False. Using a condom will help prevent AIDS but condoms can be used incorrectly or may fail.

7. False. Only latex condoms are effective in helping prevent AIDS.
8. True. Abstinence, or not having sexual intercourse, is one of the best ways to ensure that you are at a low risk for catching AIDS.
9. True. AIDS is caused by HIV.
10. False. There have been no cases of AIDS traced to kissing.
11. False. People who are HIV positive are carrying the virus and can infect others, even though they are not showing signs of the disease.
12. False. Every person with every type of lifestyle is susceptible to AIDS if they practice high-risk behaviors.
13. True. You can avoid behaviors that put you at risk and adopt behaviors that protect you from the AIDS virus.
14. False. People do not recover from AIDS. There is no cure for AIDS. Some people have lived with the AIDS virus for 10 or 12 years and that time may lengthen as more treatments are devised, but there is no cure yet.
15. False. In California, anyone age 12 or older can be tested for HIV without parental permission. Check the health code where you live. Call your state or county health department.
16. False. HIV can only be contracted through blood-to-blood contact or the transmission of sexual fluids.
17. True. The AIDS virus will eventually develop into full-blown AIDS.
18. False. Although exercising regularly may keep you in good physical shape, only avoiding high-risk behaviors will help avoid infection by HIV.
19. False. HIV infection affects us all, even if we don't have the disease ourselves. Insurance rates are affected, hospitals are impacted, and the ever-increasing infection rate without a cure will affect us all.
20. True. The more you know about HIV infection and the disease of AIDS, the more you can protect yourself by avoiding high-risk behaviors and learn to be compassionate to those people who are living with AIDS.

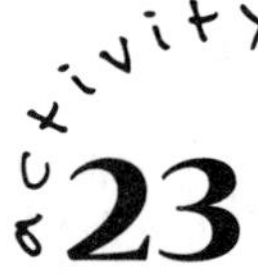

23 An Innocent Date

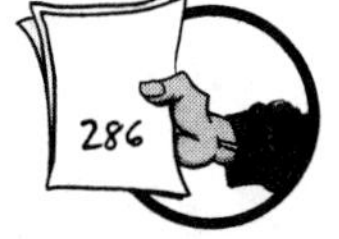

time One 50-minute class period.

purpose This activity provides students with a look at actions and situations that may put them at risk. It offers a chance for discussion and comparison of ideas and values.

materials The handout entitled "An Innocent Date."

process Read the story on the handout to the class.

Discuss the points at which Julie and Jake may have put themselves at risk. At what points are they actually in danger? As the students bring up these points, ask for reasons and arguments opposing their thoughts.

hints I have had students get into small groups and read the story together and discuss the risks and dangers by underlining the risky situations and circling the dangerous situations. The groups can then come together as an entire class and discuss the reasons for their choices.

Remember that there are no right or wrong answers in these discussions. Allow the students to point out areas of disagreement and present their reasons. Some answers are thoughtful and insightful.

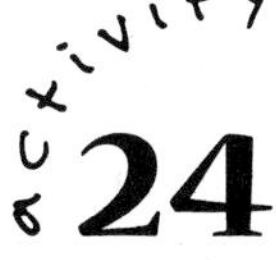

Activity 24 Why Choose Abstinence?

time 30 minutes.

purpose This activity provides students an opportunity to thoughtfully consider the benefits of abstinence.

materials The "Why Choose Abstinence?" handout.

process Give each student a copy of the worksheet. Ask them to answer the questions on the worksheet thoughtfully.

Discuss as a class the reasons for abstinence.

Sexual intercourse changes the nature of a relationship. Many times the sexual partner becomes more possessive and demanding. The relationship can become exclusive. The couple may begin to spend a lot of time alone rather than mixing with friends and enjoying social contact. Choosing abstinence allows a couple time to develop a friendship because they can spend more time having fun, talking, and building interests together.

The most obvious benefit of choosing to remain abstinent is no unwanted pregnancies. Choosing abstinence allows teenagers to enjoy the excitement and spontaneity of adolescence. They won't have to suddenly accept the responsibilities that accompany pregnancy. If they want to have a job during adolescence, they can save the money to contribute to a college fund, buy a car, or add to their cool wardrobe—not to buy formula, diapers, and health insurance, to pay off medical bills, and to prepare for emergencies. Choosing abstinence decreases the risk of contracting sexually transmitted diseases and allows teenagers to wait until they are ready and eager for the very special experience of becoming a parent.

Ask the class to think of more reasons to add to the list.

hint List the reasons for abstinence on the board as the class suggests them. Keep the list up for a few days and ask students to add to the list over the next few days as they think of more reasons.

Activity 25 Picture This!

time One 50-minute class period.

purpose This activity provides students the opportunity to picture themselves in the future in two very different lifestyles. The students can then consider which lifestyle fits the goals they may be working toward.

materials Drawing paper, colored pencils, and imagination. You might also provide magazines and glue for those students who are intimidated by drawing.

process Discuss with students the lifestyle of a person 10 years older than they are. What types of activities might that person pursue? What type of lifestyle would they have? How are they dressed? What kind of car do they drive? What does that person do for recreation?

Then discuss how the lifestyle of that same person would be different if they had a child to care for. How would their choices and opportunities change?

Hand out drawing paper to each student. Tell the students to fold the paper in half. On the left side of the paper, picture themselves 10 years from now. Illustrate the life they might have without including children.

On the right side of the paper, picture themselves 10 years from now with children. Illustrate how their lives would be different. Remind students that children require love, attention, time, and money. How would providing those things make their own lives different?

hint Don't forget that some students will want to have children 10 years from now; it is important not to emphasize that having children is a negative thing. Remind students that planning for children is the key.

activity 26 Last Saturday

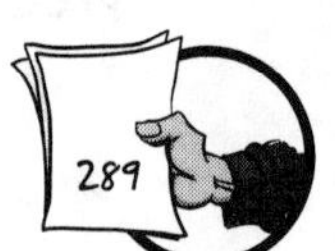

time 30 minutes.

purpose Students get a chance to look at themselves with two very different lives. Imagining life as a parent may help them see how different and difficult life could be for a teen parent.

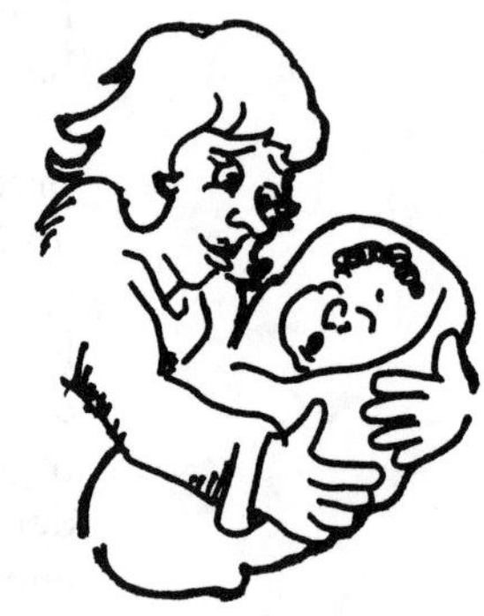

materials Each student will need the handouts entitled "Last Saturday" and "Last Saturday with a Baby."

process Give each student the "Last Saturday" handout and tell them to write down what they were doing and feeling for each hour during the entire 24-hour period. If students cannot remember what they were doing, ask them to think of a typical Saturday and record activities for that kind of day.

Discuss with students the difficulties of being a teenage parent. List the responsibilities teen parents assume and how their lives revolve around their child. Examine some of the chores teen parents must do each day and how their focus on their child can separate them from friends and the normal activities of teenagers.

Give each student the "Last Saturday with a Baby" handout and ask them to imagine themselves as a teen parent. Tell them that they are the only person able to tend to their child—no friends, no relatives, no baby-sitters. Have them imagine what they would be doing and feeling each hour of the day as a teen parent.

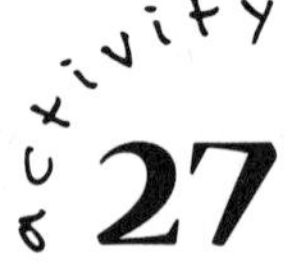

activity 27 Debate

time 45–60 minutes.

purpose Students use critical thinking skills to integrate factual information with opinion in developing arguments supporting their side of the question in debate. This activity develops public speaking skills while giving students the opportunity to share ideas and opinions on controversial topics.

materials None.

process Students debate in teams facing each other. Start by placing chairs in two half-circles, facing each other. Put both sides of the question to be argued on the board with arrows pointing to the empty seats and allow students to pick the side they want to argue. If the chairs fill up on one side, students have to sit on the other side of the room.

Explain that it is important to have people with opposing views on your team because they can often anticipate the arguments to be presented and develop a defense ahead of time. Remind students not to hold individuals responsible for their statements during the debate because they might actually be arguing a point they do not personally believe, but are trying to help their team gain points to win the debate.

Present the rules and procedures for the debate. Explain that a debate is a formal, organized argument between two opposing sides. There are two teams, each representing one side of an argument. The teams try to win by gaining one point for each new fact or idea presented. One team has an opportunity to speak and then the other has a turn. The teams alternate. Each team has an equal number of turns.

A team captain is chosen to decide who will speak on that team. The captain should be a fair-minded person who will allow each person on the team an opportunity to express his or her opinion. The captain should also be able to control the noise level of the team members so they maintain decorum during the arguments.

Rules to emphasize:

- Each person stands while speaking and deserves full attention while presenting his or her arguments. The next person to speak from the opposing team may not do so until the present speaker is seated.
- One person can earn several points by presenting many different ideas or arguments in one presentation.
- The captain alone chooses the next person to speak.
- There is no clapping, cheering, booing, or any other displays of approval or disapproval for any argument.
- A person's argument can be attacked or questioned, but the person presenting the argument cannot be attacked.
- The instructor is the referee and determines the number of points awarded for each presentation without offering any input on the argument. (This is very difficult. This activity is for the students to express themselves—not a forum for the teacher.)
- It is up to the opposing team to question any facts that seem untrue. The instructor should not corroborate any facts during the debate.

Begin the debate with a speaker from each side making an opening argument. This is merely a statement of their side of the question to be argued and gains no points. The statement should be relatively brief.

The arguments proceed, with the team that wins a coin toss choosing whether to speak first or second. The teams alternate and the instructor keeps track of the points gained by each side. The only time the instructor should speak is to explain the reason for the number of points awarded or to offer suggestions on ways to extend the topic. Offer suggestions, opening up the topic to discuss legal ramifications, religious viewpoints, moral responsibility, financial assistance, and so forth. Presenting the suggestions as topics allows both sides of the argument to get ideas without having a viewpoint imposed on them.

Allow time for a closing argument that sums up the thoughts and arguments presented during the debate by each side. Try to conclude the debate early enough so the students have 1 minute to prepare their closing argument. The closing argument should not take longer than 1 minute for each side.

POSSIBLE TOPICS FOR DEBATE

- Abortions should never be permitted versus abortions may be necessary in certain situations.
- The death penalty should never be imposed no matter the crime versus the death penalty is appropriate for certain heinous crimes.
- Should uniforms should be enforced as the dress code in public schools versus students should be permitted to choose what they wear in public schools.
- Latex condoms should be available, free of charge, to students in public schools versus students should not have access to condoms in public schools.
- Free syringes should be given to drug users versus drug users should provide their own paraphernalia for their illegal use of drugs.
- Residents in a poor community should return money found after an armored truck accident versus money found after an armored truck accident is the property of the people who found it.
- Citizens of a community should be permitted to purchase and carry guns versus it is unnecessary and dangerous for citizens to purchase or carry guns.

Any topic is good as long as it is controversial. Students can have very lively discussion and arguments on topics about which they have strong feelings and opinions.

hints Students usually get excited about this activity and continue the argument into the next class. Remind the students not to hold an individual responsible for something they presented because they might have been arguing a point they did not actually believe but were trying to win a point for their team.

activity 28 Film Discussions

time Variable, depending on the length of the film and the extent of the discussion.

purpose This activity allows students to empathize with the characters in a story. The discussion that follows provides thoughtful insight into the very real possibilities that the films portray.

materials Current, meaningful videos or films portraying teenagers of all ethnic backgrounds in various scenarios.

process There are many situational films available through teacher resource outlets that are excellent for students to watch and provide meaningful discussion. Look for catalogs from companies in your area that provide selections of films on various subjects. Watch the film or video before showing it to the class. Make sure the film presents the topic in a manner appropriate for your class and meets the criteria for your community. It is good to get a group of parents to preview films with you to ensure the acceptability of the film.

Prepare questions that get students to think about the situations of the characters in the story and how that situation could pertain to their own lives.

Many of the companies that provide films and videos have already prepared questions for discussion. Read over these questions and adapt them to your own students' needs and backgrounds.

Show the film or video after telling the students what they are looking for in the story. Get the students to share their thoughts and feelings about the characters and situations in the story.

activity 29 Parenting Skills— Egg or Flour Sack Babies

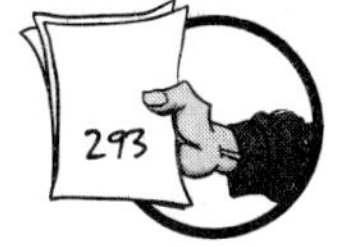

time 45 minutes to introduce the project. Five days to carry out the project.

purpose This activity provides students an opportunity to experience being a parent on a "beginner" level. Students will learn how difficult it is to provide and care for a baby—even one that does not demand very much from them.

This experience allows students to make a real connection between sex and the probability of becoming a parent. It will also help students realize just what parenting entails.

materials Students will need to provide a 5 or 10 pound sack of flour (or an empty egg). Each student should receive the eight handouts for this activity.

process Explain the parenting project. This is a project that allows students to see what it is like to be a parent and have a helpless individual rely on them for everything. Remind students that parenting is a very real possibility if they are sexually active.

Students take care of a "baby" for five days. They are expected to treat the child as if it was a real baby. They have to bring their baby to class each day for a checkup and are responsible for keeping a baby journal.

Assign the project a few days before actually beginning the project so the students can prepare their child. Students may decorate and dress their child in a positive, loving way.

If the students are bringing hollowed-out eggs, they will need some type of basket or container to protect their child. If they are bringing flour sacks, their children should be dressed and in a blanket. Baskets or baby carriers are optional. Parents should have a diaper bag containing the items their child will need throughout the day. Recommend that students borrow plastic baby bottles or use something else that can substitute. Emphasize the fact that students should *not* buy a lot of items for this project. They can make diapers out of paper towels or table napkins. Many students bring items from dolls they have at home.

On the first day of the project, have students present their child to the rest of the class. The students should tell the name of their child and the time and date of birth. Many students are very proud of their baby and want to show him or her to the rest of the class. Draw connections between the pride the students feel and the pride parents feel with their newborn child.

Check each baby to make sure it is healthy and tell students that their babies have just received their first doctor's examination. Tell students to record the fee you charge for the examination in their baby journals. Check the babies each day in class.

Remind students that they should care for their child as if it were real. If they see any other student abusing a child in any way, they can report the incident by filling out the "Incident Report" handout and turn it in to "Child Protective Services." If the incident is serious enough and has been witnessed by other students, the parent may be put on probation. The student is then monitored carefully by other students or by the teacher. The baby may even be removed from the student's care.

hint Give students points or a grade for each day they bring their healthy baby to class. This way you can check the care the parents are giving their babies by checking the condition of the babies. Explain that if their babies get "hurt" during the project, they should bring them to you. As the "doctor," you can make suggestions for repair of the babies and keep track of the students' progress.

I also provide day care in my classroom for the children. Students have to check with each of their other teachers to see if the baby will be welcome in that class or not. In those classes if the baby is not welcome, they have to bring their baby to day care and record the charges per class period or for the entire school day.

You can also prepare three-by-five cards ahead of time that assign the students an income that has to pay for any medical problems their child may have or any extenuating circumstances that may pose a problem for the child or parent for the next week. I do not have the students work as a couple in the middle school grades, although this can be done as another possibility.

The students have to bring their babies to class each day to be checked. They should also be responsible for making daily entries in a diary or journal of the care they give their baby. The journal entries should be as realistic as possible in accounting for the number of feedings, diaper changes, amount of money spent on the baby, places the baby was taken, baby-sitters, and so forth.

The students should complete the activities in the "Baby Journal" handout packet that accompanies this project.

note Students can have an even more realistic experience by using "babies" that cry when they need to be tended and record any abuse. These babies are realistic in size and weight and are provided through various companies. A commonly used company is Baby–Think–It–Over, Inc., 2709 Mondavi Road, Eau Claire, WI 54701, (715) 830-2040.

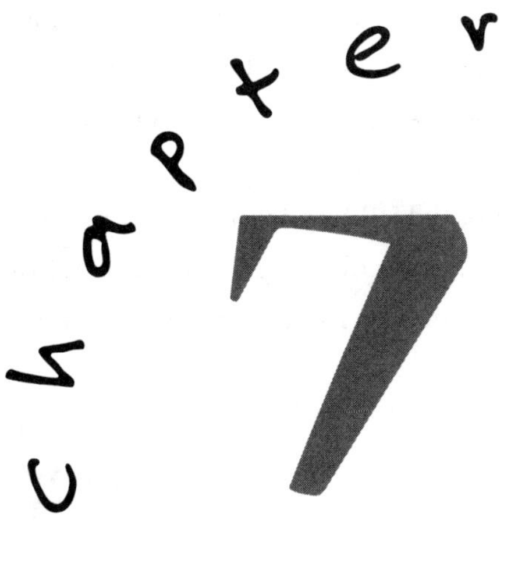

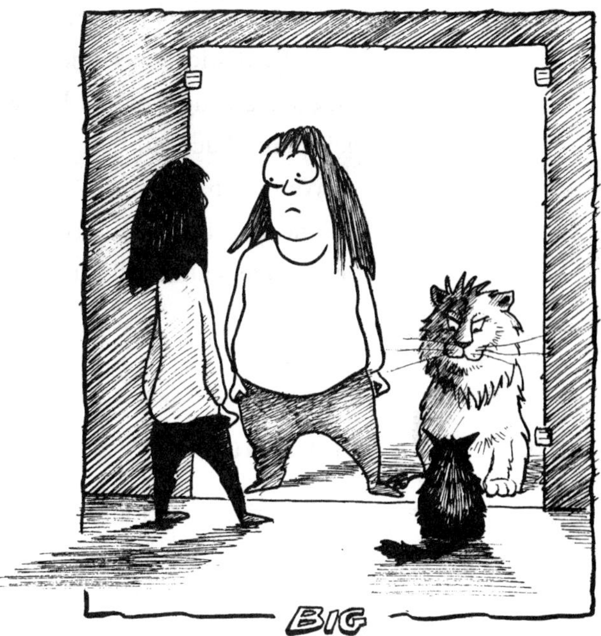

A Healthy Body

Teenagers are very concerned about their appearance and whether they meet the expectations of their peers. Teenagers feel awkward and look for advice on ways that will help them feel more accepted.

Unfortunately, there is plenty of advice available on television, in magazines, and in advertisements telling and showing adolescents how they should look and feel. The people shown are not representative of the typical teenager. The teenagers I deal with in my classes try hard to copy the actors and models, but they do not have the money, staff, or special effects to produce the same result.

It is natural for teenagers to notice and be concerned about their bodies. Their bodies are beginning to change and take on new shapes. If teenagers are given realistic guidance, they can develop their appearance in a safe and healthy way.

What teenagers eat and how much they exercise during their teen years are important factors in developing a strong healthy body that will serve them well throughout a lifetime. Teenagers sense the importance of appearance and try to control the shape and development of their bodies through severe diets or radical weight programs. Many teens deprive their bodies of important nutrition and reasonable exercise at a time when their bodies need them most.

Being responsible and taking charge of one's health and fitness is empowering. Realistic goals and a plan of action must be developed in order to achieve a strong, healthy body. Teenagers need reliable information to develop their plan of action.

We live in an age in which dieting and bodybuilding is promoted and has become a multimillion dollar industry. This chapter offers reliable information for teenagers about dieting, bodybuilding, and, most important, good health.

activity 1 Am I Healthy?

302

time One 50-minute period.

purpose Students will evaluate their own body weight using a pinch test that allows for the variable differences among adolescents.

materials The handout entitled "Am I Healthy?" for each student.

process Present the following information before getting into a discussion of body weight and responsible eating habits.

Tell the students that you hesitate to give them information about diets and eating habits because of the fear that many of them will not be happy with their body at any point. They have seen weight charts that force all body types into a rigid measurement.

Many weight charts do not take into consideration the traits people inherit from their parents. Some people can eat all day and never gain an ounce. Other people walk past a chocolate chip cookie and gain two pounds. The rate that you burn or use up food is called *metabolism.* You inherit your metabolism from your parents. You can affect metabolism to some extent by exercise but your basic metabolic rate cannot be changed.

If you eat all day and don't gain weight, then your body uses food quickly and you have a fast metabolic rate. You need a lot of fuel to make your body function. You will tend to be thin with limited deposits of fat on your body. This body type is called *ectomorph.* If you are the type that gains weight easily, then you have a slower metabolic rate. Your body uses food slowly and probably stores extra amounts of fat. This body type is called *endomorph.* You can somewhat increase your metabolic rate through exercise. The more muscle you build up, the more you will use up those deposits of fat because muscle uses more energy than fat. A person with a lot of developed muscle mass who uses food efficiently and has an athletic appearance has a body type called *mesomorph.*

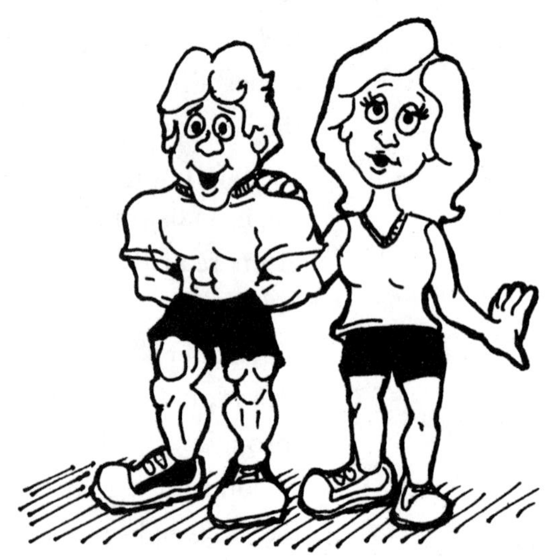

The big problem is that we live in a society that spends millions of dollars trying to convince us that being thin is the only acceptable body type. If you picture in your mind those "perfect" bodies that are in almost all advertisements, and then look around at the real world, you will realize that those people in the advertisements are unusual. The common body type is the one like your best friend or most of the other kids at school.

This constant concern about weight, combined with a poor self-image, can develop into an eating disorder. People with eating disorders live in constant fear of food and fat, and struggle continuously to hide eating patterns that have gotten out of control.

Most people eat when they are hungry, although sometimes they eat to make themselves feel better when they are hurt or depressed. A person who eats more than he or she needs or who constantly eats to try to be happier may have an eating disorder. *Compulsive overeating* results in the storage of unhealthy amounts of fat in the body. Other people may resort to bingeing. They eat large amounts of food, then purge by vomiting or taking laxatives. This type of eating disorder is called *bulimia.* The third type of eating disorder is *anorexia.* These people will simply starve themselves. People with these eating disorders are often secretive and feel ashamed and try to hide their eating patterns. If you feel that you fall into one of these three types of eating habits, you can talk to your parents or consult a physician for suggestions on regaining control of your eating habits. The doctor will be able to perform a more complete examination and be better able to determine if you have any problems.

Explain that teenagers grow in spurts. Before a 2- or 3-inch growth spurt, your body will chunk up a little by storing fat. The fat is used for extra energy as your body grows. If you have just finished a growth spurt, you may be on the skinny side because you have used up all the extra fat deposits for that spurt.

Some fat is necessary on a healthy body. According to the American Medical Association, adult women should have 15–23 percent body fat and adult men should have 12–18 percent body fat. Women naturally have more fat than men because they get pregnant. They store extra fat to help them when their body needs extra energy and nutrition during pregnancy.

Discuss the idea that people have many options in life and have some control over the decisions they make. What we eat and the amount of rest and exercise we get all make a difference in our ability to cope and feel good as we attack the problems of the day.

Hand out the worksheet and tell the students to answer the questions about the decisions they have made concerning their health.

follow-up Students can create a collage of photos demonstrating various body sizes, shapes, and weights. Have students take photos of people they consider to be healthy. Show the students several people who weigh the same amount but look different to demonstrate various body shapes and sizes. Use several body weights for comparison.

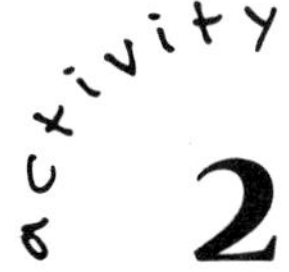

304

activity 2 A Pound of Fat

time One 50-minute period.

purpose Students will gain an understanding of the amount of exercise and reduction of calories that are needed to lose one pound of body weight.

materials The handout entitled "A Pound of Fat" for each student.

process Ask students to contribute descriptions of some of the weight loss plans they have heard about or tried. List them on the board and discuss each plan briefly. See if they can tell you what all weight loss plans must have in common in order to be successful.

Tell the students that you will give them the secret that will allow them to lose weight. Knowing this secret will save hundreds of dollars because they will be able to design their own weight loss program. The secret is that there are only two things that allow a person to lose weight and maintain a healthy body—healthy foods and exercise.

Explain that most teenagers do not need to diet to gain or lose weight. The adolescent body is changing and gains weight to prepare for a growth spurt or loses weight as the body grows in height. Dieting can interfere with that process and prevent healthy growth and development. The best way for most people to maintain a healthy weight is by being selective about the foods they eat. Tell students to make good choices about the food they eat by picking items that are low in fat and sugar and high in vitamins and minerals.

Explain that there are all kinds of fads and gimmicks that claim to make a person lose weight. Basically, weight loss or weight gain boils down to one law of science: to reduce weight, decrease the number of calories consumed and increase the daily amount of exercise. Conversely, to gain weight, increase the number of calories consumed and continue a moderate amount of exercise.

As a class, come up with a definition of a calorie. According to the Dairy Council of California, "A calorie is the unit of measure used to indicate the amount of energy contained in food. The more calories in a food, the more potential energy it contains for the body."

Explain that the key to proper weight control is to keep their calorie intake adjusted to the amount of energy their body produces, and still meet their bodies' needs for the proper nutrients necessary for good health. In other words, you can lose weight by keeping your calorie consumption the same and increasing physical activity or by decreasing your calorie consumption and keeping physical activity the same.

Give each student the handout entitled "A Pound of Fat" and have them work out the problems on the page. Go over the answers in class.

activity

3 Food Diary

305

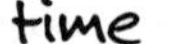 One 50-minute period.

purpose Students become acquainted with the food pyramid and the number of servings needed from each group to maintain a healthy diet.

materials The handouts entitled "Food Diary," "Food Pyramid Guide," and "Foods and the Uses to the Body."

process Hand out copies of the "Food Diary" to each student. Then explain that this activity provides a quick picture of their diet. Have the students write down all the foods they consumed yesterday from the moment they woke up in the morning until they went to bed at night. List every cookie, candy bar, French fry, and soda.

If students have a hard time remembering what they ate, have them write down what they eat on a typical day.

When they have completed the diary, have them look at the "Food Pyramid" handout. Have them compare the foods they wrote in their food diary with the foods on the pyramid.

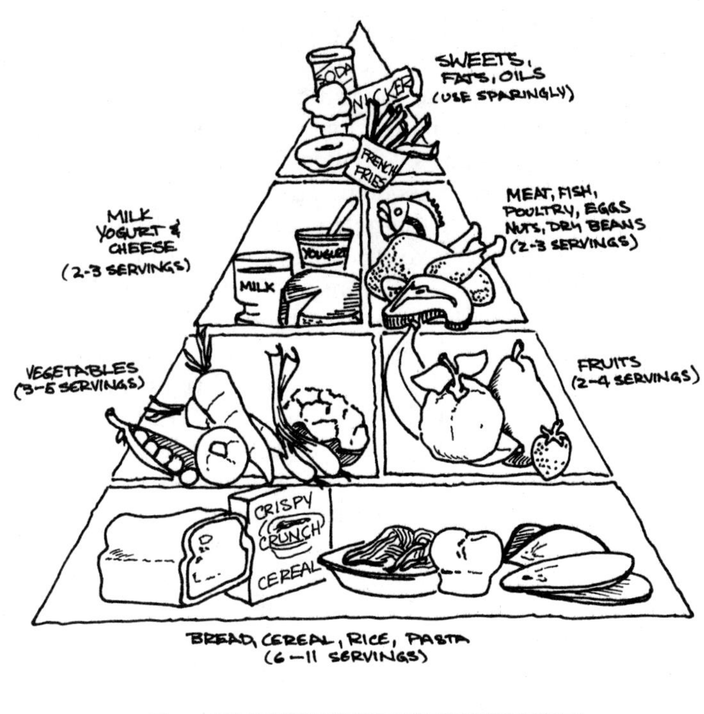

FOOD PYRAMID GUIDE

Tell them to put a check mark in the box to the right of the foods listed in their food diary according to the category the item fits in the food pyramid.

Have the students total the number of check marks they made in each column on their food diary and compare that number with the suggested number of helpings in the Food Pyramid picture.

Ask the students how they measure up. Are they getting the suggested amounts of each type of food or are they low in a couple of categories?

Have them look at the "Foods and Uses to the Body" handout.

Explain that each of the food categories serves an important need in your body. The breads, grains, and pasta group, called *complex carbohydrates,* are energy foods. They provide the main source of fuel used to make it through the day and are a better source of energy than *simple carbohydrates,* which consist of sugars. Tell the students that if they are going to participate in a physically demanding activity, eat a plate of pasta the day before so they have the energy to make it through the event. It takes about 12 or more hours for the body to process the food and have the fuel available.

Fruits and vegetables provide the body with water, roughage or fiber, and vitamins and minerals. The body is approximately 80 percent water, so it is essential to take water into the body through food. Roughage, or *fiber,* is the part of the plant made of cellulose that the body cannot digest. This undigested material acts as a scouring pad as it passes through the intestines, cleaning away material that has adhered to the walls. The fiber and the loosened material forms solid waste and is excreted from the body. The vitamins and minerals are substances that help the body function normally. Vitamins and minerals help people see better, make hair shiny, keep the skin clear, and help in production of hormones and other necessary body chemicals.

Dairy foods contain calcium for building strong bones and teeth. Bones provide the framework for the body, and strong bones support strong muscles. Dairy products also contain vitamin B_2, which converts food into energy.

The meat group provides the protein necessary for growth and repair of soft tissue. That means that if someone is trying to develop bigger muscles, he or she must eat foods high in protein in order to supply amino acids, which are the building blocks for those muscles.

Fat is an essential part of the body. Fats, called *lipids,* are used by every cell in the body. Fats help in getting some vitamins into the bloodstream so that the body can use them. Howerver, fats should be consumed in moderation.

Water makes up the greatest part of every cell in the body. Water helps the body digest food, transport nutrients, and pass waste.

The only category of food on the pyramid that has little or no use is the "extras" foods. These foods are high in sugar and fats. Some fats cause high cholesterol that builds up in blood vessels and eventually blocks the blood from flowing through that area. If the area that is blocked happens to be your heart, a heart attack results. Doctors can now detect blocked arteries and help to prevent heart attacks, but they can only repair damage. It is up to each person to prevent any damage from occurring by limiting intake of fatty foods. An adult needs only 15–25 grams of fat per day.

Sugar supplies empty calories. Sugar provides little to the body and greatly contributes to the development of unnecessary fat. The sugar in cake, sodas, and candy (you know the whole list . . .) races into your bloodstream to provide a sugar high. Some people think that eating a candy bar before a big race will improve their performance. Wrong! The high received from sugar is short-lived. It is then followed by a sugar low that leaves someone even more exhausted than before. Too much sugar can lead to obesity, which is a contributing cause of heart disease, diabetes, and some types of cancer.

activity

4 My Activity Level

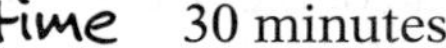

308

time 30 minutes.

purpose This activity teaches students to measure their caloric intake and compare it to their caloric output.

materials The handouts entitled "My Activity Level," "Sample Calorie Chart," and "Caloric Output for Exercise."

process Give each student a copy of the "My Activity Level" handout. Explain that they will measure the amount of calories they consume during a normal day and then compare that to the number of calories their body uses in a normal day.

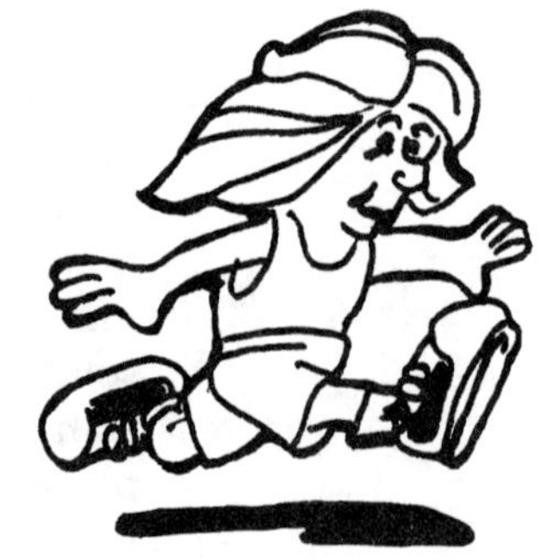

Tell the students to keep a record of everything they eat and every activity they do for one 24-hour period. Have them list the foods they eat on the left-hand column of the chart and the physical activities they have done in the column on the right-hand side of the chart.

Tell the students to use the "Sample Calorie Chart" handout to record the calories they consumed and to use the "Caloric Output for Exercise" handout to record the calories used during exercise.

Have the students total each column separately and circle the larger total.

Tell students that if the totals are about equal, they will maintain their weight. If more calories were used than consumed, they will lose weight. If more calories were consumed than were used, they will gain weight.

It is advisable to lose no more than about 2 pounds per week when dieting. That means using up 7,000 more calories per week than are consumed. To do this, they can increase their normal amount of exercise and decrease the number of calories eaten.

Losing weight slowly ensures that the weight will remain off. Losing weight quickly causes the body's metabolism to slow down and people may actually gain weight when they return to their normal daily routine.

activity

5 Design a Diet

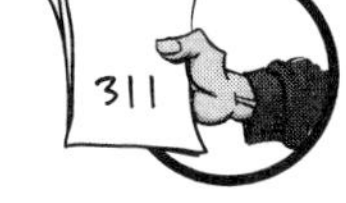

time One 50-minute period.

purpose Students develop an understanding of the food pyramid and the number of servings necessary to provide a healthy diet.

materials Each student will need the "Design a Diet" and "I'm the Cook" handouts. Copies can be made of the "Food Pyramid Guide" and the "Foods and Uses to the Body" handouts provided for Activity 3 in this chapter.

process Give each student the "Design a Diet" worksheet and copies of the "Food Pyramid Guide" and the "Foods and Uses to the Body" handouts. Tell the students to develop a healthy, pleasurable diet for one day that meets all the needs of their body as presented in the "Food Pyramid Guide." Keep in mind the required number of servings for each food group.

Allow time for the students to complete the assignment. Then have students exchange papers with a friend or partner. They can check the diet designed by the other person and make suggestions that may enhance the diet. Have them check to make sure the diet meets the required number of servings established by the "Food Pyramid Guide."

follow-up Propose that the students really test their skills as a dietitian by designing a menu for one meal and preparing it for their family. Remind them that part of the preparation of a meal includes the cleanup afterward.

Tell the students that the foods they choose should fill all the food groups in the food pyramid to have a well-balanced meal. They should be aware of the color of the food and its presentation in order to make the meal attractive. Explain that it is a real art to prepare an attractive *and* healthy meal.

Students can plan the meal on the worksheet provided entitled, "I'm the Cook," and have it signed by a parent or guardian for verification. I often give extra points to students who meet this challenge.

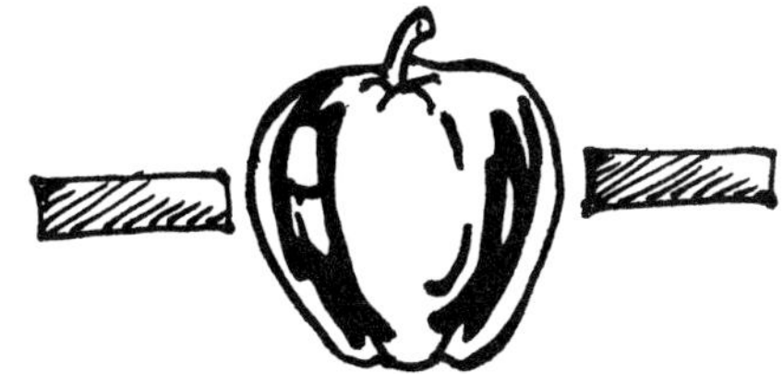

activity 6 Target Heart Rate

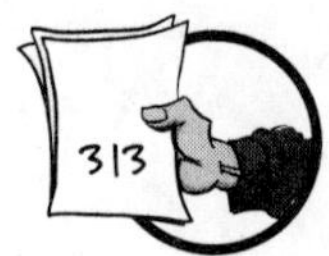

time One 50-minute period.

purpose Students will learn that in order to gain strength in any given muscle, they must "overload" that muscle as they exercise. They will determine the point of overload for their heart.

materials The "Target Heart Rate" handout for each student and room to do exercises such as running up stairs, running around a track, or climbing on chairs in the room. You will also need a lot of patience for this activity. It gets loud during the exercises and confusing while computing the target heart rate.

process Define the term *target heart rate.* The target heart rate is the rate the heart should beat in order to gain strength in the heart muscle. The stronger that muscle, the less it will have to work and the less it will get tired and weaken.

Explain that all muscles work on the *overload principle.* The following is a suggestion for use in presenting this concept to the students.

Look at your biceps muscle—that big bulge in your arm between your shoulder and your elbow that occurs when you flex your arm. You can practice doing "curls" to build strength in this muscle by resting your elbow on a firm surface and flexing your arm up while holding a weight. You can build this muscle in two ways. You can lift a 100-pound weight 5 times and hope you don't strain a muscle, or you can lift a 5-pound weight 100 times. Either way, you will be taking the muscle to a point of exhaustion and then working it just a bit further. It is only at the point of exhaustion that you begin to strengthen that muscle. All the activity that went before was good for circulating your blood and getting air into your lungs and muscles, but it did not build strength. You can only build strength by taking a muscle to a point of exhaustion and then pushing it further.

Using more repetitions with a lighter weight is the most beneficial for adolescents. Their bones are still growing, and using a heavy weight can sometimes injure the ends of the long bones where growth occurs. So don't try to be too macho and impress people with your strength. Wait until your growth is complete and then show off.

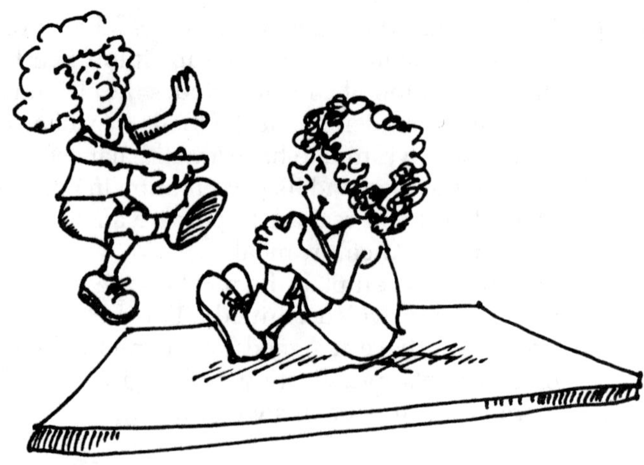

Let's apply this overload principal to the heart, which is also a muscle. You need to exercise your heart just like the other muscles in your body. You do this by making it beat harder through active exercise such as running, swimming, riding a bike, or roller skating. You must get your heart to a point of exhaustion so you can build strength. This point of exhaustion for your heart is the target heart rate. There is a formula that you can follow to figure out your own target heart rate.

You will need to take a resting heart rate for the formula. Sit or lie down for a few minutes until you feel relaxed and at ease. While in a resting position, take your pulse. Count how many times your heart beats in 10 seconds. Multiply that number by six to find your resting heart rate for 1 minute.

Resting heart rate for 10 seconds = ___ multiplied by 6 = ___

Tell students to use the answer when it is called for in the target heart rate formula. Go slowly through the equation on the handout, making sure that each student is following directions. Have students work with a partner to check each other's progress with the equation. Each person will be doing his or her own formula. Talk the students through the equation on their handout sheet slowly.

Now comes the active part. Have students see if they can reach their target heart rate. Have them run in place, jump, or climb stairs for 2 minutes. Tell them to really work hard at whatever they do. They will be active for 2 minutes. Time the activity.

At the end of the workout, have students take their pulse for 10 seconds. If their pulse is the same or higher than what they calculated as their target heart rate, then they have achieved their target heart rate and are beginning to build strength in their heart. Remind students that they need to sustain that rate for 20 minutes while exercising and to work out two or three times a week.

hint Have extra copies of the worksheet available. Many students want to take this home for their parents to use.

activity 7 Investigate Food

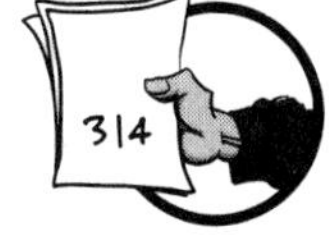

time 10 minutes to explain, 30 minutes for discussion after the worksheet is completed.

purpose Students become more aware of marketing techniques and realize the target group aimed at by most advertisers.

materials The "Investigate Food" handout for each student.

process Tell the students they are going to be assigned to watch Saturday morning television for 2 hours! Along with catching up on the latest cartoons, their assignment is to monitor and record the number of commercials during those 2 hours.

Give each student the worksheet and tell them to record their findings on the worksheet. They can work with friends and family members to do this investigation.

They will have to make a trip to the supermarket sometime during the weekend to answer some of the questions following the television commercial survey.

Have students bring their completed work to school to discuss their findings.

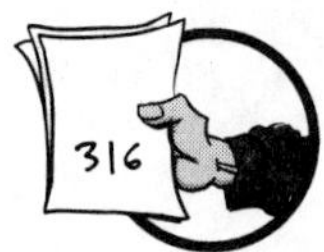

activity

8 Become a Smart Consumer

time One 50-minute period.

purpose Students will be able to read the nutrition facts food label on packaged foods and be able to interpret the meanings.

materials As many dried food, canned food, and frozen food containers as possible and the "Become a Smart Consumer" handout for each student.

hint I ask all the students to bring in one empty food container for this lesson.

process Introduce this activity by asking students to pick out the five packaged foods from the displayed containers that they think are the healthiest. Then have them choose the five foods that they think are the least healthy.

Ask the students to describe the criteria they used to determine the concept of healthy. Write their ideas on the board.

They often will present the idea that healthy food items contain the least amount of fat and sugar or the highest amount of vitamins and nutrients. Work toward a definition of healthy that everyone can agree on. Then look at the foods that were chosen. Read each one's nutrition facts label and order them according to the definition.

Explain how to read nutrition facts labels to the class. Give each student a food product and have them refer to the label on that food as you interpret the facts on the label.

Give each student a copy of the handout and have them answer the questions concerning the information that appears on the nutrition facts label of five different foods.

hints If you prefer less confusion during the investigation phase of the lesson, divide the class into groups of five students. Each student will have a product and be responsible for reporting to the group on its nutrition label. Have the students answer the worksheet cooperatively in their groups.

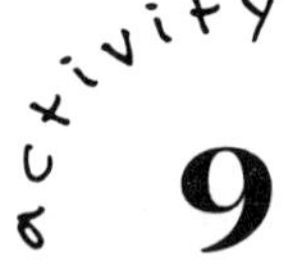

318

9 Fast Food Fun

time One 50-minute period.

purpose Students gain experience in evaluating some popular fast foods.

materials The "Fast Food Fun" and the "Fast Food Guide" handouts. You may also need to have the "Food Pyramid Guide" handouts provided for Activity 3 in this chapter. The "Fast Food Survey" handout is included for the follow-up activity.

process Introduce the lesson by asking students to tell you their favorite fast foods. You can even take a survey to find the fast foods that are the most popular with your students.

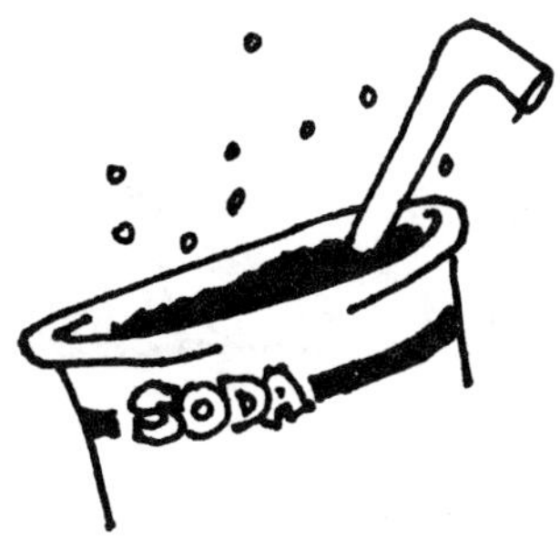

Look at the history of fast food. It all started in 1955, in Des Plaines, Illinois, when the first McDonald's was opened. Americans are busy people and this type of food fit nicely into their busy schedules. Then we discovered French fries and combined them with sodas, and a new way of eating was established.

Most of these foods can be prepared quickly because they are grilled, fried, or deep-fried. This adds a lot of fat to the foods. Americans have developed an affinity for the good taste that fat adds to the flavor of the foods. But additional fat in the diet causes health problems. In the past 75 years, our fat intake has increased 31 percent and our sugar consumption has increased 40 percent, according to Jacobson and Fritschner in their book, *The Fast Food Guide.*

Affluence, working parents, and increased mobility added to the American dependence on the fast food industry. The restaurants are clean, efficient, and predictable so that consumers do not have to deal with unnecessary stress by worrying about the menu, the presentation, or the taste of the food. It is the same across the country. If you have a Big Mac in Alaska, it will be the same as a Big Mac in Florida.

As consumers demanded more variety, more types of food chains filled the need. It is now estimated that half the money spent on eating out is in fast food establishments. Fast foods are even being supplied to schools for breakfast and lunches because they are less expensive and easier than making the food at the school.

Fast foods are a big part of the American diet, so we need to be knowledgeable in our use and consumption of fast foods. These foods need to supplement a good, well-rounded diet and not become the main source of nutrition. As good consumers and healthy individuals, we need to study the nutritional values of the fast foods we eat.

Hand out the "Fast Food Guide" taken from *The Fast Food Guide,* by Michael F. Jacobson, Ph.D., and Sarah Fritschner. Compare the nutritional values of each of the foods mentioned by the students. Discuss the findings.

Hand out the worksheet entitled "Fast Food Fun" and have students discover the answers to the questions by checking the "Fast Food Guide" handout.

Have the students work with a partner to survey people in the school and friends and neighbors outside of school to discover the most popular fast foods in your community. When the data have been collected by all the students, combine the findings in class to develop an overview of fast foods.

follow-up Students can write and print a fact sheet showing the findings of their survey. The students can present the nutritional value of fast foods and write a comparison of fast foods to foods with better nutritional values. This fact sheet can then be made available to the students in the school.

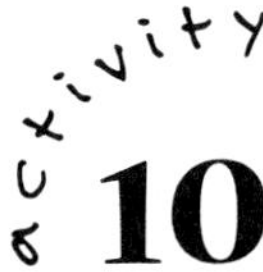

10 Workout!

time 30 minutes to present and explain the material. Two 45-minute class periods after the initial presentation.

purpose This activity helps students plan a personal fitness program. Students will better understand the need and reasons for various types of exercise.

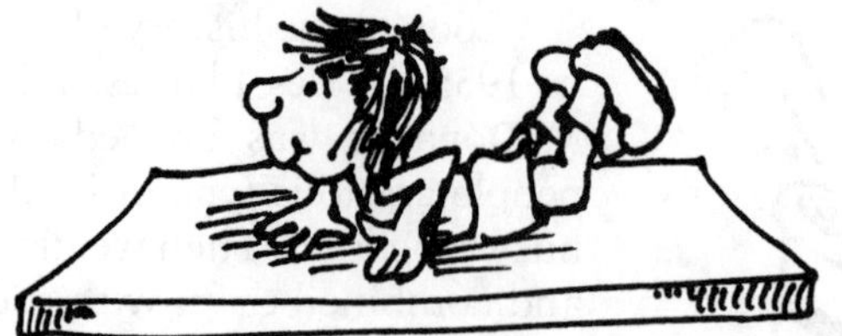
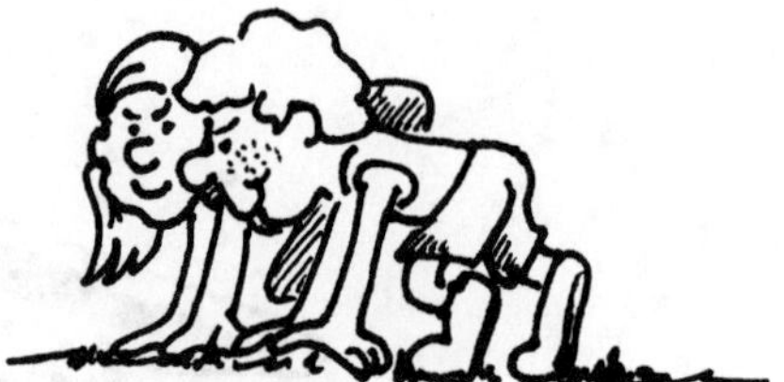

materials Writing materials or a computer and printer and the "Workout!" handout. Copy the ideas presented to make a booklet for each student.

process This activity helps students design a personal program of physical exercise that they can do on their own, and that supplements a good diet, to make their bodies healthy and fit.

Open the lesson with a discussion of the need for physical fitness. Brainstorm positive aspects of being physically fit and list the reasons on the board.

Use the following suggestions to explain the proposed workout: *Aerobic exercise* helps your heart and other muscles use oxygen more efficiently. It is an active type of exercise that forces you to move a lot and to breathe heavily. A side benefit is that as you are exercising aerobically, you are stimulating your entire body, burning fat, and strengthening your heart and other muscles. *Anaerobic exercise* is used mostly for strengthening muscles. One muscle is used in a slow and sustained movement against another.

The secret in sticking to a planned program is to design a fitness program that gives you the most benefits with as little pain and as much fun as possible. Take time each day to be active and do something that you enjoy.

The first 5 minutes of your activity should be used for warm-up. Stretch your muscles, walk, or slowly begin your activity without placing a lot of stress on your body. A warm-up of your muscles and joints greatly reduces the risk of injury during exercise. The warm-up is used for preparing your muscles and joints for activity while gradually increasing your heart rate.

The active or aerobic part of the workout is devoted to some type of *active* body movement. You can swim, play basketball, ride a bicycle, roller skate, run, or climb mountains. The more active the better. You can change your activity from day to day but you should work out three to five times a week and be active enough to achieve and sustain your target heart rate for at least 20 minutes.

Use the last 5 minutes after working out for a cool-down period. Gradually slow your activity level and stretch your muscles to prevent injuries and stiff muscles. Allow your heart rate to slow gradually to a normal rate.

Ask students to talk to coaches and physical fitness educators and bring in several exercises that can be presented to the class. You can have students work in groups of five or six people and have each person explain and demonstrate one of the exercises to the rest of their group.

Have the groups then pick five warm-up or stretching exercises and five additional aerobic exercises. Each group should share its ideas with the class. I allow them to present one idea, and then move on to the next group until all the new exercises are presented.

Give the students the handout and have them work alone to develop a schedule of exercise for a week. They can vary the exercises so that they do not get bored and so that they are not working the same muscles each day.

follow-up Students work in groups or as a class to compile a workout booklet containing all the recommended exercises with a description of each. Have the artists in the class illustrate each exercise. Copy the completed booklets and give one to each member of the class.

activity 11 Homemade Gym

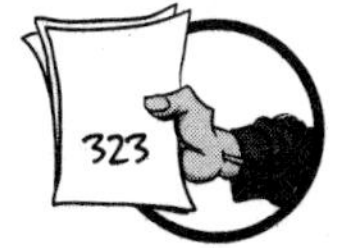

time 20 minutes to introduce the assignment.

purpose Students discover that they have all the gym equipment they need at home ready to be used.

materials Students will need to supply their own materials at home, or the students can bring materials from home and construct their projects in class. As an alternative, use the "Rube Goldberg Gym Equipment" handout.

process Suggest that we often feel that the *best* equipment will help us to perform better. Sometimes good equipment does make a difference but many times, especially as we begin a sport, it is not that important.

Tell the students that they are going to create or invent their own gym equipment out of everyday, household products. Keep in mind that safety is an important factor in determining whether to make your own gear.

Some ideas:

- You don't need fancy chrome dumbbells for weight lifting or exercise. Use two full 15-ounce soup cans—one in each hand. If you want the weights to be heavier, get bigger cans and fashion handles out of duct tape.
- Instead of buying a stationary bike to put in front of the television for a workout, get your own bicycle and make a stand that supports the back axle so the wheel is not touching the ground.
- You can swim long distances in a very small swimming pool by attaching long bungee cords to a belt that you wear and then to the side of the pool (or fence behind the pool). Swim against the resistance.
- You can substitute running up and down real stairs for that expensive stair climbing machine.
- Jog, run, or walk around your street instead of insisting on a treadmill. You may meet people as you travel and have more fun.

Students can either make their piece of gym equipment and bring it into class or they can design a piece of equipment on the worksheet provided.

hint Have a size limit on projects brought into class or students will bring in their bicycles.

activity 12 The Ultimate Me!

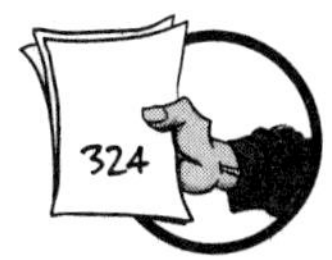

time One 50-minute period.

purpose Students take a look at the realistic type of body they would like to work toward.

materials The "The Ultimate Me!" handout, colored pencils or markers, drawing paper, magazines, glue, scissors, and imagination.

process Tell students that they are going to imagine their physical bodies as they would like them to be.

Tell them to draw or cut out pictures from magazines to create an image of themselves in peak condition. Use this image as a goal. Remember that in setting goals, choices need to be realistic and achievable. Give them the time to do the project.

Students can then share in small groups their methods for reaching their goal.

activity 13 What's Available?

time 20 minutes.

purpose Students become aware of the fitness facilities available in their neighborhood or town.

materials The "What's Available?" handout and access to newspapers, phone books, college directories, or public recreation facilities bulletins.

process Give each student the handout and have them work in groups of two or three to find as many listings as possible for fitness activities in their community.

After the students work in small groups, bring them together to share some of the available activities they found. Tell students that many times a person can find out about what is available by talking to friends.

Ask the students to pick out the facilities that are inexpensive and require no membership or dues.

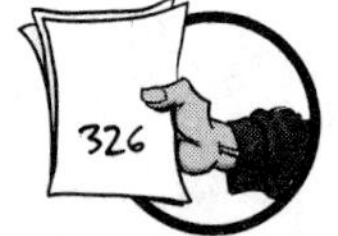

activity 14 Hygiene

time One 50-minute period.

purpose Students become aware of good personal hygiene practices. They will be given a chart to record their daily personal grooming habits.

materials The handouts entitled "Good Grooming Habits" and "Preparation for a Date."

process Introduce this topic by explaining that as young people enter adolescence, their bodies change rapidly. Because of the physical and hormonal changes occurring, their body will need more care and attention in order to control offensive body odor and acne. Adolescents need to practice good grooming techniques.

Tell students that it is time for them to accept the responsibility for their own cleanliness and to develop habits that will remain with them for life.

Personal grooming is important because people's appearance is often what other people notice first. Your appearance—clean hair, brushed teeth, the type of clothes you wear, your posture—give people a message about you. Ask the students what message their appearance portrays to others.

Offer the "Good Grooming Habits" worksheet as a checklist that should be completed each day in order to practice good personal hygiene.

Discuss with students how to properly do each of the items on the list. Ask students for advice that they can offer their friends. Remember that the reason you need to discuss this topic is that some students just do not know how to perform each of these daily habits adequately.

Have the students then complete the worksheet "Preparation for a Date."

activity 15

I Can Change

time 15 minutes to give instructions.

purpose This activity can be used alone by the student to improve personal hygiene habits and behaviors.

materials The "I Can Improve" handout, one copy for each personal hygiene habit that the students wish to improve and extra handouts.

process Introduce this activity by explaining that we all have personal habits we can improve so that we present a better image of ourselves to others, which allows us to take pride and have confidence in our appearance. Old habits are hard to break, however.

This activity offers some steps to follow to break old, undesirable habits and to help shape new habits.

Give each student the worksheet. Tell them to think of a personal hygiene habit they would like to change or improve on. They can use a new personal grooming skill they would like to learn such as how to shave or how to apply makeup.

Use the worksheet and follow the steps to learn a new grooming habit. Have extra copies of the worksheet available for students who want to use this technique to learn new habits later in the year.

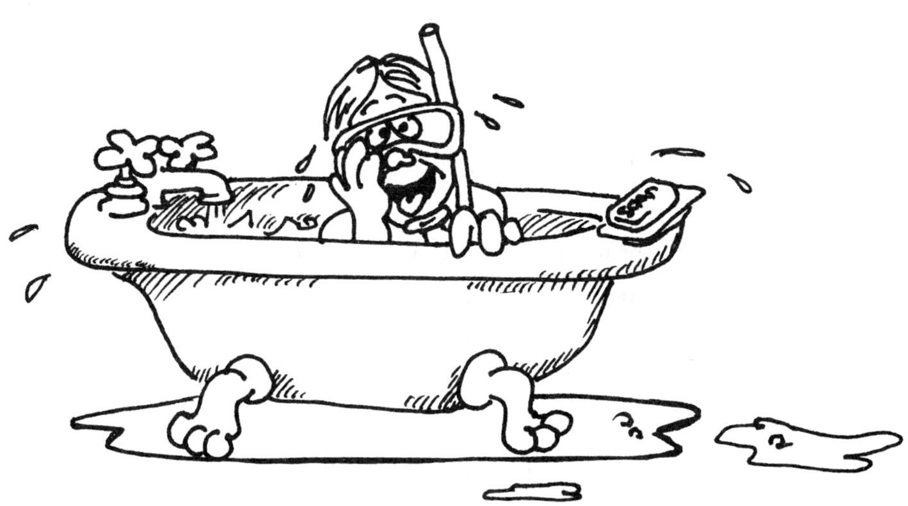

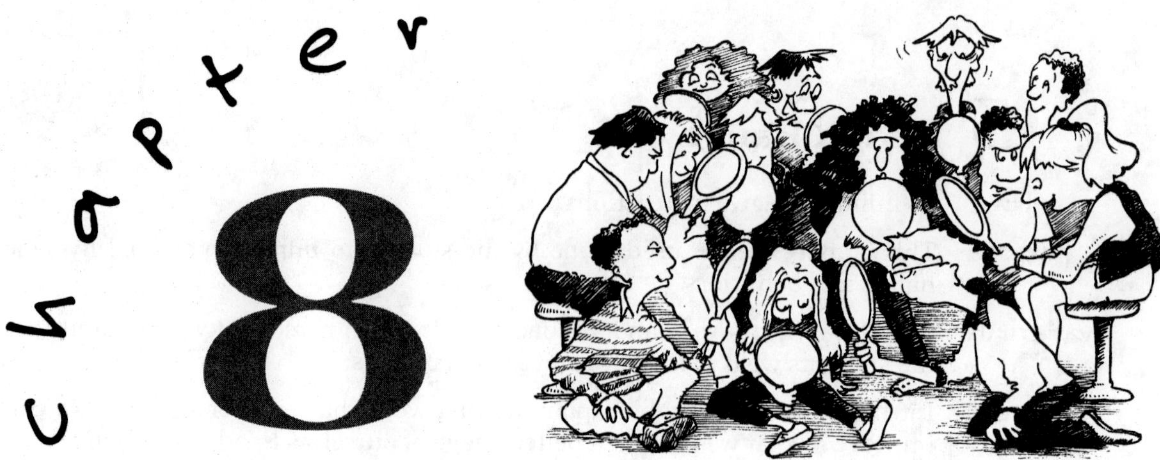

Chapter 8

A Closer Look

Adolescence is a difficult time for kids. They are confronted with serious decisions about drugs and sex at a much younger age than their parents were. Many adolescents today are being raised by parents and grandparents who experimented with drugs during the sixties and find it difficult to keep their own children from that same experimentation. Adolescence tests young people's values and limits as they try new things. They are taking those inevitable steps toward becoming an adult.

Teenagers think they are safe—that nothing can happen to them. It is always the other person who gets into trouble because they were dumb or "that" kind of boy or girl. Students need to realize they are all vulnerable and subject to pressure and stress. We are all constantly under siege from all directions and need to look within ourselves to resist those pressures.

Teenagers are continually exploring their limits and learning to function in a larger world than they experienced as children. They rely more on their peers for understanding and support, which often causes problems at home. Parents feel as though they are losing control and losing the little child they once knew. All of this contributes to misunderstandings and conflict. As teenagers experience more frustration and confusion, they often become resentful of parental involvement and rebel. Common directions for expression of resentment and frustration are sex, drugs and alcohol, tobacco use, and delinquent behavior.

This chapter provides activities that enable students to take a good look at themselves and at the risks that confront them. They will be given the opportunity to determine whether they might be at risk for using harmful substances and then, if they are, how they can protect themselves.

TEACHER REFERENCE MATERIAL

Information on Harmful Substances

A drug is any chemical substance put in the body that causes changes in the mind or body of the user. The drug can be swallowed, inhaled, injected, or rubbed into the skin. Some drugs are used legally as medicines to fight or prevent disease or infection. Drugs are considered illegal if they are misused or abused. A legal prescription for medication can be misused if it is taken too often or for the wrong reasons. A drug is abused if it is taken for reasons other than medical ones and causes impaired reactions in the user. Some drugs are called "gateway drugs" because they seem harmless but lead the user to experiment with more serious drugs. Although they seem harmless, the use of gateway drugs can have serious consequences.

Alcohol

Alcohol is widely abused by kids because it is cheap and easily available. It is also one of the most deadly drugs available to the youth of today. The leading cause of death among teens in the United States is alcohol-related traffic accidents.

Alcohol is an addictive drug. The addiction is caused as the individual's body becomes dependent on the drug. Alcoholism strikes all age groups and is considered to be an inherited condition. In other words, if you have parents who are alcoholics, you are at an increased risk of becoming an alcoholic.

Advertising promotes many false images about alcohol. It has become associated with celebrations, fun, and good times. It is a drug that is taken for granted and yet it causes heartbreak, suffering, and loss.

Alcohol is absorbed quickly into the bloodstream from the stomach and small intestine. The body can deal with about 7 grams an hour by breaking it down in the liver or removing it from the body by perspiration, exhalation, or urination. If alcohol is taken into the body at a faster rate that it can be broken down, the level of alcohol will rise in the blood. As the blood alcohol level increases, the drinker will experience changes in body control and function.

Alcohol is commonly sold in 1-ounce servings. This means that one beer contains about the same amount of alcohol as a shot of whiskey—it is just diluted in more liquid. A wine cooler can get you just as drunk as a mixed drink if you drink it in the same

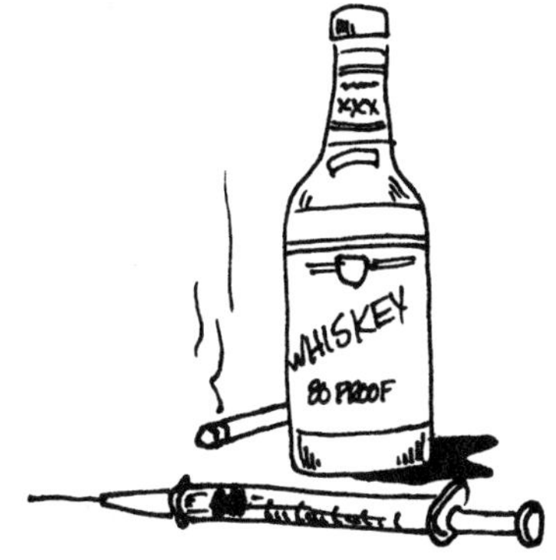

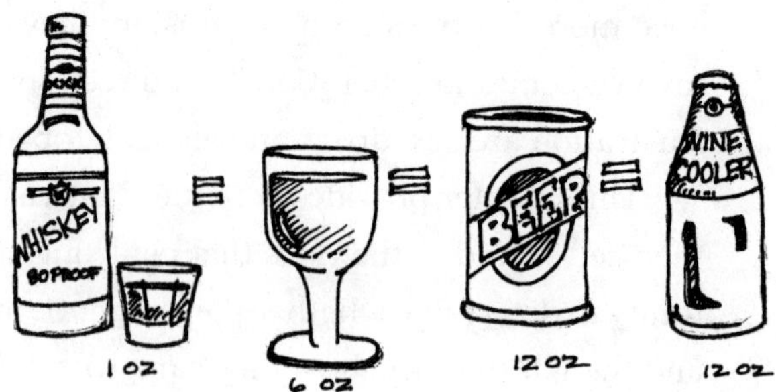

amount of time. Don't fool yourself into thinking that you can't be an alcoholic because you just drink beer—it's all the same.

Look on the label of a bottle of whiskey or rum—or any hard liquor. Usually on the bottom of the label is the "proof" of the liquid inside the bottle. The proof will tell you what percentage of that liquid is alcohol. One half the proof of that beverage will be the percentage of alcohol in the beverage. So if the vodka is 90 proof, it contains 45 percent alcohol. If grain alcohol is 200 proof, it contains 100 percent alcohol—and is extremely dangerous to drink in large quantities or quickly.

Tobacco

Many teenagers start using tobacco because they think smoking looks grown up and sophisticated and chewing tobacco makes them seem macho like professional athletes. Tobacco is used by many cultures as a form of hospitality or even in religious ceremonies. The use of tobacco has a long history.

Tobacco is a plant. The leaves are dried and cured to make cigarettes, cigars, and pipe tobacco. Tobacco leaves can also be made into chewing tobacco or ground into snuff, both of which are placed into the mouth. However it is used, tobacco contains some very harmful chemicals.

Nicotine is a poison and is the addicting chemical in tobacco. It is also used as an insecticide to kill bugs. One or two drops of pure nicotine can kill a human. Nicotine is the substance that makes you feel dizzy, headachy, and nauseated once it gets to your brain. The nicotine in tobacco is one of the most addictive substances legally available. Studies show that quitting smoking is as difficult as quitting heroin—a narcotic drug.

Tar is also found in tobacco and is a sticky, dark brown goo that stays in the lungs if inhaled. The lungs fill with tar, leaving little surface area free for the exchange of oxygen and carbon dioxide—the primary function of the lungs. When tobacco is placed in the mouth, the tar sticks to teeth and soft tissue in the mouth.

Carbon monoxide is a poisonous gas and is in tobacco smoke. It has no color or smell but can make a person sick or even kill them when taken in large amounts.

Many people don't realize the extreme danger of tobacco use. Advertisements make tobacco use look attractive. Tobacco companies have spent a lot of money promoting the advantages of smoking while covering up the disadvantages. It has been estimated that almost 2,000 people die each day in the United States from diseases that are directly linked to tobacco use.

The harmful substances found in cigarette smoke travel from a pregnant mother's lungs into her bloodstream and from there into a developing baby. A baby born to a mother who smokes regularly during her pregnancy is twice as likely to be born with a lower birth weight than a baby born to a woman who does not smoke. It is estimated that 1 in 10 infant deaths is due to smoking, because a baby with a low birth weight is at greater risk for complications.

Tobacco affects you directly by giving you bad breath and making your clothes and hair smell bad. The smoke trailing up past your face dries your skin and causes wrinkles. It permanently stains your fingers and teeth, and makes your voice raspy and deeper. Smoking costs hundreds of dollars a year that could be spent on something more beneficial. With so many terrible side effects, why would anyone choose to smoke?

A good resource for information on tobacco is *Tobacco, Biology and Politics* by Stanton A. Glantz, Ph.D., Health EDCO, 1992.

Marijuana

Marijuana is a popular drug among teenagers. It is usually smoked in hand-rolled cigarettes called "joints." Marijuana or "pot" is considered to be safe by most teens, but it is an addictive drug. Users experience physical withdrawal when they try to quit. Because it is smoked, they risk lung disease and cancer, the same as with regular cigarettes. Traces of marijuana are stored in the brain and reproductive organs for a month or more after use.

Marijuana used in small amounts can make you restless or put you in a dreamy state of relaxation and give you bloodshot eyes. Many people complain about getting a case of the "munchies" because pot causes an increase in appetite. Using pot in larger doses can cause you to experience strong smells or illusions. Your emotions may change rapidly and you may hallucinate or feel a loss of identity.

Teenagers who use marijuana on a regular basis tend to have less energy and lose interest in school or in achieving their goals. They may experience a loss of memory and generally "drop out" of life. They tend not to grow up emotionally because they hang around people with low expectations. Regular users often withdraw from society.

Other forms of marijuana include hashish and hashish oil. These are usually stronger than marijuana and are smoked in pipes or mixed with tobacco in cigarettes. The effects are similar to marijuana but can be more intense because of a higher concentration of the chemicals that make you high.

Stimulants

Stimulants include legal and illegal drugs that make a person feel more energetic, stronger, and more confident. Some of these drugs include prescription medicines such as amphetamines and methamphetamine. Diet pills can fall into this category.

Cocaine and "crack" are stimulants and probably the most addictive drugs available. They are illegal drugs that are inhaled, injected, or smoked. These drugs can be fatal because they make your heart beat faster and harder until you have a heart attack or a seizure.

The problem with cocaine and crack is that most users have no control over the potency of the drug they are taking. The cocaine may also be "cut" or mixed with various ingredients. It may be cut with baking soda, sugar, or even rat poison—any white powder.

After the period of excitement and confidence experienced when you are high, you may experience extreme depression. The depression is dangerous because some people become so distraught they commit suicide.

Narcotics

Heroin, morphine, and codeine are narcotic drugs that are extremely effective in medical use for relieving pain. They are taken in pill form or injected into a muscle and produce a feeling of euphoria—a feeling of happiness and well-being. Narcotics are also sold illegally and can become addictive quite easily.

Hallucinogens

Hallucinogens include LSD, PCP, peyote, and psilocybin mushrooms that are all taken by swallowing or smoking. These drugs cause a distortion in your senses so you experience things that do not actually exist. Extremely small amounts can produce drastic effects and cause hallucinations that can be experienced years later as "flashbacks."

PCP is the most dangerous of all hallucinogens because it can have extreme effects on people's perception. Users may become violent and psychotic, causing injury to themselves and others. It can cause users to become extremely strong and violent and believe that nothing can harm them. They may be experiencing a reality completely different from that of other people around them.

Inhalants

A trend that has been popular lately among teenagers is inhaling fumes from aerosol cans to produce a high. When inhaled, the fumes in the can may produce a rapid heart beat and breathing rate, nausea, lack of coordination, and more. If used over a long period of time, they can permanently damage the brain. Inhalants have caused death by suffocation because they replace the oxygen in your lungs with harmful chemicals.

All these substances can be tempting to a teenager. They are young and ready to try new things. But these substances are dangerous. Their bodies are growing and changing rapidly and are more vulnerable to these substances than those of a grown adult. Teenagers are also at a time when they want to be included and be part of the "gang" and do what everyone seems to be doing. They need to realize that they must stand up to dangerous pressures and take responsibility for their health and safety. Remind students of their goals and have them ask themselves whether using these substances will help or hinder them in reaching those goals.

Students will be pressured by people they admire, care about, and trust. Ask students to look at the values they learned as a child when making choices. Evaluate and question the pressures they are confronted with. Look at the consequences of the choices and then decide what the best decision is. Encourage them to talk to people they admire and trust and follow the advice that supports them in reaching their goals.

activity 1 Friends and Family Maps

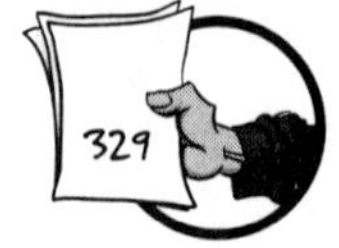

time One 50-minute period.

purpose Students look at the behaviors of their friends and family members and evaluate the effects of those behaviors on their risk factor for using harmful substances.

materials Either blank paper or the "Friends and Family Diagram" handout.

process Students have many people who influence them to take risks. Some of those people might be their family members and friends. Explain that students need to be aware of the obvious pressure placed on them by other people. But sometimes pressure and permission to take risks are not easily detected.

Explain that this activity is completely private because students will be looking at very personal information to determine their risk factor. Students do not need to share the information and can take the papers with them as they leave.

Have students make a friendship diagram by placing their name in a circle in the center of the page. Ask them to consider their friends and think about each person and the relationship they share. Then place those friends in circles around their name, with their best friend's name in a large circle and friends of lesser importance in smaller circles. These circles should be placed according to the amount of time spent with each person. The more time that is spent, the closer the circle should be to their name; the less time, the farther away. Connect their friends' circles to their circle with a line.

Now make a family diagram in the same manner. Think of all their family members and relatives. The more they admire and care for the person, the bigger their circle should be. The more time they spend with that person, the closer their circle should be to theirs.

Next, consider each person on both diagrams. Indicate his or her use of harmful substances in the following manner:

Lightly shade in the circles of anyone who uses alcohol.

Place stripes across the circle of anyone who uses tobacco products (smoking or chew).

Place stars in the circles of anyone who uses any type of drugs other than medication prescribed by a doctor.

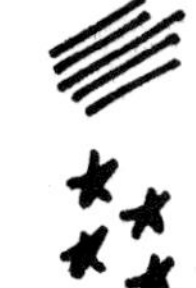

Have the students consider the diagrams. If they did not have to shade, stripe, or star anyone in their friendship or family diagrams, they have no harmful influences to their health. They are in a low-risk category for using any of these substances.

If they did shade, stripe, or star any of the people in their diagrams, consider the influence of the people concerned. If the people are in a big circle or are someone they spend a lot of time with, the effects of their influence will be greater. Have students evaluate the influences with which they are confronted. Have the students list some of the substances they might be at risk for using.

Explain that even though the person may never try to get them to use those substances, the fact that they are using them gives students implicit permission to use. If every person in a family smokes, the chances are high that the student will also take up the habit because it is considered the normal thing to do in that family. The same thing happens with friends. Individuals tend to follow their friends' lead so they feel accepted into the group.

Tell students that just because they are at risk, it is not inevitable that they will ultimately succumb to these habits. Being made aware of the risk may help them decide not to follow the habits presented by friends and family. Sometimes, the student will have to use considerable effort and determination to avoid those habits. If they need help in avoiding the use of harmful substances, they need to get support from people they trust or from support groups available in the school or community.

activity 2 Priorities

time 15 minutes.

purpose This activity gives students a look at their goals and what they want to accomplish in life, and presents a quick look at the consequences that can result from using substances that are harmful and dangerous.

materials A piece of lined paper and a pencil or pen.

process Have students think of a least six things they would like to accomplish in life and write those things on the lined paper.

The students can share some of their ideas with the class. Discuss some of the steps that must be taken to be successful.

Tell students to keep those goals in mind. Tell them to pretend they have just received news from a doctor that they will die in 6 months because of the harmful effects of tobacco or drug use.

Have students write what they will do in those last 6 months. How does that terrible news change their decisions and their priorities?

follow-up This activity can also be used as an essay assignment. Follow the same directions but have students describe their feelings and the changes they would make in their priorities.

activity 3 Ten Years from Now

time 50–60 minutes.

purpose Students see how their future might change if they use substances that are harmful to their health.

materials Drawing paper and colored pencils or markers.

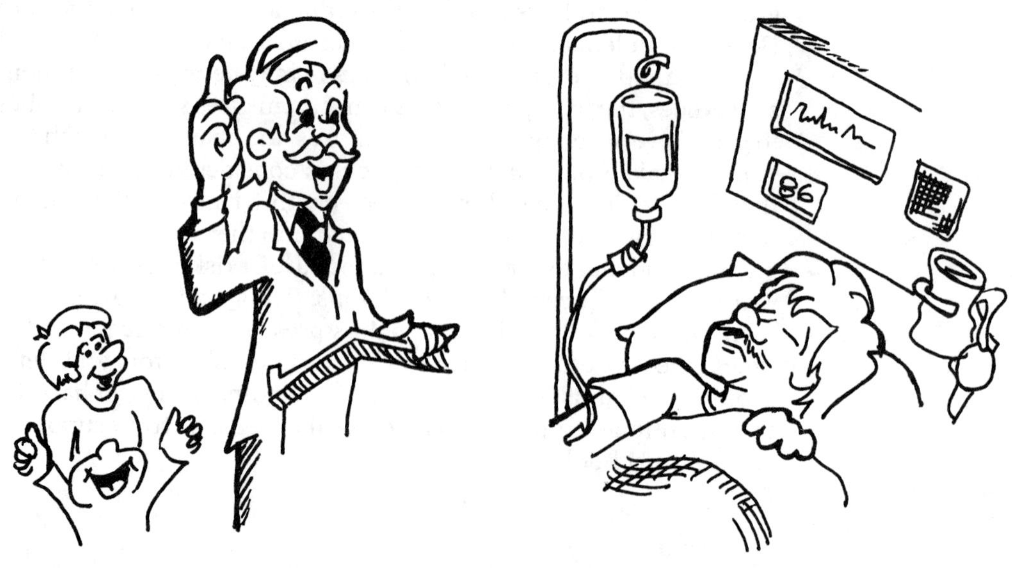

process Ask students to picture themselves as adults 10 years in the future. Think about their appearance, their home, and the people around them. Ask them to picture the career they would choose.

Tell the students to divide their paper into halves. Have them draw themselves living that lifestyle 10 years in the future on the left-hand side of the paper. Give the students 15–20 minutes to complete their drawing.

Ask the students to draw themselves on the right side of the paper 10 years in the future after spending those 10 years as a heavy drinker, a heavy smoker, or a user of illegal drugs. Think of how that future on the left side of their paper would change. Would they still be able to accomplish the same goals? Would they even care about the future?

Give the students about 15 to 20 minutes to complete their second drawing.

hints Be prepared for a lot of talking during this assignment. Students need to compare their pictures and ideas with the other students in class. I often have the students volunteer to share their pictures in small groups or with the class when the assignment is complete.

This activity can lead to some heated discussions of what is possible and not possible while using drugs, alcohol, and tobacco.

activity 4 Your Risks

330

time 30 minutes.

purpose Students learn the various stages of drug, alcohol, or tobacco use and are able to identify various support groups and agencies in the community.

materials The handout entitled "Your Risks" for each student. Each small group will need to have access to a local phone book.

process Use the following information in a presentation to the students.

Drugs can be tempting. People you know who use them look like they are having a good time and don't seem to be dependent on the drug. Addicts are not always losers and bums like those that are stereotyped in movies. Some people who are addicted to drugs and alcohol are professional people with good careers. Appearances can be deceiving, however. Depending on drugs and alcohol can put that career in jeopardy.

The use of drugs and harmful substances follows a similar path leading to addiction. Alcohol, cigarettes, marijuana, cocaine, and the others all seem so harmless at first, but users go through four definite stages as they become more dependent.

EXPERIMENTATION You are curious to see how the substance will affect you. Most people first try a drug (including tobacco and alcohol) with a friend or family member. The younger you are when you experiment with drugs, the more you increase your risk of dependency in the future.

MISUSE You begin to use the drug occasionally or at regular intervals. Many teenagers drink every Saturday night at some party and don't see that as a danger. You may use the drug to cope with certain situations—to feel more at ease on a date or to look cool.

ABUSE The use of the drug becomes more frequent as you think of more excuses to use the drug. What was occasional use becomes a habit, and some people depend on the drug to make it through the day. Eating and sleeping habits may be affected and relationships may suffer.

ADDICTION You are now hooked on the drug and need it on a regular basis. You can't stop using the drug. Many people deny that there is a problem. They feel they are still in control and can stop whenever they want to. A physical dependency may have formed that causes illness and physical pain if the person tries to stop using. At this point, the addicted person will need professional help to break the addiction.

Have students work together in small groups to answer the questions on the worksheet. Each person should fill out his or her own worksheet so that the information is available if needed.

Students will use the local phone books to find the telephone numbers of various support groups and agencies in the community.

activity 5 Addictions

time About 10 minutes to explain on the first day and about 15 minutes to discuss on the second day.

purpose Students gain a better understanding of the strength and power of an addiction and better appreciate the willpower needed to break away from an addiction.

materials None.

process **DAY ONE** Discuss with students the topic of addiction. Explain the difference between an addiction and a dependency on a substance. Ask the students to explain the difference before giving them a definition.

Dependency is a person's desire for a substance. I use the example that I have coffee ice cream every night and really crave it. I would panic if someone told me that I would never be able to have coffee ice cream again but there would be no adverse physical reactions to withdrawal from the ice cream.

Addiction is a physical need for the substance as well as a strong desire for it. Take away cigarettes from an addicted person and he or she shows physical signs of withdrawal along with a change in behavior. A person addicted to tobacco will demonstrate a change in heart rate, may sweat, may have tremors in the hands, and may become nauseated as well as becoming irritable and completely focused on the loss of tobacco.

Ask the students to think about a substance or habit that they cannot do without. They might feel a sense of panic if told that they could not use that substance or continue the habit. Some examples might be drinking soda, chewing gum, eating candy, watching TV, or using hair spray or makeup. None of these things are necessary for our existence, but some of us may have become extremely dependent on them.

Challenge the students to test their ability to overcome an addiction. Ask them to choose one substance or habit they feel they cannot do without and break their dependence on it. They will go for 24 hours without using the substance or engaging in the habit. Have them report on their progress the following day in class.

DAY TWO Ask students to raise their hands if they were successful in breaking their dependence on the substance or habit for 24 hours. Ask the successful students how they overcame their dependence and how they felt during the time. Did they find that they focused on their loss more than usually? Were they irritable? Did they substitute another substance or act for the one they broke away from?

Ask the unsuccessful students why they were not successful. Some students will say they forgot or did not even want to try. Explain that the same thing happens with people facing addictions. It might be too much effort to try to summon the willpower needed or they conveniently forgot and found themselves practicing their addiction out of habit.

Some students may say they made an attempt but that they gave in at the last moment. Again, tell students this happens to people with addictions. This activity illustrates the fact that a tremendous amount of willpower is necessary to overcome an addiction.

Point out that the students only had to do without for 24 hours. They could see an end to the experiment. People facing addictions will have to continue fighting their addiction for the rest of their life.

follow-up Ask students to write a description of their feelings and struggle to overcome their dependency for the 24-hour challenge.

activity 6 Red Flags

time One 50-minute period.

purpose Students will identify behaviors that might lead to the use or abuse of alcohol, tobacco, or drugs or lead to a risky sexual situation in a story about a typical teenager.

materials Each student needs a strip of red construction paper and a strip of yellow construction paper approximately 3 by 6 inches.

process Tell students that you are going to read the story of "A Day in the Life of Timmy Teen." They should listen carefully to the story.

After reading the story, give each student a strip of red construction paper and a strip of yellow construction paper. Tell them you are going to read the story out loud once more. This time, however, they will listen for situations that might lead Timmy Teen to use alcohol, tobacco, or drugs or might lead to a risky sexual situation. When the students hear something that might be risky, they will hold up the yellow strip of paper. If they hear something that sounds more than risky—actually dangerous—they will hold up the red strip of paper.

Explain that there are no right or wrong answers to this activity. The answers will depend on their own ideas of what might be considered risky and what might be dangerous.

Read the story again, this time stopping for the yellow and red markers held up by the students. Discuss each situation as a class and determine the class opinion on each incident. Allow for and encourage discussion and disagreement but have students explain their opinions.

Some questions and topics for discussion:

- Is Timmy Teen a typical teenager? Explain your position.
- Who and what are the bad influences for Timmy? Explain your answer.
- Who and what are the good influences for Timmy? Explain your answer.

- What will Timmy have to overcome in order to reach his goals for the future? Explain your position.
- What are some of the good and bad situations that occur to real students every day in school? What can be done to improve the situation?

A DAY IN THE LIFE OF TIMMY TEEN

Timmy Teen awakens to a bright, fresh, colorful fall morning. The wind is blowing a crisp, cold breeze through the open window. Tim stretches awake, enjoying the first few quiet moments before his older brother gets up and begins to grump around the house.

Timmy really loves his older brother and wants to be more like him, but he decides that he will not be as grumpy two years from now when he is his brother's age. He wishes his brother would not go out drinking so much on the weekend because even though Mom and Dad don't know about it, the drinking sure seems to upset their normally happy routine. His brother is always grumpier after a night of drinking.

Timmy pushes these thoughts out of his head as he rolls out of bed and begins to dress for school. He puts on his new jeans that are extra baggy, just like the cool guys wear at school. He chooses the T-shirt with the beer can on the front even though he knows that his mom hates this shirt. After his turn in the bathroom, Tim decides to skip breakfast and run to the bus stop early so that he and the guys can get to the mini-mart before the bus comes.

His best friend, Joe, introduces Tim to the new kid who just moved in down the street as they race toward the mini-mart. Tony, the new kid, looks cool but seems a bit too eager to prove himself. Timmy watches as Tony sneaks around the market to the aisle where the liquor is lined up in neat rows on the shelves. Before Tim realizes what has happened, Tony has grabbed Joe and together they are racing out of the store. Tim follows close on their heels. They get to the bus stop and fall down laughing and pushing at each other even though Timmy is not quite sure why.

The bus arrives in a cloud of smelly exhaust that kicks up the leaves drying in the gutter. The three boys climb on the bus and find their way to the backseat. It is only then that Tim realizes what happened at the market as Tony pulls out a small, flat bottle filled with an amber liquid. Joe grabs the bottle of whiskey and twists off the cap as the sweet smell fills the rear of the bus. Joe puts the bottle to his mouth and takes a long swallow. He offers the bottle to Timmy, encouraging him to join in the fun. Timmy hesitates, but takes the bottle.

Finally, the bus reaches school and everyone tumbles out of the bus and runs to their classrooms. Tony and Joe are laughing and pushing at each other as they wave good-bye to Tim. They tell Tim to meet them at lunch behind the gym, away from the curious eyes of the other students and the teachers.

Tim gets to his first class and just has time to wave to Marie, across the hall. Tim sits through his morning classes, daydreaming of the date with Marie next Friday. This is going to be their three-month anniversary and Tim is trying to think of a way to make this date memorable and special. Tim talked to his brother about what he could do and his brother wasn't very helpful. He told Tim to get a six-pack of beer and then gave him a couple of condoms. Timmy knows that Marie doesn't want to have sex but he kept the condoms anyway. Maybe if they could find a nice quiet place and be alone for a while she would feel more at ease. Timmy knows that they love each other and he really wants to show Marie just how much he cares for her.

The bell for lunch interrupts Timmy's thoughts. Tim races out to the gymnasium to look for Tony and Joe even though he promised Marie he would eat lunch with her. He will think of some story to tell her later.

Tony and Joe swagger out to the gymnasium a few minutes later with two other guys who are lighting up cigarettes from cheap lighters, their hands shielding the flame against the wind. The group of boys acknowledge Timmy as they all huddle together to protect themselves from anyone who might be watching. These guys are wearing baggy jeans and it makes Tim happy that he thought to wear his baggies today. The lunch period passes with a lot of bragging and bad jokes as the boys finish the bottle that Tony has stashed in his jacket and pass the cigarettes around for warmth.

Timmy finishes the day at school with a headache and a feeling of relief that he did not get caught at lunch.

Tim arrives home and as he slams the kitchen door, he hears his dad yell from the living room. "Tim, there's a good football game on this afternoon. Grab me a few beers and come in and watch the game with me." Tim has a soda with his father as his father drinks the beer, and together they discuss the game.

Before he knows it, Mom is calling them for dinner. The food is set on the table but they don't sit down together to eat. Mom has to go to her aerobics class. Dad is going to eat watching the game. His brother is out with his friends, and Tim is left to take his food to his room. He has a lot of homework to do and can eat while he listens to "heavy metal" music and works. He doesn't mind being alone. He eats dinner alone a lot. He even prefers it—he doesn't have to listen to his brother and his parents fight. He seems to be spending more and more time at home by himself lately.

Timmy finishes his homework, then decides to work on a few activities in his health workbook from school. He reads the part about setting goals and is proud of all the goals that he has set for himself and decides to really work to achieve them. His mother checks on him at about 9:00 p.m. and tells him all about her aerobics class. They laugh about the new woman in class who tripped using the stair step machine. Tim wonders what Marie would look like in those tight leotards and sexy workout clothes. He wonders if she does any type of exercise and decides to ask her tomorrow. Suddenly he realizes that he did not see Marie all day—she is going to be mad!

It is late, but he decides to call her anyway. As he listens to the phone ringing, he makes up a story about staying late with a teacher at lunch. He hopes she believes him.

About midnight, he recalls his day, feeling pleased with himself that he didn't get caught while he was with Tony and Joe. He decides that he really likes Tony because of all the excitement and the thrill that he felt at lunch—he was really one of the guys today. Marie believed his story about having to stay after school with the teacher so, all in all, it was a great day. He gets ready for bed wondering where his brother is and when he will be getting home. Tim hopes he isn't drunk again.

activity 7 Feelings Continuum

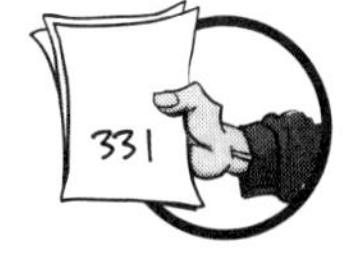

time 30 minutes.

purpose This activity gives students the opportunity to become aware of their feelings about various important events in their lives. This activity allows students to validate their own reactions in comparison with others.

materials The "Feelings Continuum" and the "Checklist of Traits" handouts.

process Tell students that they are going to evaluate their feelings about different special events in their lives. Remind students that there is no right or wrong answer for this activity. They will just prioritize their feelings.

Hand out the "Feelings Continuum" worksheet and have students take about 10 minutes to prioritize the way they feel on the continuum as to how painful or joyful each of the events may have been for them. They may discuss the placement of their feelings on the continuum with those students sitting around them.

While working in small groups, have students decide on three different ways to deal with painful experiences they can present to the whole class. Make a list of those ideas on the board and discuss them.

Discuss some painful situations that might occur, using made-up or real experiences from your own life. Have the students describe appropriate ways to handle the situation. Review the effects of various choices and the consequences that occur because of those choices.

Draw a correlation between being angry, withdrawn, or depressed and the possibility of using alcohol or drugs to cover those feelings. Explain that expressing or sharing feelings allows other people to offer help and support. Instead of brooding, think of positive ways to solve problems and to relieve hurt feelings, which provide closure to the situation.

Have students check off the traits on the "Checklist of Traits" handout that they think best describe themselves. This worksheet can be personal and kept private.

activity 8 Ad-Lib

time Two 50-minute periods.

purpose Students will develop consumer awareness as they evaluate the messages presented and tactics used by companies in promoting their products.

materials The teacher will need to videotape a series of television commercials. Try to get commercials that demonstrate the different marketing techniques presented in the lesson.

Each student needs the handouts entitled "Ad-Lib" and "Consumer Awareness" and a box of magazines, scissors, and glue.

process Introduce the lesson by suggesting that we are manipulated every day by advertisers promoting their products. Advertisers spend a great deal of time and money trying to get your attention and then convince you that their product is not only worth buying, but you can't live without it. Some ads are very convincing and memorable. Ask students to sing or recite some memorable slogans from commercials.

Afterward, ask the student if they can tell you why they can remember these slogans and jingles so easily and why they have such a hard time remembering their history lesson for a test.

Explain that some advertising is misleading and other advertising verges on telling lies about the product. You, as a consumer, must be aware of the tactics companies use to lure you.

Review the list on the "Ad-Lib" worksheet of the various techniques used by companies to sell their product. Ask students to refer to this list as they watch TV or read magazines and see if they can determine the advertising technique being used. Indicate what segment of the audience is being targeted and what the age group is of that population. Go over the list and explain the techniques used before showing the videotaped commercials.

Give students a copy of the techniques used in advertising and ask them to find one example of each technique in the magazine advertisements. Cut out or draw the example and attach it near the written description on the handout. This can also be done as a homework assignment.

Show the videotape of the commercials, stopping after each one. Discuss the techniques used to present the product. Ask students to share their favorite commercial with the class and then determine the advertising techniques used.

Give each student a copy of the worksheet entitled "Consumer Awareness" and have them evaluate three commercials or magazine advertisements on their own at home.

activity 9 Advertising at Its Best!

time This activity can easily take five days of 50-minute periods.

purpose Students will gain a working knowledge of the techniques employed by advertising agencies to attract the public to their product. Students also develop cooperation skills as they use their creative and technical talents to produce a commercial.

materials You will need a video camera and videotapes, plus any drawing paper or art materials necessary for each group to complete the project. Each small group will need the "Ad-Lib"handout from Activity 8 in this chapter and the "Commercial Guide" handout provided for this activity.

hint Have students make a list of the materials they need from you as they finish the planning stage of their project. You can then have the materials ready by the following day.

process Use the handout entitled "Ad-Lib" as a reference sheet in developing this project. Have the students work in groups of four or five to create a commercial advertising an imaginary product. Explain that they will need to pick a product to advertise, determine the population and age group they will be targeting, and decide what advertising techniques they will use in making their commercial.

They can use the "Commercial Guide" as a checklist to make sure that they have thoughtfully planned their commercial.

DAY ONE The first day should be used for introduction of the project and the organization and planning stages of production.

It might be necessary to explain the use of a *story board.* The storyboard is used by filmmakers to plan their action and script. In a short production, like a commercial, the first picture should be the display of the product and the techniques used to capture the audience's attention. The following two pictures present information about the product and continue the advertising techniques to "hook" the audience. The final picture is the image, which should leave an imprint on the mind of the audience. The script or jingles that accompany the visuals should be inserted in the appropriate pictures.

DAY TWO The second day can be used for planning and making props needed in the commercial. Student groups can also sign up for a time slot over the next two days to be videotaped.

Have another activity planned for those groups that finish filming early. I often use Activity 8 in this chapter to keep students occupied while other groups finish filming.

hint Have a time sheet ready for two class periods to schedule taping. Advise the students that they will have only 10 minutes available in which to tape. They will be taped once and should have their rehearsing and organization complete. Because the commercial should be no longer than 1 minute, most of the time is taken in setting up props, placing people, and ensuring silence for filming. I often have students film outside the room so that the students still working on their projects will not disrupt filming.

DAY FIVE Day five should be the screening of the commercials. Make a big production out of it by introducing the participants in each commercial. You might also have the class vote and present an Academy Award for the group that presented the most effective commercial.

After viewing each commercial, have the class determine the age group targeted, the population targeted, and the techniques used in promoting the product. Have the participants in each commercial be the experts who answer the speculations of the class about the commercial.

activity 10 A Convincing Letter

time 30–50 minutes.

purpose The students will gain an increased understanding of the influence of advertising and take an active role in expressing their opinions.

materials Lined paper or computers with printers.

process Ask students to pick a product advertised on television or in magazines that they consider harmful or dangerous. Make a list on the board of some of those products. Discuss how each product is harmful and the methods manufacturers use to get people to buy the product. How are they misleading the public?

Suggest that students voice their opinions on these products and advertising techniques by writing letters to the manufacturers. Work with the students to compose an assertive letter expressing the opinions of the students concerning one of the products listed on the board.

Have students pick a product they consider dangerous or advertising that is misleading and have them compose their own assertive letter to the manufacturer. You may want to send the letters and review the responses from the manufacturers with the class.

activity 11 Last Will and Testament

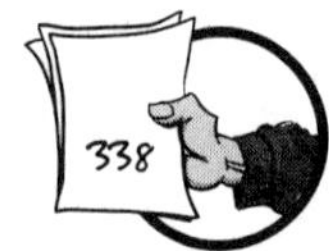

time Four or five days of 50-minute periods.

purpose Students will explore the dangers of tobacco by using research skills and reporting techniques. They will practice creative thinking skills and gain public speaking experience. The students will review the attributes of a healthy person.

materials Each group will need a packet of the 10 handouts concerning the last will and testament of Jacob M. Bayfield. Be aware that the students acting as the jury should *not* see these materials.

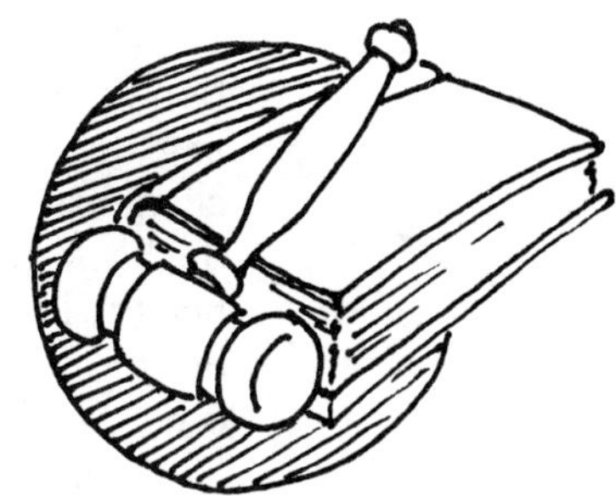

process I want to introduce this activity by saying that it is my all-time favorite and the kids love it. This activity takes a little practice but is well worth the effort.

preparation **DAY ONE** Introduce the activity by explaining that most of the students in the class will be acting as attorneys over the course of this project. Some students will be acting as jurors and will decide the outcome of the trial.

The class will be grouped into four law firms and one smaller group that will act as the jury. The attorneys in a law firm will act together to research, build, and argue a case for their client. Suggest that each member of the law firm become a specialist or expert in one phase of the case. That way each student will have a specific job to do and feel like a contributing member of the team. Each member of the law firm is essential to the final judgment awarded in the case.

Explain that the jury will be deciding the case based on the arguments presented by the law firms. The jury will have no background information regarding the case other than what the law firms present in class. It is up to the jury to make a fair and impartial decision on the case.

I have found that it is best to carefully place the students on the law firms. Make sure each firm has students who are verbal and responsible. Each team will need both leaders and cooperative workers.

The jury can be selected in several ways. I sometimes allow the students to elect one member of each firm to act as a juror. I specify that the jury members should be people who like to take notes, are good listeners, and are good at making fair decisions. The attorneys are people who like to research or argue. Emphasize the fact that the jurors do *not* get to speak during the trial, so groups should not send their most verbal member to the jury.

Another way of picking the jury is to select the members yourself as you are establishing the law firms. Students who are absent during the beginning phases of the preparation can serve as jury members.

hint Have the room set up to resemble a courtroom for this week. Give each law firm a fairly private area to work and have the jury work in an area of the room where they won't be able to hear the attorneys. I have the room set up with the groups facing each other in a circle.

Review all the information in the packet concerning cigarettes and smoking. Explain the significance of the findings about smoking and the graphs. Review the traits of a healthy person. Students should have gained an understanding of good health during the course.

DAY TWO Assign the students to their groups. Then call court to session. Explain that participants can be held in contempt of court for unprofessional conduct. Unprofessional conduct can include yelling, impolite behavior, or even losing the team papers. This promotes a serious atmosphere and allows students to get into the parts they will be playing while enforcing the need for responsibility.

Read the "Last Will and Testament of Jacob M. Bayfield." Explain that this is a scenario about an eccentric millionaire with four children who has recently died and left the will being contested.

The law firms are given their packet of handouts with background information on each of the four adult children of Jacob M. Bayfield. The students work in groups using the biographical sketches of the heirs to create a defense for the client assigned to them. They build an argument based on the facts presented in the background information that presents their client in a positive light, living a healthy lifestyle. They should also be preparing arguments, or cross-examination questions, against the other heirs, using the background information on the other law firms' clients to build their case. Remind the students that the jury will know only what is presented to them by the law firms during the trial.

While the attorneys organize and decide who will research and argue each phase of the case, the jury needs to prepare a booklet with the names of each of the four clients on the top of a page of note paper. They should separate each client's page into *positive facts* and *negative facts* to facilitate note taking. They will also be researching, designing, and drawing a poster that will denote their idea of a healthy person. They need to look at all the aspects of healthy living and picture those in the poster. They will be working on this while the other students are preparing their cases.

DAY THREE The attorneys continue building their cases while the teacher visits each law firm to cross-examine the participants about their client.

I encourage students to take the facts in the background information and stretch those facts, embellishing them with additional ideas and imagination to fit their needs. This creates an atmosphere of suspense among the law firms because each firm is wary of what might be asked. The teacher should ask questions to each law firm that will prepare the students for the day of the trial. Encourage the students to think beyond the information presented in the background sheet and to be creative. Ask questions that will cause the students to think on their feet to defend their client while presenting more negative images of the opposing clients.

Some students can make evidence that will implicate other clients in unhealthy lifestyles.

DAYS FOUR AND FIVE This is the beginning of the trial. Begin by reading the "Last Will and Testament of Jacob M. Bayfield." Then proceed to the first law firm. They make their presentation to the jury, bringing out all the positive and healthy traits about their client. They should try to convince the jury that their client should win the judgment.

After the presentation of the first client, each law firm will get a chance to cross-examine with two (or more) cross-examination questions. These questions should be created in advance and should point out the negative or unhealthy aspects of the client being presented. In this way, the jury will hear both sides of a client's case.

Proceed to the next client and follow the same procedure. Continue until all the presentations are made and all the firms have had a chance to cross-examine all the clients. Allow students to follow up cross-examination questions with other questions that are on the same topic to allow the attorneys to get at the facts.

After the argument phase of the trial is complete, allow each firm about 1 minute to make closing statements, which summarize the reasons their client should win the judgment.

Excuse the jury to a private area where they can talk over the case and pick a winning client. The jury should return to court with a foreperson who will read the verdict and give the reasons for their decision. I often award the winning law firm extra credit points as a reward for their winning verdict.

conclusion Probably the best way for the students to gain closure on the project is to ask the jury members to give their impressions of individual classmate's presentations during the trial. Which students were believable and did a good job of speaking and why? It is very powerful for the students to hear praise from their own classmates. Allow for positive opinions from other students in the class about the speaking ability of their peers.

instructor's job The instructor is very busy during the preparation phase of the trial cross-examining and stimulating students' imaginations and creativity. As the actual trial is going on, the instructor acts as the judge, making sure that the teams speak in turn and that order and propriety are upheld in court.

I use the opportunity to write comments on the presentations made by the various law firms as a way of offering feedback and establishing a grade. I give the comment sheets to the law firms at the end of the trial.

hint It is possible to have the law firms grade each other and gain more power in the classroom as they offer opinions on the preparation and performance of themselves and their classmates.

activity 12 Blood Alcohol Levels

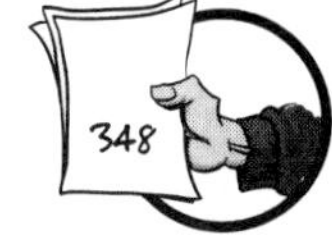

time One 50-minute period.

purpose Students learn to identify the effects alcohol has on the brain and on behavior. Students learn techniques they can use to check their blood alcohol levels when consuming alcohol.

materials The "Blood Alcohol Content Wheel," "Levels of Intoxication," and "Questions Concerning Alcohol Consumption" handouts, one brad (paper fastener), and scissors for each student.

process Introduce the activity with information about alcohol.

The amount of alcohol in a person's blood is called the blood alcohol level. When a person drinks alcoholic beverages, the alcohol in the drink is absorbed through the lining of the stomach and small intestine into the bloodstream and circulated to all parts of the body. When the alcohol reaches the brain, a person's judgment is affected. The individual is slower to react and has more trouble interpreting messages from the senses.

A person's blood alcohol level increases with each drink. If the person is quite large, it will take more alcohol to get him or her drunk. The body acts like a sponge—the larger the sponge, the more liquid it can absorb.

One drink is approximately 1 ounce of alcohol. Most beverages contain alcohol in 1 ounce amounts. One beer contains about 1 ounce of alcohol, the same as one wine cooler or a shot of whiskey. Mixed drinks, however, may contain several types of alcohol and, therefore, contain several ounces of alcohol.

Give each student a copy of both pages of the "Blood Alcohol Content Wheel," a brad, and scissors. Have them cut out and assemble the wheel according to the directions.

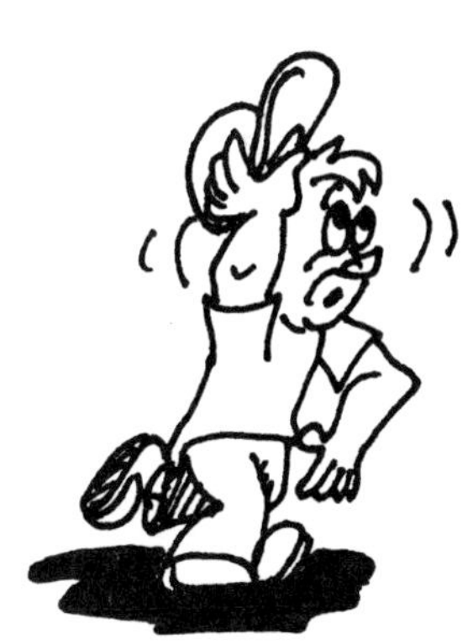

0.08–0.10
Legally drunk, slurred speech

Have the students use the wheel to find the blood alcohol level for various drinking scenarios.

Give students these directions for using the wheel. To find the blood alcohol level of a person weighing 100 pounds and having consumed 3 ounces of alcohol in an hour:

- Find the number 3, indicating the number of ounces of alcohol consumed, on the outer wheel. Then find the weight (100 pounds) on the underneath wheel. Match up the two numbers by placing the 3 directly over the 100.
- Holding the wheels in place, look in the long, thin window at the number pointed to by the arrow. It should be pointing to 0.08. That is the blood alcohol level of a person weighing 100 pounds and consuming 3 ounces of alcohol in one hour.
- The larger window at the bottom of the wheel indicates the blood alcohol level of the person after various periods of time who doesn't consume any additional alcohol.

Use the wheel along with the "Levels of Intoxication" handout to indicate the behavior a person would exhibit with a certain blood alcohol level.

Have students use the wheel or the chart to answer the questions on the "Questions Concerning Alcohol Consumption" worksheet.

answers

1. Benjamin is legally drunk and it will take four hours to be under the legal limit.
2. Sadie is legally drunk.
3. Celia is legally drunk even though she has only been drinking beer. Remember that each beer has about one ounce of alcohol, just like other drinks.
4. It will be about 8 hours before Celia is below the legal limit.
5. Ask someone what the legal drinking age is for your state.
6. How many drinks can you have and still be sober?

13 Refusal Role-Play

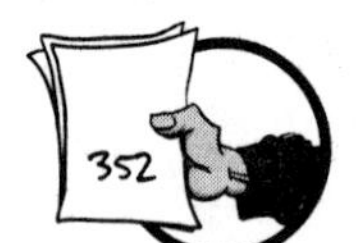

time Two 50-minute periods.

purpose Students will learn refusal skills as they practice refusing drugs and alcohol in various situations.

materials The "Refusal Role-Play" and "Practice Refusals" handouts for each student.

process Discuss the steps a person takes in making a friendly refusal. Give some examples by acting out a friendly refusal. Remind students that they need to practice refusals if they are going to be able to effectively avoid dangerous situations. Below are the steps to a friendly refusal:

- Include the word "no" in the refusal.
- Repeat the refusal using several different methods.
- Tell briefly why you are refusing—explain the problem.
- Provide an alternative.
- Walk away. After suggesting another activity, change the subject or walk away.

Have each student get a partner. Each person will tell the other something he or she really enjoys doing that would be difficult to refuse. One person tries to talk the other person into doing what he or she likes to do most. The other person must refuse, using the guidelines presented.

Give each student a copy of the handouts and have them work with their partner on refusals to the situations presented on the worksheet. Students can also write a script of their own incorporating a friendly refusal.

If you have time, the students can act out some of the refusals.

Students can use the worksheet entitled "Practice Refusals" to practice answering common methods that friends might use to encourage them to do something inappropriate. Remind students they have to refuse.

activity 14 Drugs and You

354

time One 50-minute period.

purpose Students gain a better understanding of the uses and dangers of various types of legal and illegal drugs.

materials The "Effects of Drugs on the Body" and "Drug Description" handouts. If students are working in small groups, they will need markers and large pieces of butcher paper.

process Make three headings on the board or on butcher paper. The headings should be *Prescribed Medication, Crossover,* and *Illegal Drugs.* Have students brainstorm the reasons for using prescription drugs and illegal drugs.

Discuss how prescription and illegal drugs could be considered crossover drugs. Marijuana is considered an illegal drug and yet it is used in the treatment of glaucoma and in relieving pain. Prescribed medications are often abused and taken for reasons other than those prescribed.

Then give each student a copy of the handout entitled "Drug Description." Categorize all drugs into one or all of the three lists. Remember to include alcohol and tobacco.

Describe briefly how many drugs work in the nervous system. The dendrites of one nerve cell meet the axon of another nerve cell in an area called the *synapse.* Where the two nerves meet, there is a space that is normally filled with natural chemicals that either inhibit or excite the impulse as it jumps from one cell to the other. If these chemicals are blocking the impulse, the body reacts by becoming sleepy or slowing down. If the chemicals excite the impulse and speed it up, the body reacts more quickly and with more strength. For example, adrenaline is pumped into the system when you are afraid and excites the impulse so you can react quickly by fighting or fleeing.

When people introduce other chemicals into their system, the system is changed according to the chemical introduced. Alcohol introduced into the synapse of cells actually slows down, or inhibits, the impulse so reaction time is slowed. The individual cannot make clear decisions because the information being carried by the nerve cells is interfered with and the messages are jumbled. This can happen with most drugs. Hallucinogens can interfere with the impulses being sent to such a degree that the person will experience things that are not actually occurring.

This is a simplified version of the action of drugs on the nervous system but it gives some explanation of how drugs interfere with the normal functioning of the brain and the messages traveling to and from the muscles. See the following illustration.

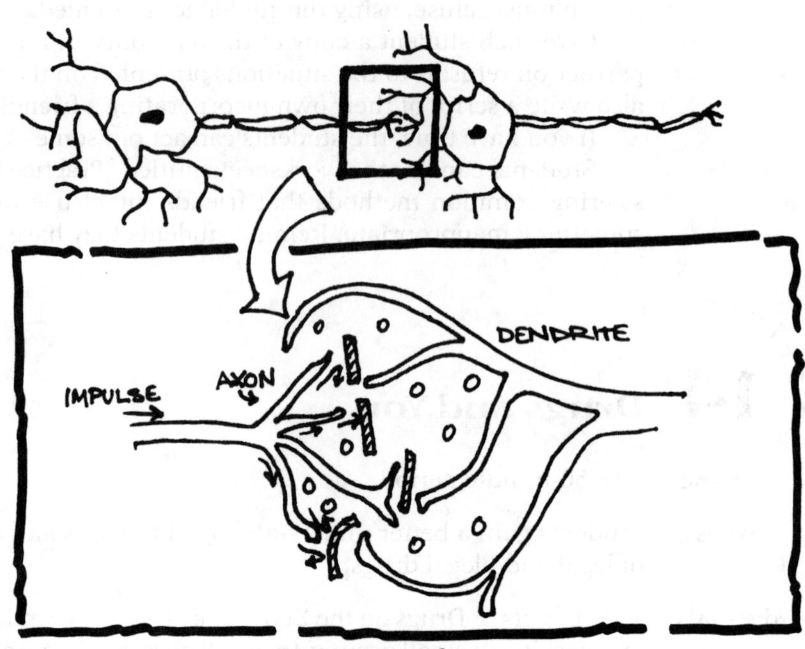

activity

15 Understanding Dependency

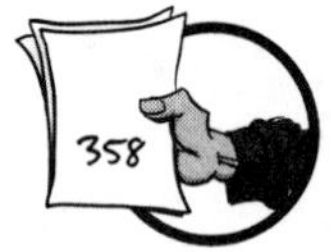

time One 50-minute period.

purpose Students will gain an understanding of chemical dependency and addictions and be able to indicate the stages of addiction. Students will test their own stage of dependency or addiction.

materials The "Identifying the Signs of Dependency" handout for each student.

process Explain that no one really wants or intends to become dependent on a chemical substance, but it happens to all kinds of people, from teachers and doctors to children. There are all kinds of addictions: alcohol, smoking, illegal drugs, prescription and over-the-counter drugs, work, eating, and gambling.

One of the indications of an addiction is that you no longer have control over the behavior. The high you get from the behavior or the chemical substance actually clouds your thinking, making you believe that it is improving your life and your ability to function.

It is difficult to recognize a behavior or use of a substance becoming an addiction because it develops over a long period of time, from a harmless action into something that can be detrimental to your normal existence.

The stages of addiction are:

- *Experimentation.* The person tries the behavior or substance for fun, or to fit in with his or her friends. It may cause him or her to relax more and feel more in control or more popular.
- *Occasional Use.* The person may use the behavior or substance for specific activities because he or she recognizes the lift or comfort derived from it.
- *Habitual Use.* The person recognizes the need of the behavior or substance to get through the day. He or she makes plans to use the substance or do the behavior and may become attracted to people who share the same need.
- *Addiction.* At this point, the person has lost control over the substance or the behavior. He or she continues to use in spite of the risks and dangers to others and to himself or herself. The person may continue the practice secretly as it consumes time and energy.

Some of the warning signs of an addiction or problem may include one or several of the behaviors described below:

- Personality changes—the person may become withdrawn or want to be left alone; he or she may have mood shifts or may become depressed.
- Absenteeism or tardiness—the person may develop a pattern of missing school or work; when he or she does attend, long breaks may be needed to escape.
- Work suffers—the person's quality of work may suffer because he or she no longer cares as much about the results of the work. The person may be unable to meet deadlines or do the work correctly and may not produce the quantity of work he or she used to do. Handwriting and ability to communicate may suffer.

Hand out the copies of the"Identifying the Signs of Dependency" questionnaire and tell students they can test themselves for possible addictions or may take copies home for use with family or friends. Remind students that this questionnaire is not a scientific test but merely one method of indicating a possible problem.

Tell students that if they decide that they may have a problem with addiction to some substance or habit, they will need to decide if they want to break that addiction. It is difficult to overcome an addiction alone. People need support from professionals, family, and friends. There are community agencies and groups that understand the process of overcoming addictions and can help. Have students contribute phone numbers and agencies available in their own community where help could be obtained for addictions. You might want to include other hotlines, agencies, or clinics that would be helpful to students in all kinds of emergencies.

hints I copy the addresses and phone numbers for agencies and hotlines concerning abuse, addictions, sexually transmitted diseases, and runaways as well as other relevant crisis lines and print them up on wallet-sized cards. I hand them out to each student and have extras available.

Check with community services in your area. Many services will produce a publication or a card that has all the free public services available. These cards are usually free and can be obtained in bulk for distribution.

activity 16 Building Character

time One 50-minute period.

purpose Students identify the building blocks of character and offer suggestions for ways they can develop those ideals in their own lives.

materials None.

process Have the class define the word *character.* Suggest that there is a crisis in society concerning character. Discuss the validity of such a statement and ask students to brainstorm things they see in the news, in school, or in their own lives that they consider a contributing factor to the loss of character in society. Below are some suggestions for discussion:

- rise in youth violence
- increase in dishonesty and tolerance of that trend
- growing disrespect
- increase in peer cruelty
- rise in prejudice and hate crimes
- deterioration in polite language and behavior
- decline in work ethic
- decline in personal and civic responsibility
- rise in self-destructive behavior and a decline in self-respect
- decline in ethical literacy
- decline in moral values and standards and acceptance of that

Propose some universal building blocks for developing character in individuals. These are universal truths that cross all boundaries and religious beliefs. If each person were to develop these character traits to their fullest, there would be no crisis in society.

Those building blocks of character are:

- trustworthiness
- responsibility
- respect
- fairness
- caring
- citizenship
- courage

Have students define each of the components in building character.

Read the story about the "Brink's Truck Wreck" and discuss how each of those components to building character is represented in the story.

hint The "Brink's Truck Wreck" is a true story about an incident in the Los Angeles area in 1996. Have students write a story about what they would have done in that situation and a justification for their action. You might want the students to write their ideas before you present the building blocks of character and then discuss their feelings. Allow for and encourage interaction between students with differing points of view.

THE BRINK'S TRUCK WRECK

A Brink's truck had just made its final collection and was on its way to the bank to deposit millions of dollars in cash collected from businesses in town. The armored car was fully guarded with an armed driver and two armed guards when it hit a pothole in the street and careened out of control, crashing into the guardrail of an overpass. The truck flipped over, stunning the guards and ripping the side of the truck open. The bags carrying hundreds of thousands of dollars in coins were thrown from the truck and burst open as they hit the ground, sending coins flying everywhere. The coins flew over the guardrail of the overpass onto the street of the neighborhood below. The stacks of paper money were scattered into the air and millions of dollars were carried by the wind to the neighborhood below the overpass.

Some local boys from the neighborhood were playing stickball in the street and heard the screech of brakes and the grinding metal as the Brink's truck was torn apart in the crash. They lived in poor houses below the overpass where they were constantly tormented by the noises and fumes of the traffic that flowed above their heads. Every family in the neighborhood was struggling to survive, having each member contribute by doing odd jobs downtown, collecting bottles and newspapers for recycling, and generally scavenging for every cent that came their way. These people lived in tar paper townhouses with little or no heat. The cars parked in the street were old and scarred by broken windows, lopsided bumpers, and big patches of rust.

The boys playing stickball ducked when they heard the crash of the Brink's truck and then had to cover their heads as they were pelted with coins raining down on them from above. Coins poured like water and pooled in mounds at their feet. The boys looked up carefully in astonishment only to be showered by paper money fluttering out of the sky. It was like a dream. It was unbelievable. They called to friends and family to help. All the people in the neighborhood ran to the street with bags, pots and pans, and whatever they could grab to collect and hold the money. Kids and adults ran from the scene with pockets and shirts bulging with money. The guards had recovered by now and yelled from the overpass for the people in the street below to put the money down and return to their homes.

The people from the poor neighborhood either did not hear or did not care. They had never been given a chance like this. This was money from heaven being bestowed on people long overdue for a break. They scrambled, bit, and grabbed for the money. They ran back to their houses and got bigger bags and more family members to help as the guards stood helpless, watching from the overpass.

In the end, when the wreck was cleaned up and the remaining money was counted, the Brink's company estimated their loss at five million dollars. They pleaded with the people in the poor neighborhood to return the money voluntarily but because the numbers on the bills were not registered, the company had no way to prove that any money confiscated was from the wrecked truck. They were helpless to retrieve the money.

POSTSCRIPT

Several days later, a single mother with three young children came to the Brink's company and returned over $100,000 in coins and bills that she and her children had gathered from the street. When asked why she had returned the money, she stated that she and her children knew that it was not theirs and they were returning it to the rightful owners.

This story has been fictionalized but was based on a true incident that occurred in the winter of 1996.

QUESTIONS FOR DISCUSSION

- What would you have done?
- If your child came home with pockets full of money and no way to trace it, would you make them return the money?
- Was it legal for the people to keep the money?

- Was it right for the poor people to keep the money?
- Who ultimately pays, both financially and morally, for this event?
- How does this event affect all of us?
- What would you do if you found a wallet with $100 in it? What would you do if you saw a student at lunch drop a dollar?
- What would you do if you were failing a class and the teacher left the room during the final exam?
- Use the building blocks of character to support your ideas.

activity 17 Fake Final Exam

time 30 minutes.

purpose The students review the materials presented during the unit and have fun demonstrating their knowledge. This activity helps bring closure to a unit.

materials Have questions prepared in advance that cover the most important concepts you want to review from the unit just covered. Have some kind of reward prepared—copy and cut out the reward certificate provided on the "Reward" handout or give a piece of candy or a special privilege—whatever you think will appeal to your students.

process Tell students that you are going to give a "little final exam." After they calm down, explain that this is your own special exam and will not be graded but instead students will be rewarded for correct answers.

Explain that you will read the question and the students will respond by raising their hand if they think they know the answer. You will call on the person that you see first with his or her hand in the air. If the student answers the question correctly, he or she will win a reward. Remind students how much their parents like them to bring home awards—they will tape it to the refrigerator and display it for years!

Ask each of the prepared questions and allow the students to answer. I even help the students answer. Remember that the main objective is to review the material. Discuss the answers and award the certificate or prize and have the class applaud the participant. Half the fun of this activity is in recognizing students' knowledge.

Many times a student can answer one question correctly but may not do well on a whole test. This activity allows that student recognition and a sense of accomplishment for the knowledge that he or she does know. Try to make sure that every student gets a chance to participate with a correct answer.

activity 18 Class Evaluation

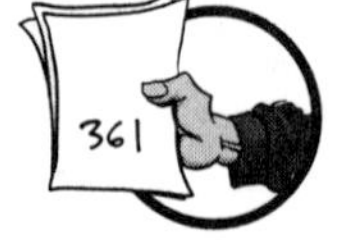

time 15–20 minutes.

purpose The students have a chance to think about the class and evaluate the worth of the material presented. This gives students a sense of power because they are evaluating the class or teacher's presentation. The students feel valued.

materials Students need some lined paper or the "Class Evaluation" handout. Each student should be given the "Thoughts to Take with You" handout.

process Have the students review the activities presented in the class. Ask students to be honest in answering the questions concerning the class. Tell them that their input is valuable because the activities are adjusted according to the feedback received. You need to know what they feel is valuable and what is unnecessary. Give some examples of how you have changed the class as a result of the information received from student evaluations.

hint I allow students to offer their thoughts on the evaluation anonymously because they can feel free to be truthful without any recriminations. I often have them complete the evaluation after I have told them their final grade so they do not feel that their grade will be affected.

I have found that students feel more involved in the process when their opinions are valued and actually used in making decisions. Also, this is a great way to bring closure to the class. Students may have some difficulty leaving this class where they have so freely shared their experiences and beliefs. Asking students to help you prepare the structure of the class for the next group allows students to realize that it is time to move on and provide the same opportunities for those who follow.

IN CONCLUSION

Educators are faced with an overwhelming task of shaping the future through the ways they touch the minds and hearts of their students. It is not an easy task. Students today come from a variety of backgrounds and experiences. Students need to be taught the skills and given the tools to overcome the problems and challenges they face.

Educators can help students do this by helping them build confidence and develop skills that will contribute to their success in the future. Classrooms should be places where the students can share and feel connected. Each student needs to feel that he or she is important and belongs. Teachers can encourage independence and help students find a meaning and purpose in their lives. Teachers should recognize and support each student's individual interests, heritage, and talents.

Build a classroom community based on respect, trust, and cooperation. Set an example for students with your own exemplary demonstration of the values and lessons that you present. Model the behavior you want students to achieve. Really listen to your students. Respect them as you want them to respect you and each other. Allow students the opportunity to take risks and to realize their mistakes are stepping stones and learning experiences that result in eventual success.

Allow yourself to like and enjoy each student. Each student has a desire to be seen as a worthwhile human being. Find the fun in every activity and enjoy it with the students. Make your classroom a safe haven where even you can have fun as you create an atmosphere for growth and development. Remember that kids are like the rest of us. They are in transition. They are on a road of growth and development that will be good and bad at times. Help students recognize and reach for the best in themselves by helping them recognize behaviors that will enhance their futures.

Most of all, have fun as a teacher. Take care of yourself so that you can give your best to the students you serve. Enjoy the students every day and watch as you help the future unfold before your eyes.

handouts

Appendix

NAME ____________________

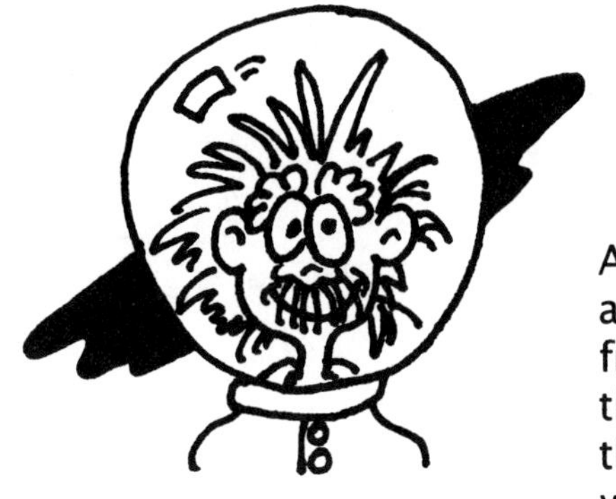

Time Capsule

A time capsule is a collection of items that represent a certain time in history. Make a list of the items from your life that will best represent you and your times to your great-grandchildren. Remember that the items you choose will be your picture to them of who you are.

Below is the capsule. Draw or write in the items you want to use to describe you and your life.

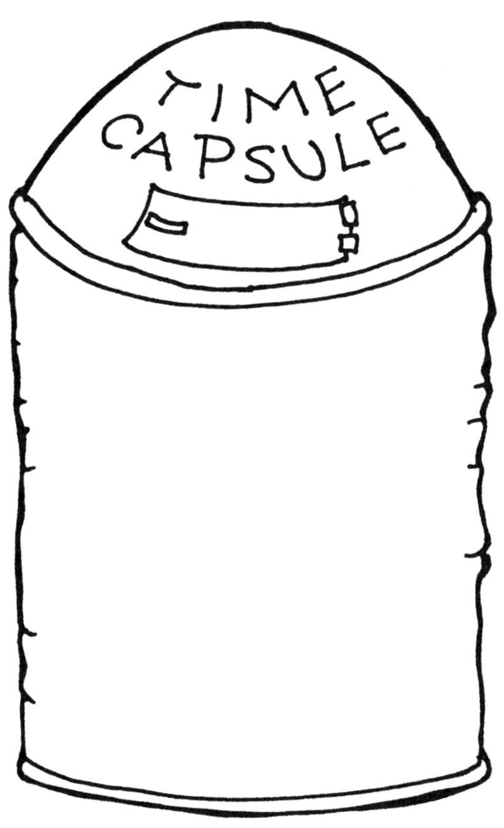

NAME ___________________________

Venn Diagram

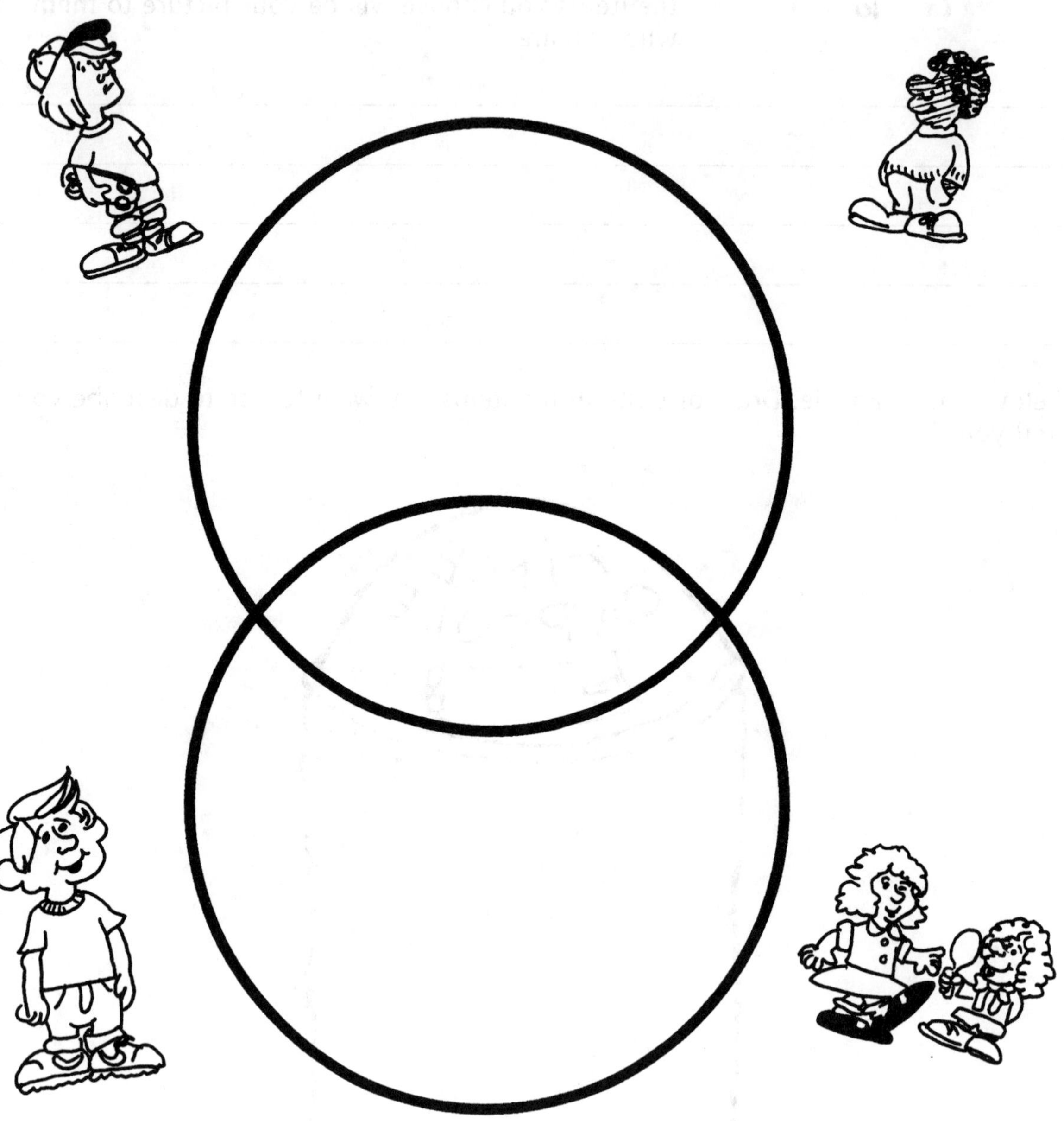

NAME ______________________

One of a Kind

Part One:

Look closely at your peanut. Answer the following questions about your peanut.

1. What color is it? ______________________
2. How many peanuts do you think it contains? ______________________
3. About how long is it? ______________________
4. Note any lines or marks that make your peanut different from all the others.

____

____

5. What did you name your peanut? ______________________
6. Draw an accurate picture of your peanut.

Part Two:

1. How is your peanut different from all the others? ______________________
2. What did you learn from this activity? ______________________

____

3. Write a statement applying the lesson from this activity to people. ______________________

____

4. How could you be picked out of a group of people? What makes you unique?

____

____

NAME ______________________

Human Scavenger Hunt

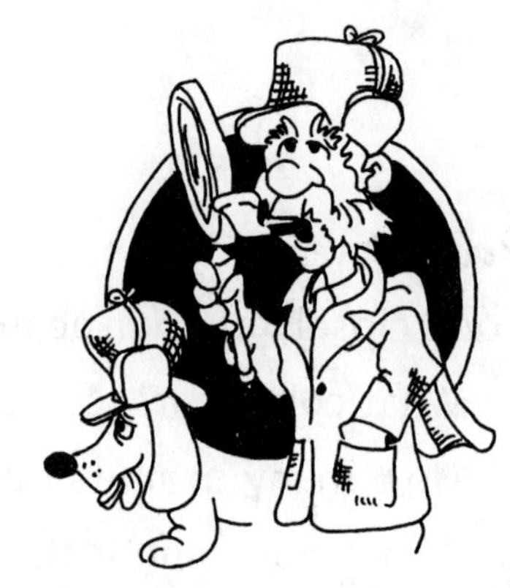

Find a person who:

1. Likes to ski on snow ______________________
2. Was born the farthest from your school ______________________
3. Has no siblings ______________________
4. Has eaten a s'more (Graham crackers with roasted marshmallow and chocolate) ______________________
5. Is good at using in-line skates ______________________
6. Has won an award in the last year ______________________
7. Likes school ______________________
8. Has recently cleaned his or her bedroom ______________________
9. Plays a musical instrument ______________________
10. Has traveled out of the country ______________________
11. Has gone camping ______________________
12. Tells a terrific story about a fish they once caught ______________________
13. Has been to Disneyland ______________________
14. Likes cafeteria food ______________________
15. Is good at math ______________________
16. Has invented a new sandwich ______________________
17. Actually eats the things he or she has cooked ______________________
18. Has a famous relative ______________________
19. Likes snakes ______________________
20. Can dance in time with the music ______________________
21. Actually is comfortable in the bathroom of an airplane ______________________
22. Can sing on key ______________________

NAME ___________________________

Life Map

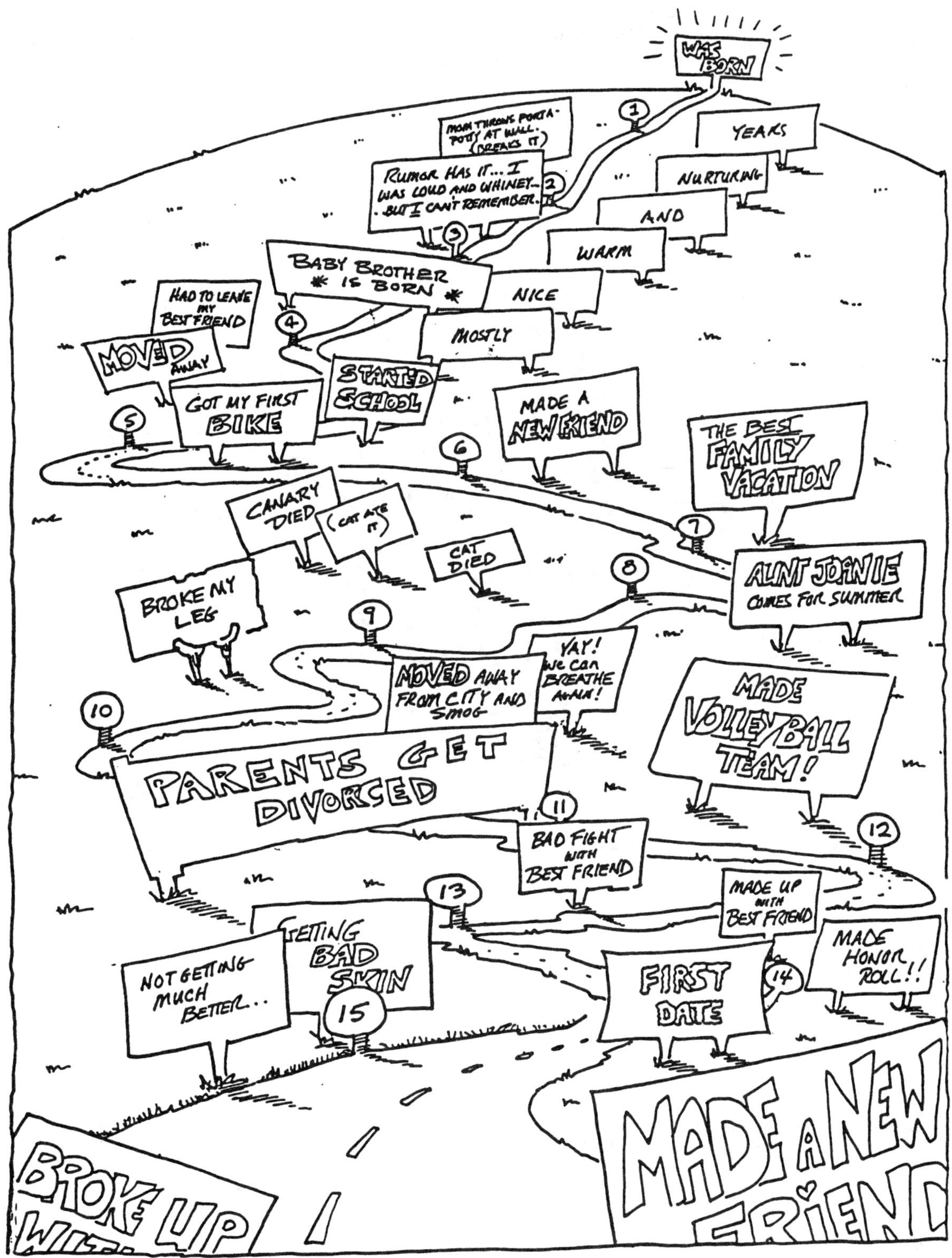

NAME ____________________

This Is How I See Myself

Read each quality listed on the activity sheet and decide how each applies to you. Write the qualities you feel apply to you the best on the left, and write those that you feel apply to you the least on the right. Space the qualities along the continuum as you feel they apply to you.

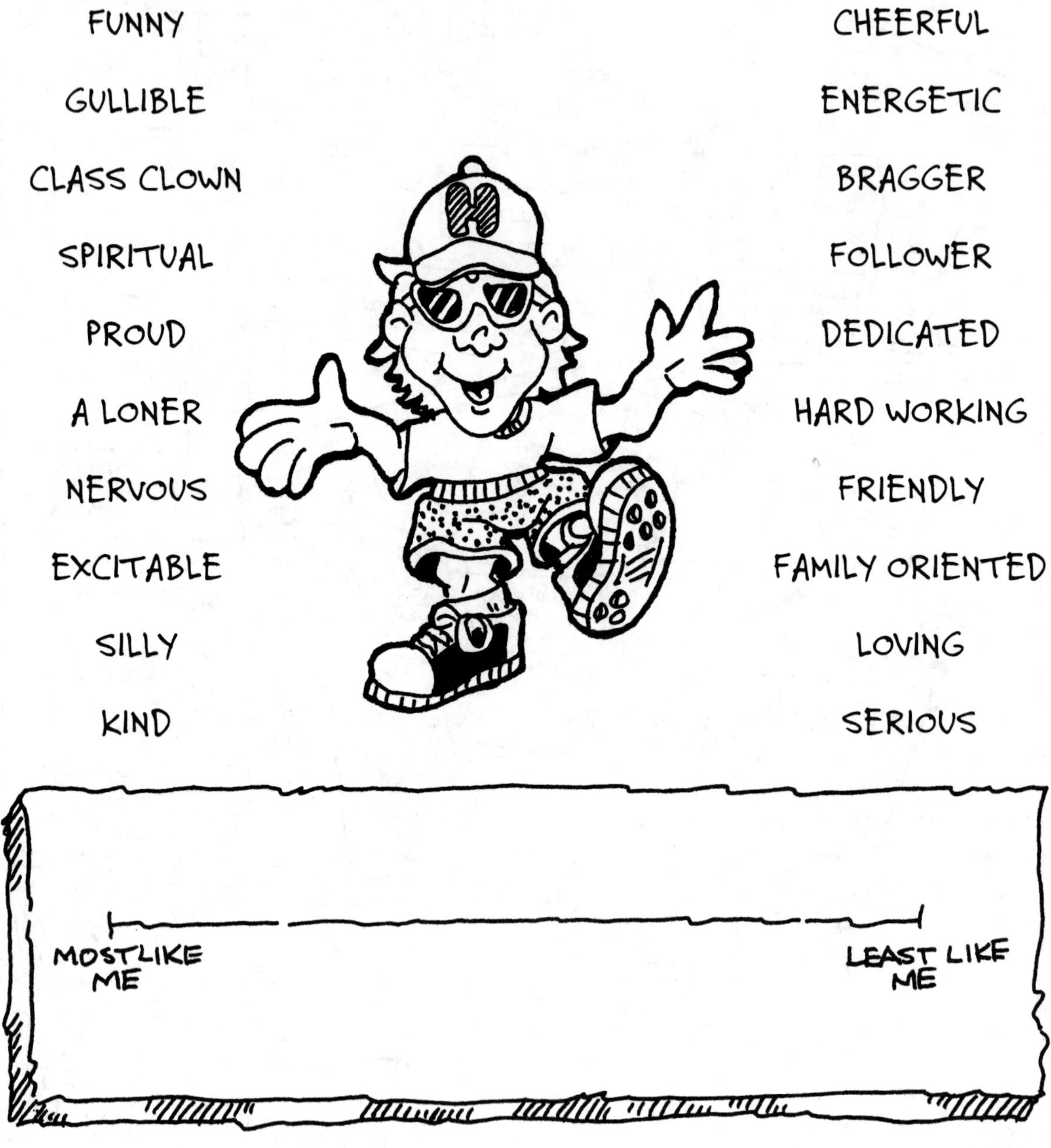

NAME ____________________

You're My Kind of Person!

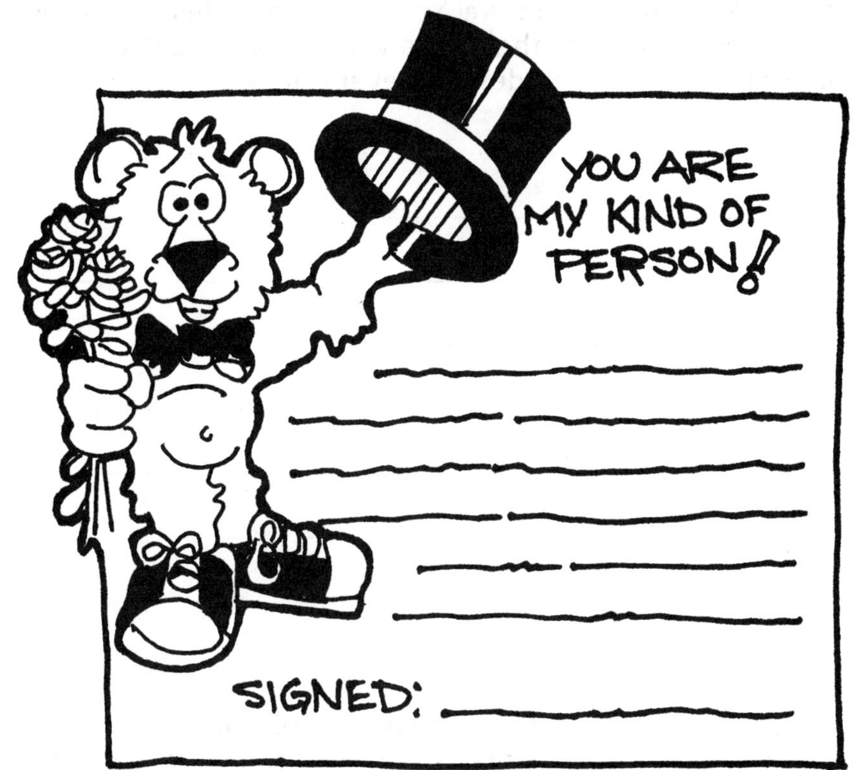

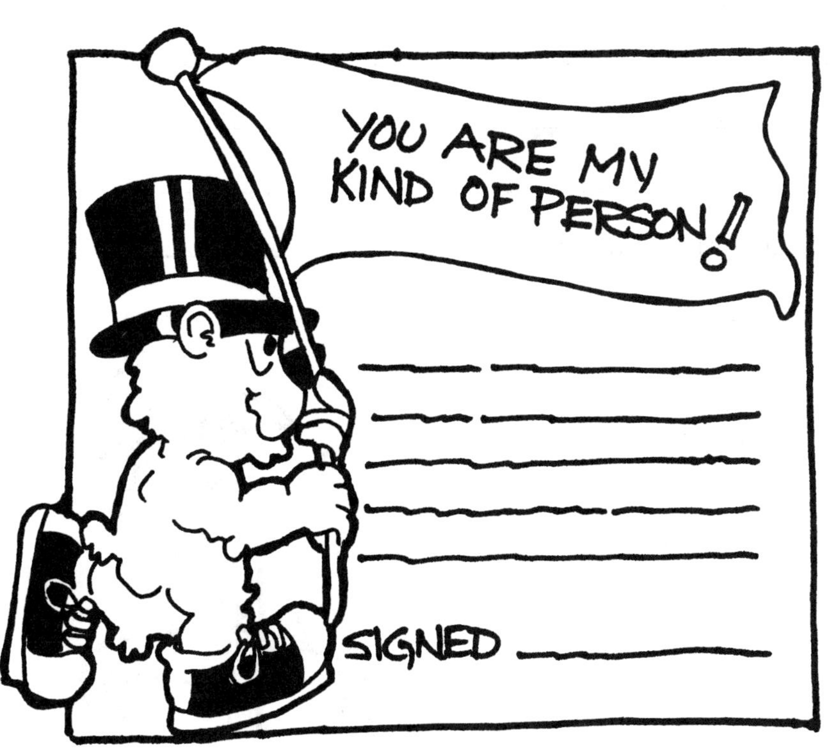

NAME ____________________

It's Important to Me!

Oh no!! Your house is on fire! You have 5 minutes to save whatever you can from the fire. Make a list of the things you would save if you only had 5 minutes before the roof crashes in and destroys everything.

The items a person feels are most valuable and precious can help define that person's values. Look at the list you made and tell why you saved those particular items.

Describe your feelings about the choices you made.

What do you think your choices say about you?

NAME ______________________________

This Is How I Feel

Complete each of the following sentences in your own words.

1. I feel best when I am ______________________________

____

2. I am happiest when ______________________________

____

3. I feel most safe when ______________________________

____

4. I enjoy spending time with ______________________________

____

5. People who care about me often think ______________________________

____

6. People who don't know me very well might think ______________________________

____

7. My feelings are hurt when ______________________________

____

8. I probably hurt other people's feelings when ______________________________

____

9. I struggle most when ______________________________

____

10. I feel most successful when ______________________________

____

11. Before I die I would most like to accomplish ______________________________

____

NAME ___________________________

12. The three words that best describe my personality are ___________________________

____

13. My most important possession is ___________________________

____

14. The most important person in my life is ___________________________

____

15. The one thing that I would like to help others do is ___________________________

____

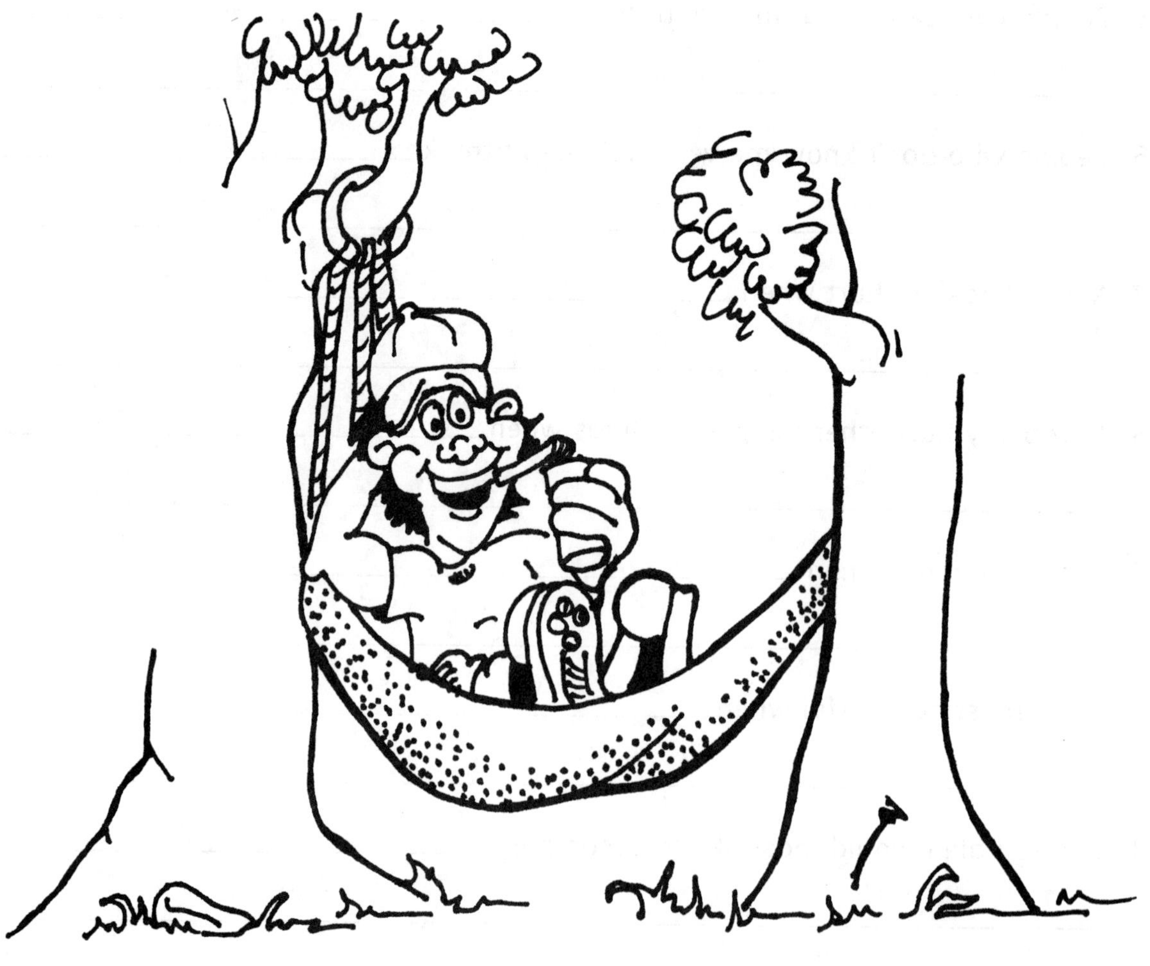

NAME ____________________

Promote Yourself

This is your chance to brag! You are going to promote your best qualities, talents, and skills as if you are applying for work. Show off!

Use whatever method of advertising you want to promote yourself. Write a script for a radio announcement, design a billboard, draw a poster, compile a collage of magazine pictures, or write a television advertisement that will show your best qualities.

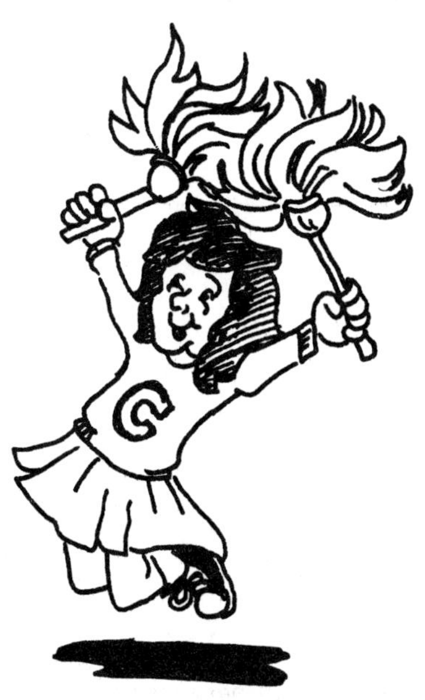

NAME ____________________

An Important Party

You are hosting a party and you may choose 11 people to attend. You may choose any 7 people in the world that you admire, but you must also choose 4 people that you do not like. Remember to use initials or code if you do not want to share your dislikes with the class. Seat everyone, including yourself, around the table. Be able to explain why you invited each person and why they are seated in the order you chose.

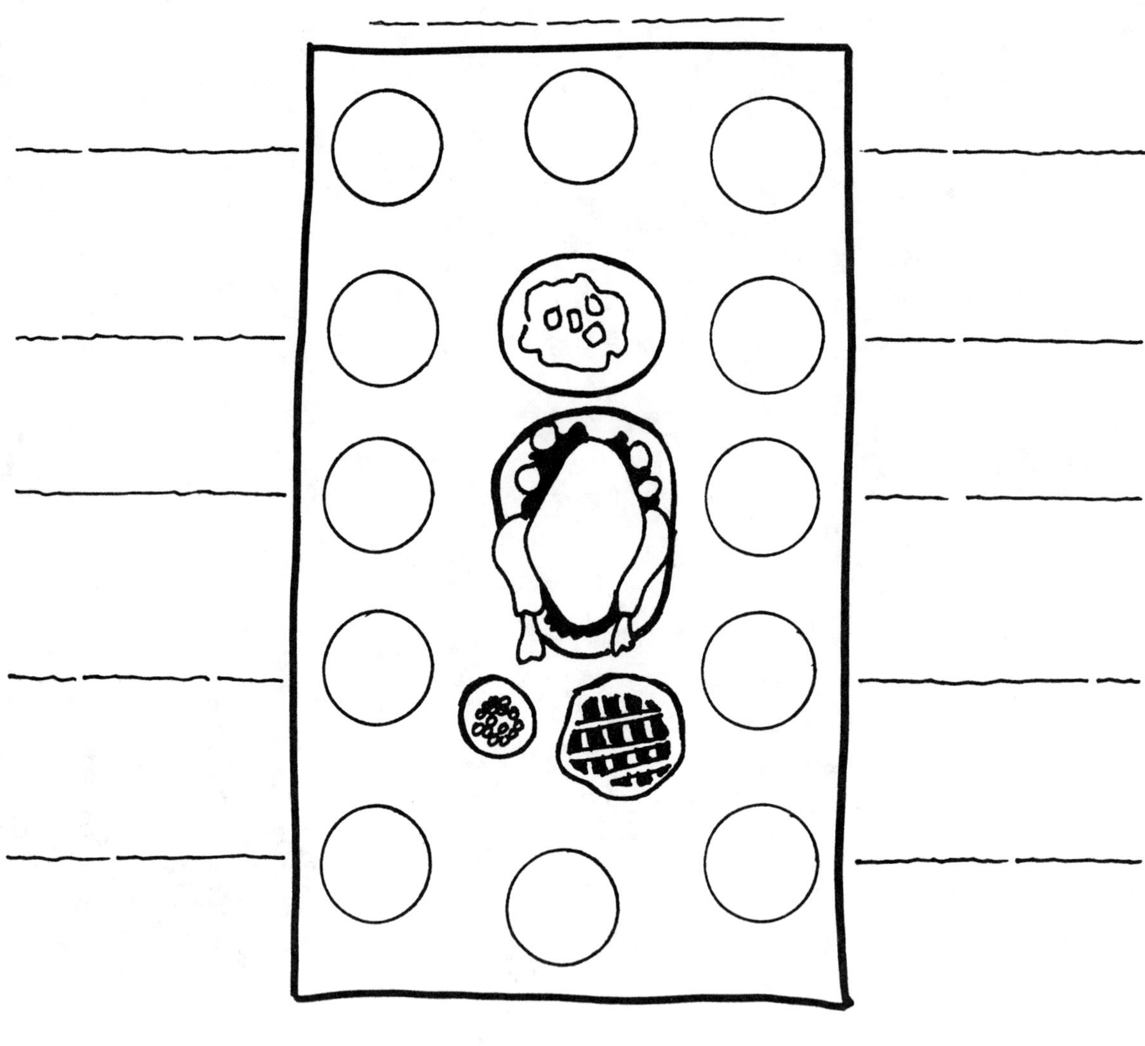

Adapted with permission from *Prevention Skills for Youth,* ETR Associates Training Department. Santa Cruz, CA, 1987–1998.

NAME ______________________________

Questions about Your Party

1. Who is sitting on your left? ______________________________

   Why did you place them there? ______________________________

   ____

2. Who is sitting on your right? ______________________________

   Why did you place them there? ______________________________

   ____

3. Are you sitting near people you do not like? ______________________________

   Why or why not? ______________________________

   ____

   ____

   ____

4. Describe your feelings about how the party will go and discuss what problems might arise.

   ____

   ____

   ____

   ____

5. What can you do to make sure your party is successful?

   ____

   ____

   ____

   ____

   ____

NAME ____________________

Build a Firm Foundation

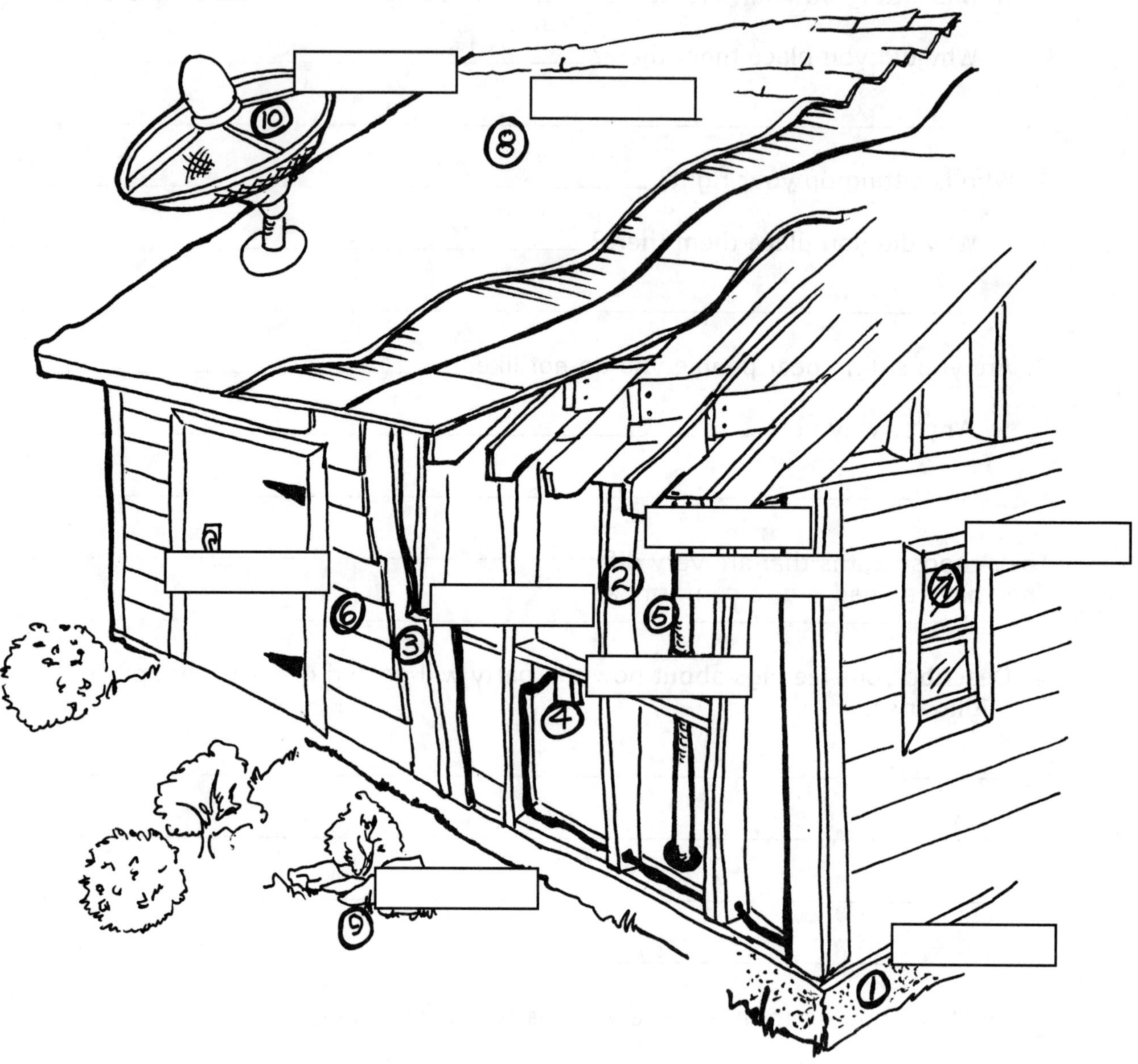

NAME ______________________________

Birth Order Factors and Personality Traits

First Born

They are disciplined more strictly and develop strict consciences (strong feelings of right and wrong).
They are likely to be rigid and intolerant of others who do not meet their standards.
They are overachievers, especially in intellectual pursuits.
They go to school longer than children born later.
They may be more jealous and express more anger than middle or youngest children.
They are tense and driven.

Middle Children

They are diplomatic and good negotiators.
They are more friendly and able to maintain better relationships in life than the first born.
They have an easier time with their parents, because the parents are more relaxed and less demanding.
They look for assistance from others.
They discover that competition can be fierce when the older child is of the same sex.
They choose paths that are very different than that of the first born.
They have a need not to conform, as a contrast to a conservative older brother or sister.
The center birth position seems to affect girls more strongly than boys. The most difficult position seems to be the middle of three girls. The easiest middle position is that of the middle child of the opposite sex.

Youngest Children

They are charming, good companions, playful, and lighthearted.
They expect others to take care of them.
They have so many teachers and role models that they are likely to learn to walk, talk, and read at an earlier age than did their brothers and sisters.
They may be driven by the need to keep up with older brothers and sisters.
They may lose self-confidence if older siblings present too much of a challenge.
They may avoid real tests of their abilities and try to wriggle out of difficult situations.

Only Children

They seem to have a lot of self-confidence because of the absence of competition.
They are dominant and verbal and strive for perfection. They are not jealous, because their position in the family has never been threatened.
They are eager to please the authority figure.
They are overachievers.
They have a close relationship with their parents, even into adulthood.

From an article by Loretta M. Bierer, *Parents* magazine vol. 55, no. 3. March, 1980, pp. 52–55.

NAME ______________________________

BIRTH ORDER INTERVIEW

NAME →					
NUMBER OF KIDS IN FAMILY					
BIRTH ORDER					

IS THIS PERSON . . . .

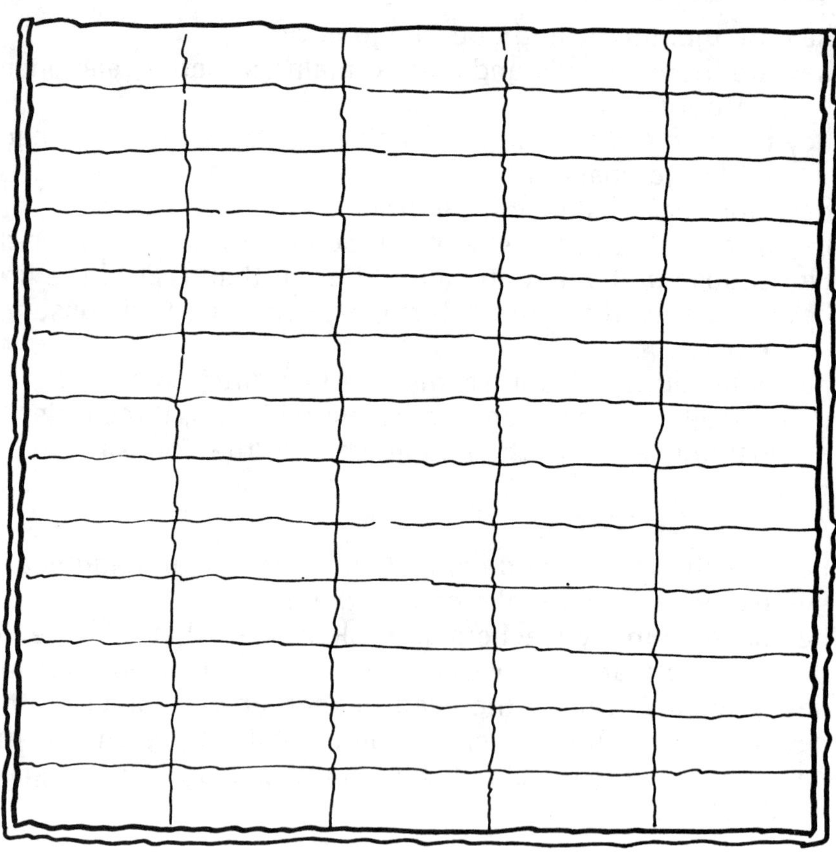

COMPETITIVE					
LEADER					
ACHIEVER					
MORAL					
OPEN-MINDED					
JEALOUS					
EASILY UPSET					
FRIENDLY					
EASY GOING					
LIKES TO BE DIFFERENT					
ACCEPTING OF HELP					
SELF-MOTIVATED					
CONFIDENT					

CONCLUSIONS:

NAME ______________________________

Meeting Needs

BIRTH ORDER	SPECIAL NEEDS SOCIAL, EMOTIONAL, ETC.	METHODS OF MEETING THOSE NEEDS
ONLY CHILD		
FIRST BORN/OLDEST		
MIDDLE CHILD		
LAST BORN/YOUNGEST		

NAME ______________________________

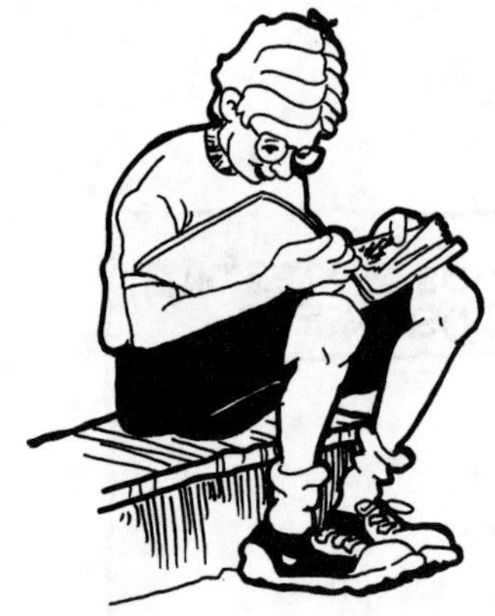

I Have Responsibilities

If you want to:	You have to:
Go to the store by yourself	______________________________
	______________________________
Stay out late with a friend	______________________________
	______________________________
Have a party with the opposite sex	______________________________
	______________________________
Be treated like an adult	______________________________
	______________________________
Be treated with respect by other kids	______________________________
	______________________________
Have many friends	______________________________
	______________________________
Receive praise for doing well	______________________________
	______________________________
Be a leader in your group	______________________________
	______________________________
Do well on your homework	______________________________
	______________________________

NAME ______________________

Sit next to a friend in class ______________________

____

Play in a game at school ______________________

____

Hang out with friends at the mall ______________________

____

Talk on the phone ______________________

____

Ask for help in class ______________________

____

Study for a test with a friend ______________________

____

Be chosen for activities at school ______________________

____

Have a terrific future ______________________

____

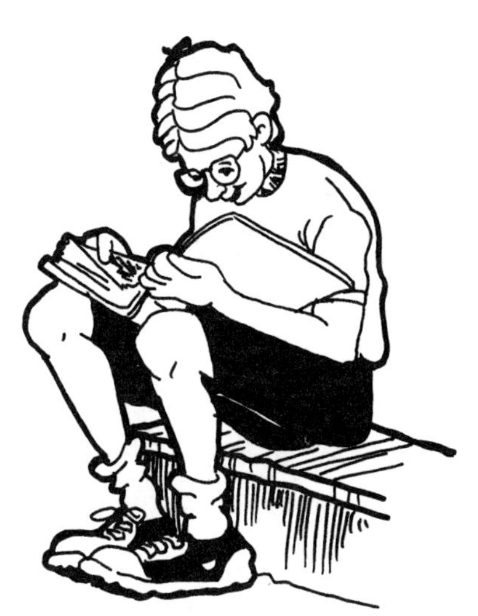

NAME ______________________

This Is My Life

By ______________________

Paste or draw your baby picture here.

Paste a recent photograph here.

____

Date of Birth

BIRTH

Draw your best friend in childhood.

NAME ______________________________

Tell the story of what happened when you were born. You may need to ask parents or friends for their recollections.

What is your happiest childhood memory?

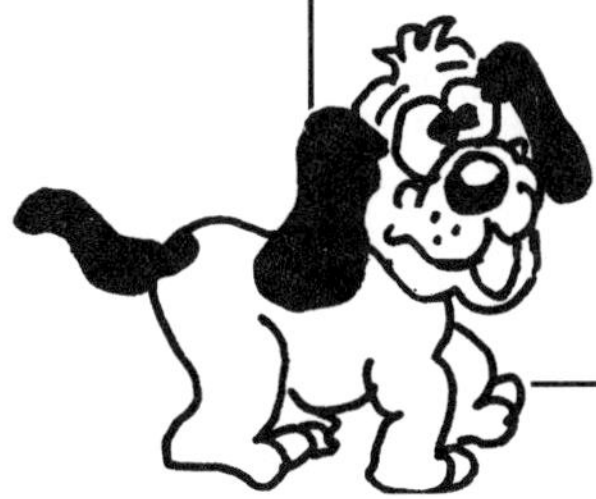

Draw a picture of the floorplan of your dream house.

Draw a map showing where you want to live.

What was your favorite toy?

NAME ____________________________

Describe the types of education you plan to achieve.

What types of jobs will you hold?

Describe the work you enjoy most.

Who will be the important people in your adult life?

Draw a picture of yourself as an adult.

NAME ________________________________

Place an X on places you would like to visit.

Place an O on places you have already visited.

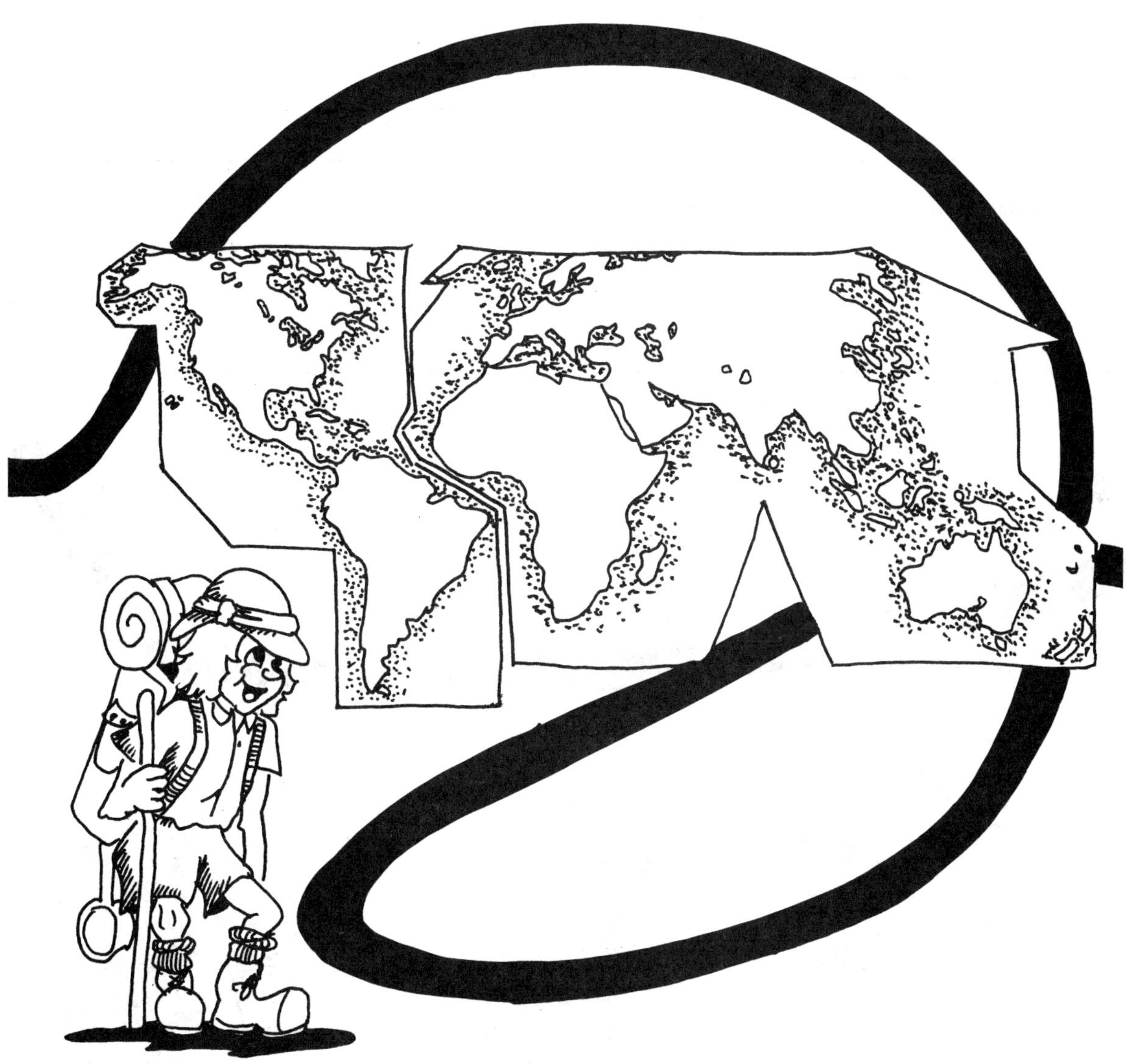

NAME ______________________________

What or how will you contribute to the world?

What do you want people to write about you when you die?

What do you want people to remember you for?

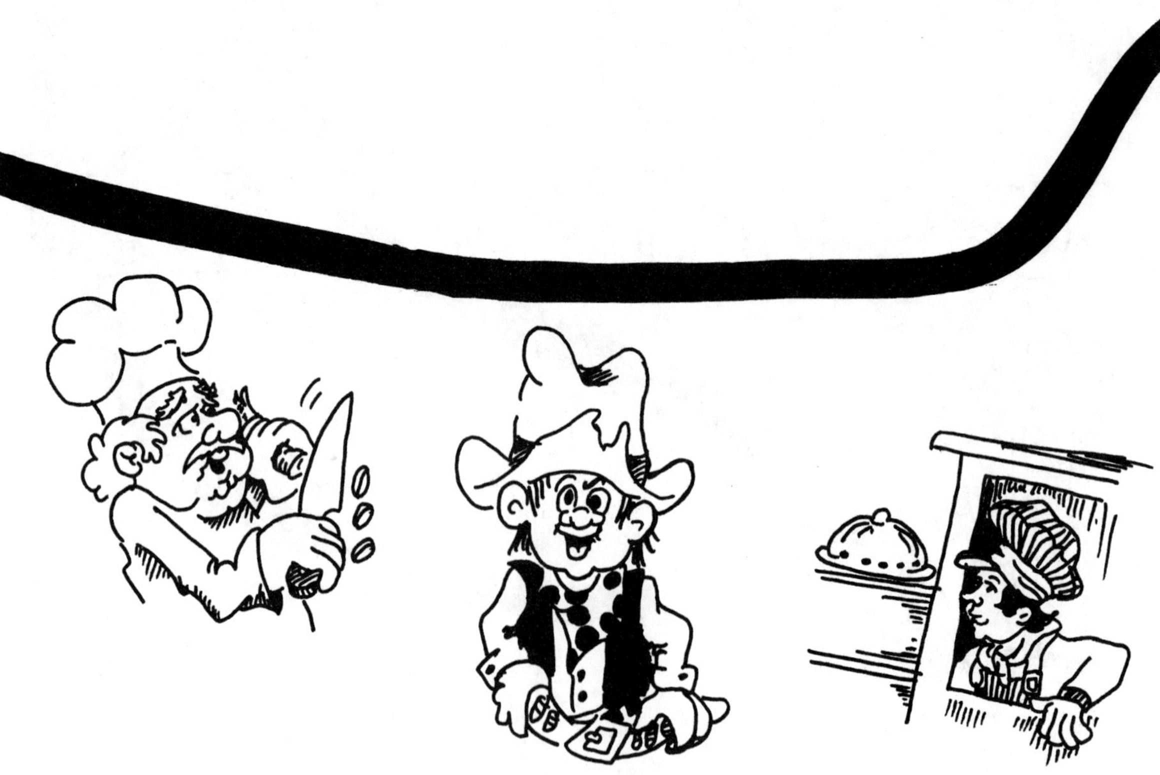

NAME ______________________________

What would you like the future to be like?

What can you do to make that future a reality?

NAME ___________________________

What is the most important thing in your life?

What do you want to acccomplish in your lifetime?

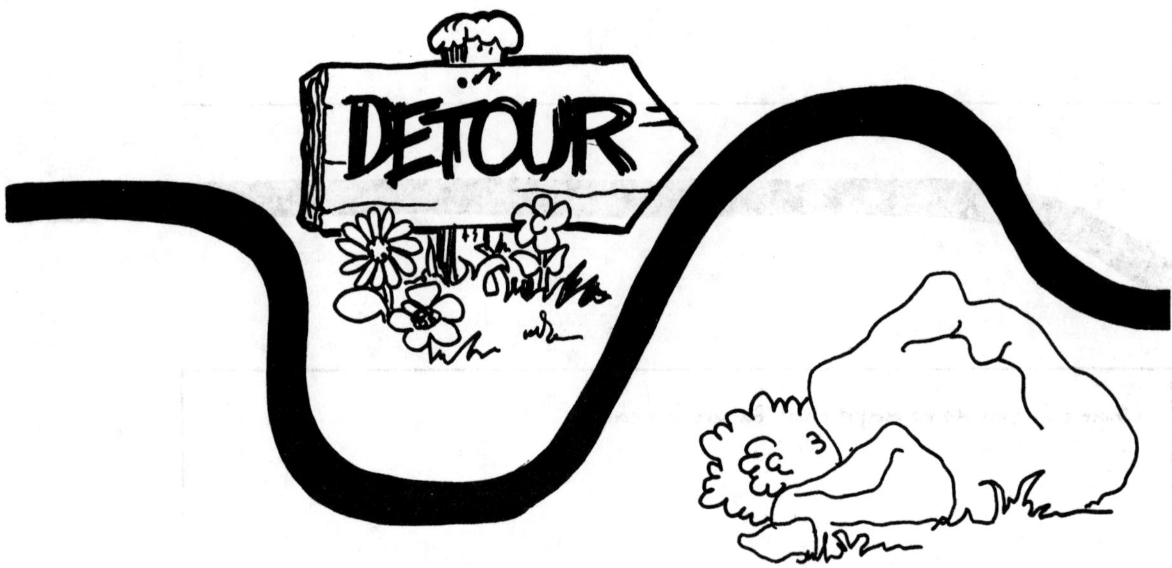

What will You look like when you are old?

NAME ______________________________

Make a collage that best represents your whole life.

What do you think will be an obstacle to your success?

What will you do for fun as an adult?

NAME ________________________________

Oh Look! It's Me!

Pretend that you can see yourself sitting in the shade against a tree. You seem to be sitting thoughtfully, kind of daydreaming. I want you to describe yourself. What do you look like? Describe in detail all the important things about your physical body that make you different and unique from everyone else.

NAME ______________________________

After you finish the physical description of yourself sitting under the tree, describe what you think you are thinking about. What are the most important things to that person under the tree?

____

____

____

____

____

____

What are the strong and admirable points of the person sitting under that tree?

____

____

____

____

How could your thoughts and beliefs about yourself make a difference in you life?

____

____

____

____

Henry Ford once said, "Whether you think you can or think you can't—you are right." Develop a positive view of yourself. Be kind to that person under the tree.

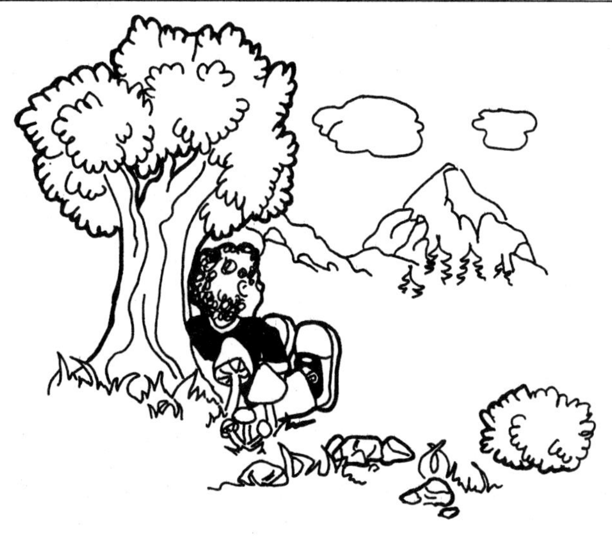

NAME ____________________

Getting to Know You

Answer the questions on the left side of the page. Hide your answers by folding the page, then exchange papers. Place your answers on the right side of their paper and compare answers.

1. What animal are you most like? ____________	1. What animal are you most like? ____________
Why? ____________	Why? ____________
____________	____________
2. What type of food would you like to be? ____________	2. What type of food would you like to be? ____________
Why? ____________	Why? ____________
____________	____________
3. What color represents your feelings? ____________	3. What color represents your feelings? ____________
Why? ____________	Why? ____________
____________	____________
4. What famous person would you most like to be? ____________	4. What famous person would you most like to be? ____________
Why? ____________	Why? ____________
____________	____________
5. What musical instrument would you like to be? ____________	5. What musical instrument would you like to be? ____________
Why? ____________	Why? ____________
____________	____________

NAME ______________________________

Make a list of five things you have in common with your partner. You may use information not found in the answers to the questions.

1.

2.

3.

4.

5.

Make a list of five things that are very different between you. You may use information not found in the answers to the questions.

1.

2.

3.

4.

5.

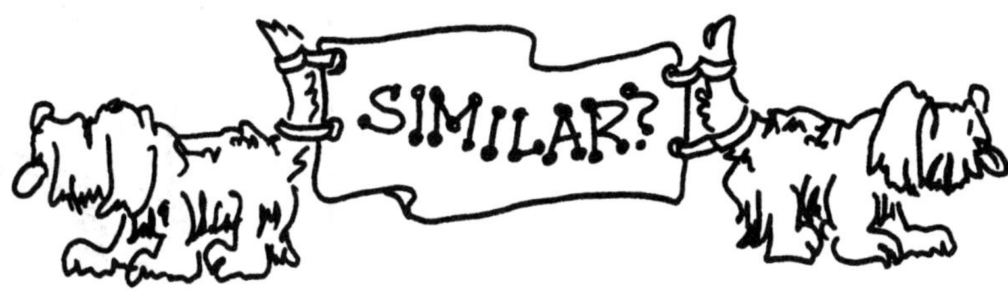

NAME ______________________________

Most Wanted

Picture a person who could be your imaginary best friend. Write a detailed description of what you would choose that person to be like. Draw a picture of that person and you, together.

My best friend would be

This is a picture of me with my best friend.

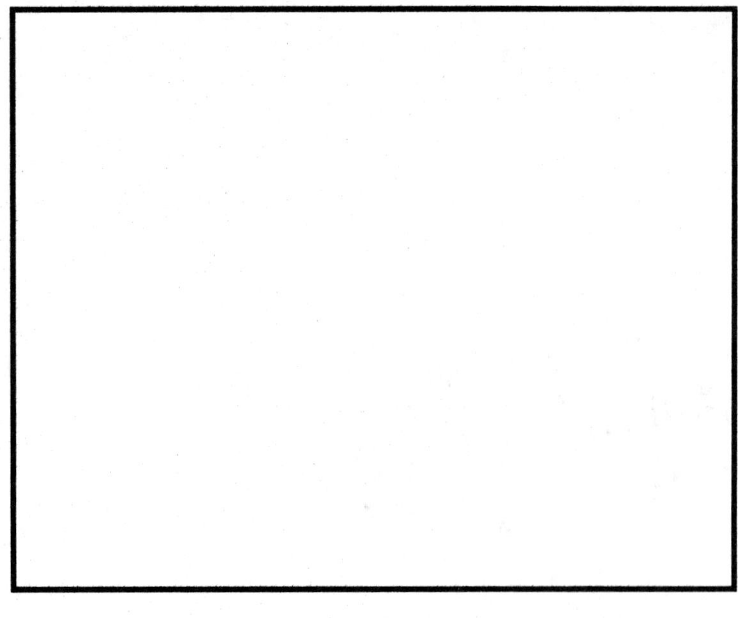

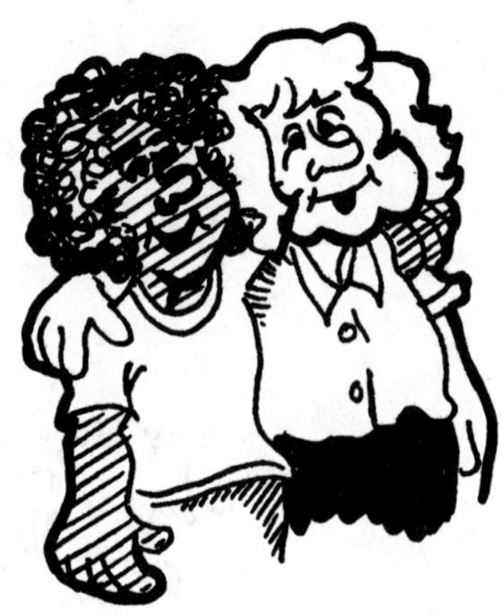

NAME ______________________

Pretend that you are going to advertise in the newspaper to find this friend and you have a limited amount of space for the advertisement. Limit yourself to 25 words or less and write that ad.

____

____

____

____

____

Do you know anybody who might fit that description? Can you meet that person if you don't already know them?

Make a list of some of the things you could say or do to start a conversation with that person. You could give them a compliment, ask about their class schedule and teachers they like or don't like, inquire about sports they might be interested in, or people you both know. Then start a conversation.

Write what you would say to begin this friendship.

____

____

____

____

____

____

____

____

____

____

____

____

____

NAME ______________________________

Circle of Support

Place your name under the person in the center of the circle. Place the names of the people who are important in your life under the people around the circle.

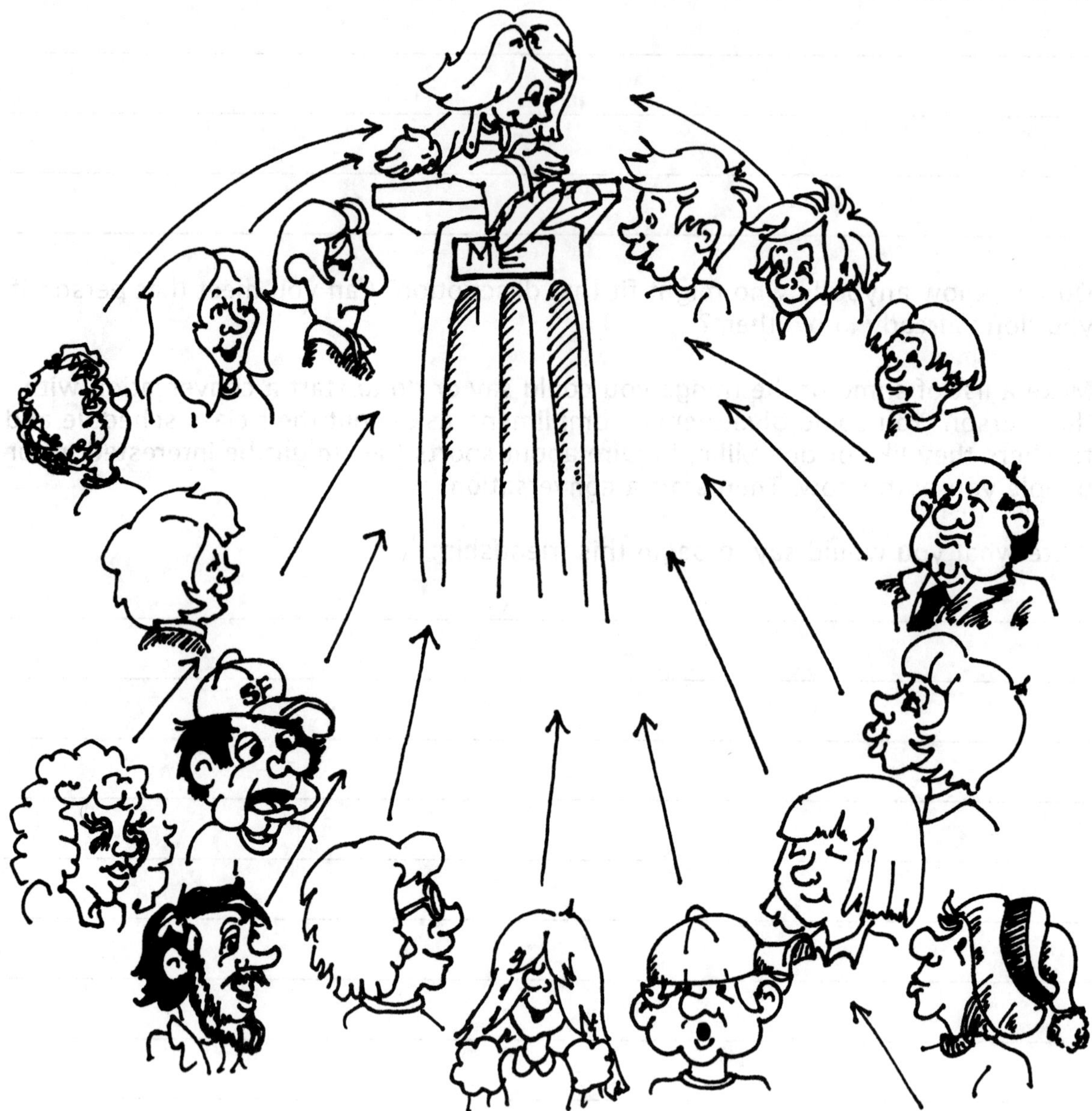

Who are the people who influence you the most in your circle of support?

____

____

____

NAME ______________________

How do your friends influence your decisions? ______________________

____

____

Who are the people you can rely on the most for help in making healthy decisions?

____

____

Who relies on you for support and guidance? ______________________

____

____

How do you influence the people around you? How does your behavior affect the people closest to you? ______________________

____

____

One of the important steps in making decisions is to think about how you are influenced. It is also important to realize how your decisions affect people who are important to you. The next time you make a decision, stop to think about who is influencing you and how your choices will affect others around you.

NAME ____________________

Friends

Write the name of a good or best friend in the center circle. Write down words that come to mind when you think about this person.

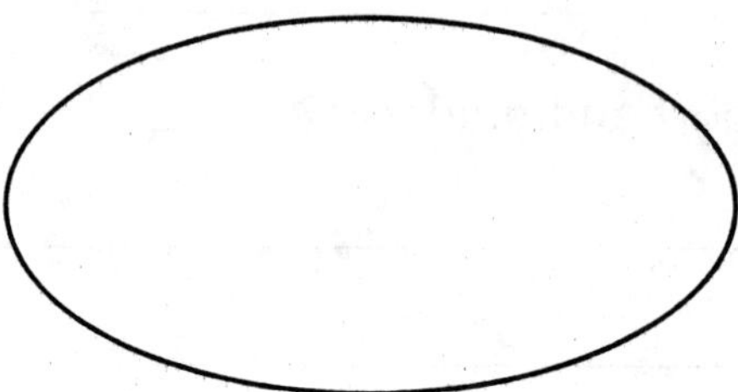

Place your name in the center of the circle below. Write down words that you believe other people think of when they think about you.

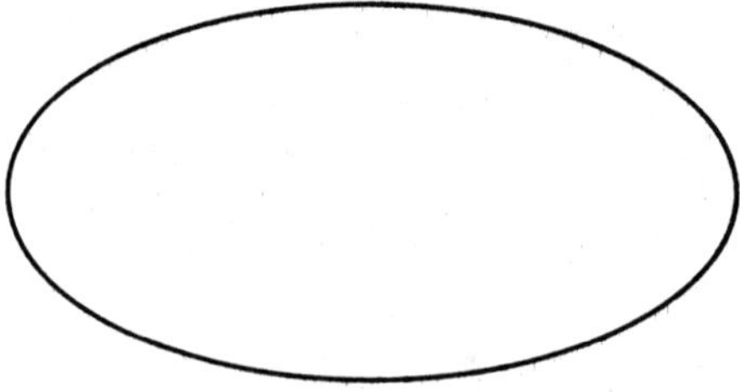

NAME ________________________________

Talk to a Parent or Grandparent

____

Name of person

1. What activity do you like to do most with a friend?

2. Do you have a friend that you have had for a long time?

   Why do you think you have stayed friends so long?

3. What do you like most about your friend?

4. Are your friends today . . .

   more important now?

   less important now?

   just as important today as when you were younger?

5. Do your friends influence your decisions?

   If they do, give some examples.

NAME ______________________________

Friendships versus Values

Place a check mark in the box that indicates how you would react to a friend asking a favor. Indicate how this might create a conflict.

YES	NO	MAYBE	
			Lend him or her $50 Conflict: ______________________________
			Lie to cover for him or her Conflict: ______________________________
			Loan him or her your new sweater Conflict ______________________________
			Ditch school with him or her Conflict: ______________________________
			Help him or her with homework Conflict: ______________________________
			Cheat for him or her on a test Conflict: ______________________________
			Settle a fight with his or her date Conflict: ______________________________
			Talk his or her parents into a trip with you Conflict: ______________________________
			Compliment him or her on a really bad haircut Conflict: ______________________________
			Visit him or her every day in the hospital Conflict: ______________________________

NAME ______________________________

YES	NO	MAYBE	
			Talk to him or her every night on the phone Conflict: ______________________________
			Hang around with only him or her at school Conflict: ______________________________
			Go to a dance with him or her Conflict: ______________________________
			Shoplift because he or she is doing it Conflict: ______________________________
			Take drugs with him or her Conflict: ______________________________
			Get cigarettes for him or her Conflict: ______________________________
			Set up a date for him or her Conflict: ______________________________
			Stop a fight he or she is in Conflict: ______________________________
			Get up at 4:00 a.m. to go fishing Conflict: ______________________________
			Invite him or her on your family vacation Conflict: ______________________________

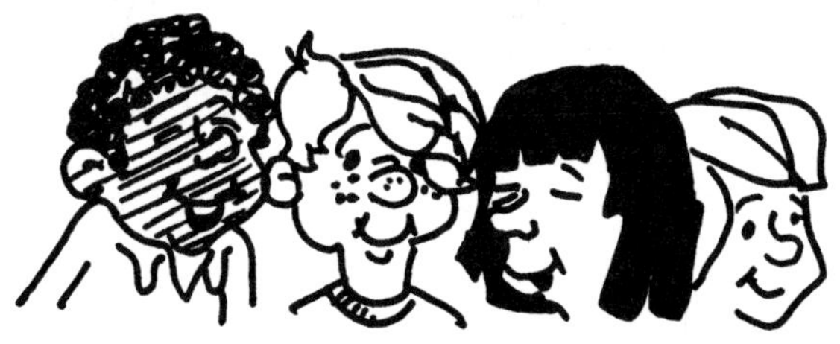

NAME ___________________________

Peer Pressures

GOOD

BAD

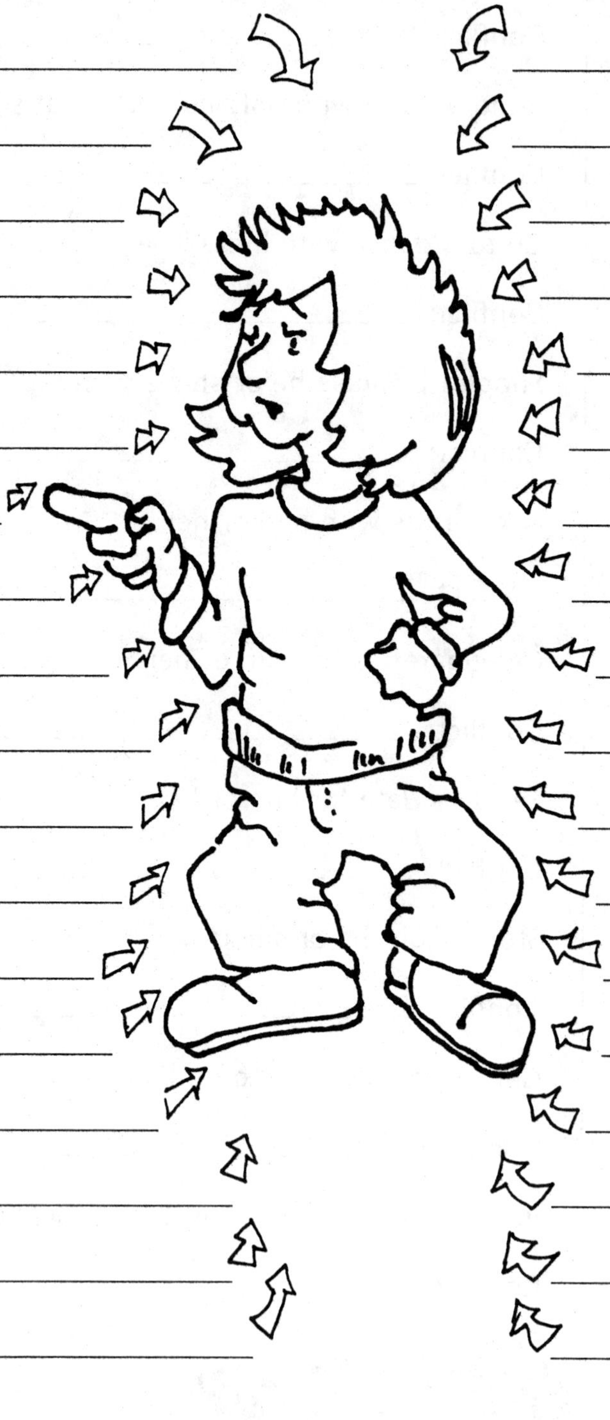

NAME ______________________________

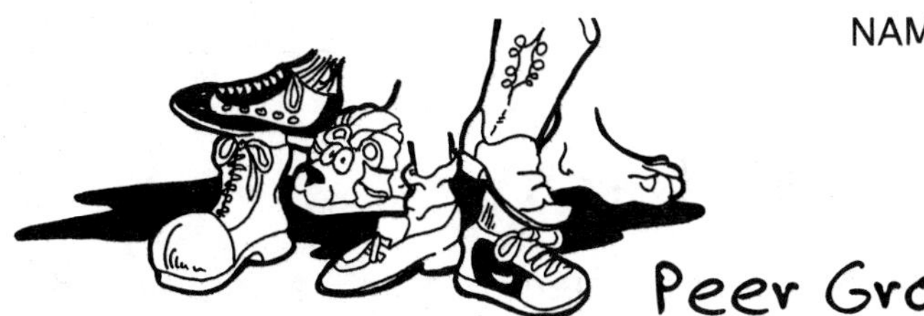

Peer Groups

Look around your school at various groups of teenagers. All these groups impose standards and pressures on the people in the group. Answer the following questions about one of the groups you observe.

1. The name of the peer group that I observed is ______________________________
2. What do most people think about the members of this peer group? ______________________________
3. What seems to be really important to the people in that group? ______________________________
4. Where do the members of this group hang out? ______________________________
5. What risks do these people take? ______________________________
6. How do people dress if they are a part of this group? ______________________________
7. What would you have to do to join this group? ______________________________
8. What type of behavior is *not* allowed in this group? ______________________________
9. How does the group influence each member? ______________________________
10. What do members gain from being in this group? ______________________________
11. What contributions does this group make to the whole society? ______________________________
12. What pressures are put on members because of their membership in the group? ______________________________

NAME ____________________

My Role Model

To some extent, we all pattern our behavior after different people we admire and respect. Think of a person you use as a role model while answering the questions below.

1. What do you admire and respect about this person?

____

____

2. Why did you pick this person as a role model?

____

____

3. What special skills does this person have?

____

____

4. What do you think is important to this individual?

____

____

5. How are you like this person?

____

____

6. In what ways would you like to be more like this person?

____

____

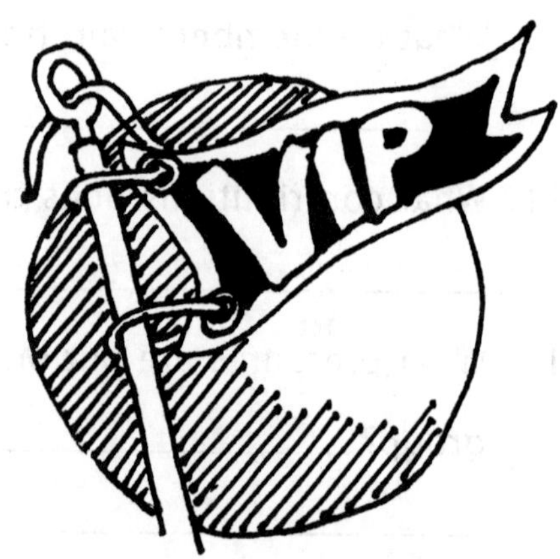

NAME ______________________

Boaster Poster

Make a collage illustrating the things you admire about a person you have chosen for a role model. Use magazine pictures, newspaper words, photographs, or your own drawings to make your collage.

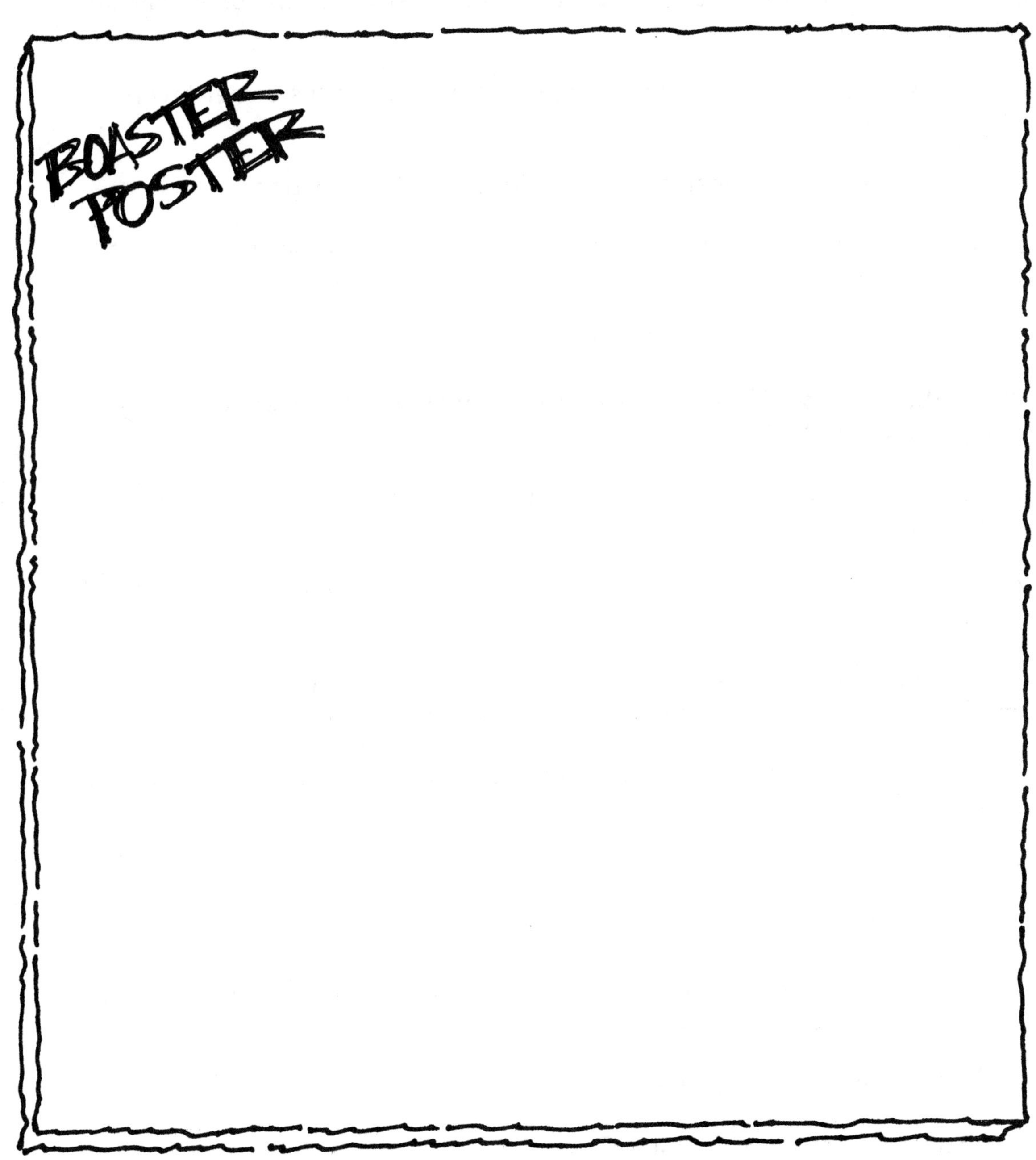

NAME ____________________

Questions for Teens

It is often difficult to take time out of our busy lives to communicate with those people we care about most. Please take the time to sit down and get to know this young person better. First, see how many questions you can answer about them without help; then talk about the questions and answers to the ones you cannot answer.

1. What kind of music does this teenager enjoy? Who is his or her favorite musical group?
2. Who would this teenager have voted for in the last election?
3. What type of food is his or her favorite? What is his or her favorite fast food restauraut?
4. Who is this teenager's best friend?
5. Are there any people who pick on this teen at school? What is his or her opinion about bullies?
6. List three subjects this teenager is taking at school. What are his or her grades in these subjects?
7. What is his or her favorite class? Who is his or her favorite teacher? Which teacher is really annoying?
8. How much has this teenager grown this year? What is the style of his or her clothing? Where does he or she shop most for clothes?
9. What subject would be easiest for this teenager to talk about? Which is most difficult?
10. What are the two biggest problems this teenager has?
11. Who was this teen's last crush?
12. What is his or her favorite book or movie? How much does this teen read? Does he or she like to read?
13. What was his or her proudest moment?
14. What is this teen most afraid of?
15. What makes this teenager really happy?

Questionnaire from *Instructional Patterns: Curriculum for Parenthood Education*, "Exchange of Information and Feelings by Parents and Teenagers," pp. 131–133, the California State Department of Education.

NAME ______________________

16. What is this teen's greatest strength?

17. What would this teen most like to do for a whole day?

18. Where would this teen like to travel if money was no object?

19. What would this teenager like to achieve in life?

20. What are this teen's long-term goals?

What comments or questions would you like to add?

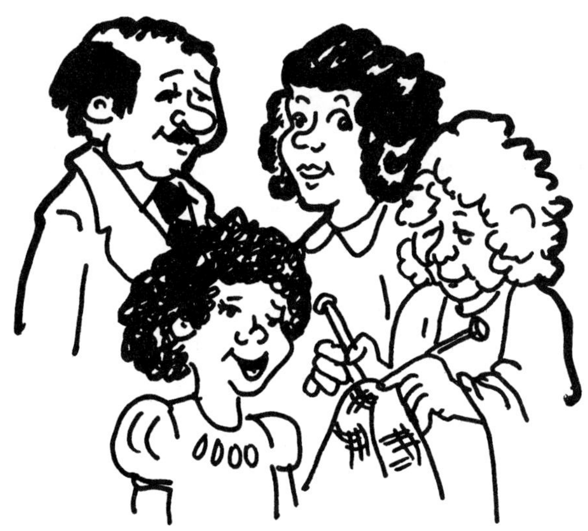

NAME ____________________

Questions from Teens

It is often difficult to take time out of our busy lives to communicate with those people we care about most. Please take the time to sit down and get to know this person better. First, see how many questions you can answer about them without help; then talk about the questions and answers to the ones you cannot answer. This information is for you only and will not be turned in at school.

1. Name this person's favorite movie or movie star.
2. If this person is married, how did he or she meet their partner? Was it a long or short engagement?
3. Relate one of this person's favorite memories about his or her childhood. Relate one he or she has about your childhood.
4. What type of food does he or she like most? What is his or her favorite fast food restaurant?
5. How does this person feel about politics? Is he or she active in community affairs? Is he or she members of the PTA?
6. What is this person's biggest worry? How does he or she deal with it?
7. Who does this person admire and respect?
8. Is this person good in sports? Art? Music?
9. What type of music does he or she enjoy? Which musical group does he or she listen to most?
10. What types of problems take most of his or her time?
11. What was this person's room like as a teenager?
12. What was the one thing his or her parents always told him or her?
13. How much is the gas or electric bill each month?
14. What is his or her hardest job as an adult?
15. What was his or her greatest dream as a teenager?

Questionnaire from *Instructional Patterns: Curriculum for Parenthood Education*, "Exchange of Information and Feelings by Parents and Teenagers," pp. 131–133, the California State Department of Education.

NAME ____________________

16. What were his or her goals when he or she was young? Has he or she reached them? Have the goals changed? Why?

17. How would this person spend a pleasant evening?

18. What would this person want most for a gift?

19. How did his or her parents discipline them?

20. What does he or she wish most for you?

What comments or questions would you like to add?

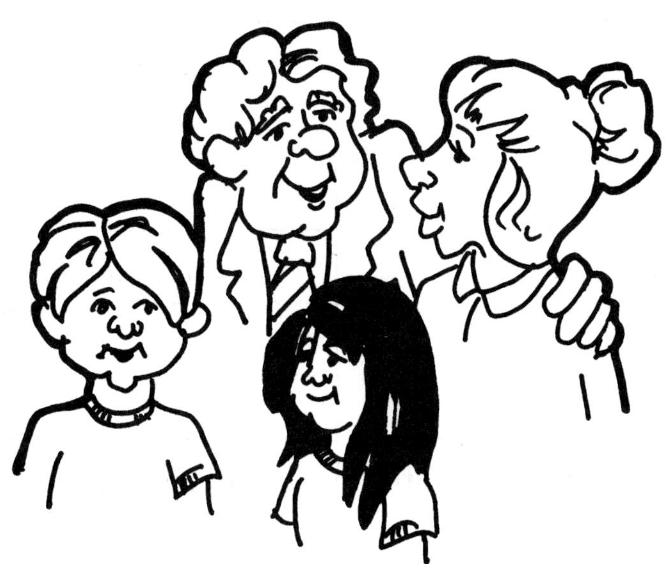

NAME ____________________

What Friends Think

Fold this paper down the center. Ask someone who really cares about you to answer the questions on the left side of the page. Without looking at his or her answers, answer the questions on the right side of the page. Compare the answers.

Please be thoughtful and sincere in answering the following questions about this adolescent.	This side is for your answers. Be honest in answering.
Write three positive words to describe this young person:	Write three positive words to describe yourself:
What do you consider to be this person's strengths?	What do you consider to be your strengths?
What is this person's greatest ability or talent?	What is your greatest ability or talent?
What will you always remember fondly about this person?	What do you think people remember most about you?
When do you like this person most?	When are you most likable?
What has been this person' greatest accomplishment?	What has been your greatest accomplishment?

NAME ____________________

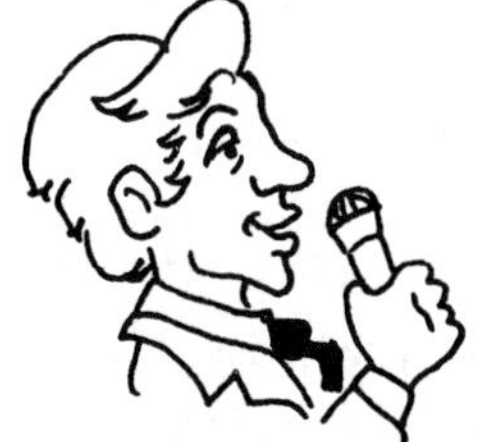

Age 30

Answer the following questions, keeping in mind the way you would like to live at age 30.

1. What type of job or career will you have? ____________________

____

2. List several skills you will need for this job. ____________________

____

____

3. List the skills you have now that will help in this line of work.

____

____

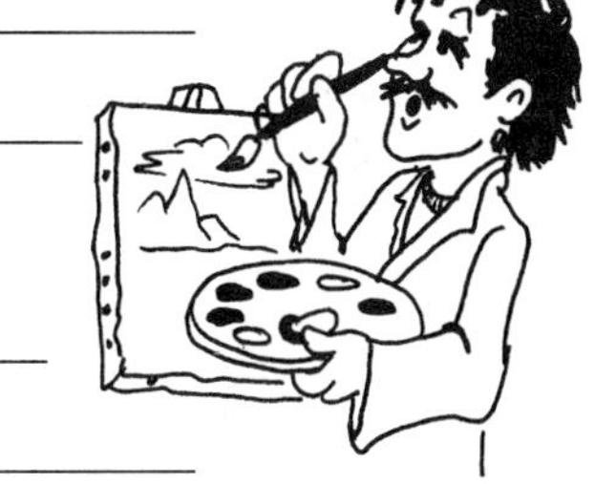

4. What subjects in school will help you in this line of work?

____

____

5. List some of the things you like about this job. ____________________

____

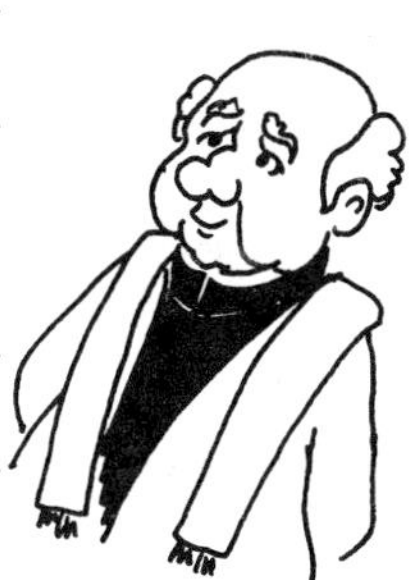

6. What would an employer look for when hiring someone for this job? ____________________

____

7. What steps do you need to take to achieve this career?

   Education: ____________________

   Physical or personal skills: ____________________

   Number of years working toward this job: ____________________

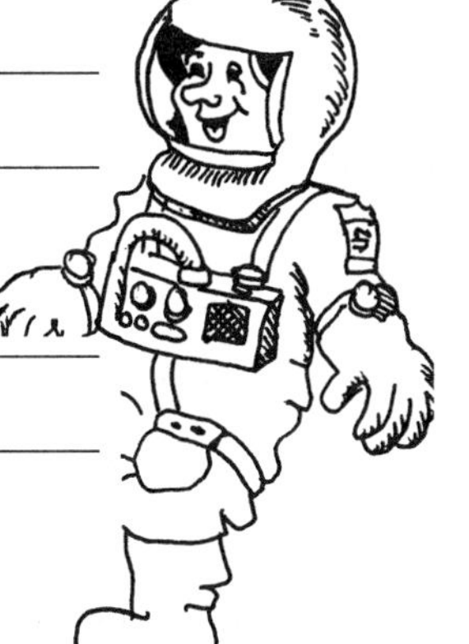

8. What could you be doing now to prepare yourself for your chosen line of work? ____________________

____

Carol Bershad and Nancy DiMella, *The Changer and the Changed* (Santa Cruz: Network Publications, 1983), p. 40.

NAME ______________________

A Typical Day

Diagram a typical day in your life. Include items such as school, sleep, chores at home, sports, clubs, meals, television, social activities, and personal activities.

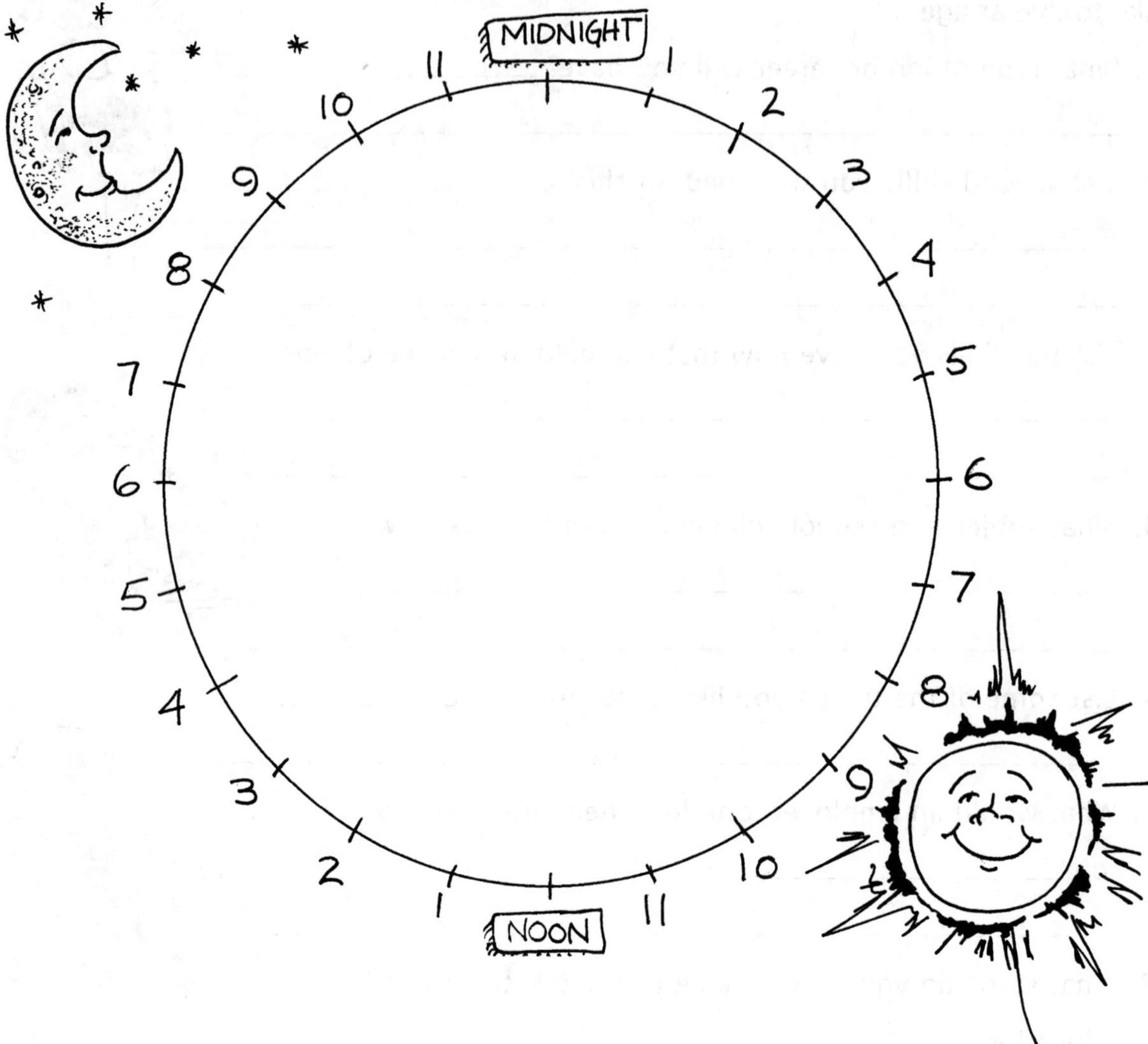

Answer the following questions:

1. What surprised you after seeing how you spend your time?

2. How could you use your time more wisely?

NAME ____________________

Be Specific

Guidelines for goals:

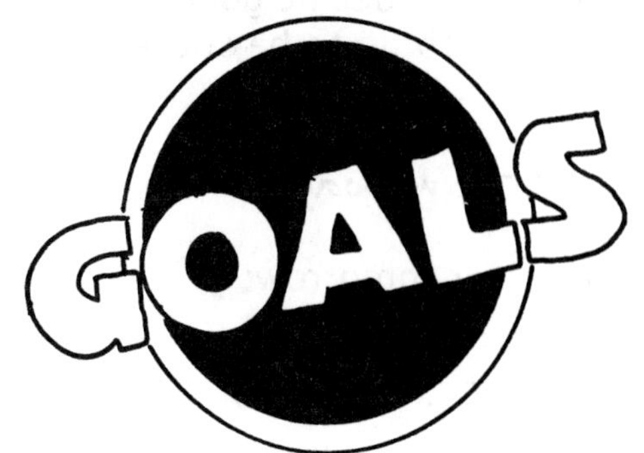

- understand yourself
- be specific in what you need to accomplish
- be positive
- be realistic
- be able to have control over the outcome
- the goal should challenge you

Rewrite the goals written below to make them more specific, clear, and manageable. Refer to the guidelines for writing goals.

1. I want to get "straight A's" in school this year.

2. I don't want to gain any more weight this year.

3. I am not going to fight with my little brother.

4. I want to be a professional basketball player.

5. I want to go to college.

6. I want better clothes.

7. I am going to be physically fit.

8. I will be good in school.

NAME ______________________________

My Goals

Write clear, specific goals for the time periods presented below. Indicate what you will have to do to be successful in achieving that goal.

Short-Term Goal

A goal for tomorrow: ______________________________

____

Actions I will have to take: ______________________________

____

Midrange Goal

A goal I will accomplish by next week: ______________________________

____

Actions I will have to take: ______________________________

____

A goal I will accomplish by next year: ______________________________

____

Actions I will have to take: ______________________________

____

Long-Term Goal

A goal I will accomplish when I graduate from high school: ______________________________

____

Actions I will have to take: ______________________________

____

NAME ____________________

Solutions to Problems

Read the situations and set a goal. Determine the problem to be overcome, and present a solution to the problem.

You tried out for the basketball team and are chosen. You realize that practice will be held at the same time you are being tutored to improve a poor math grade. You need to keep your grades up in order to stay on the basketball team, but your tutor can only work with you at the time scheduled.

Goal: ____________________

____

Problem: ____________________

____

Solution: ____________________

____

You have always been the class clown. You have found that the best way to get friends and to be admired is by making people laugh. You have been getting in a lot of trouble lately for your behavior in class and your grades are dropping. You are in danger of failing.

Goal: ____________________

____

Problem: ____________________

____

Solution: ____________________

____

NAME ____________________

Alternative Solutions

Read the situations and set a goal. Determine the problem to be overcome and create three solutions to the problem. State the advantages and disadvantages of each solution.

Jimmy has to give up playing on the school football team and go home right after school to take care of his two younger brothers. His mother died a year ago and his father just got a new job that requires longer hours away from home. Jimmy's grades are dropping and he feels the pressure of the responsibility placed on him. He misses hanging out with his friends.

Goal: ____________________

____

Problem: ____________________

____

Suggestions for solutions: ____________________

____

1. ____________________

   Advantages: ____________________

   Disadvantages: ____________________

2. ____________________

   Advantages: ____________________

   Disadvantages: ____________________

3. ____________________

   Advantages: ____________________

   Disadvantages: ____________________

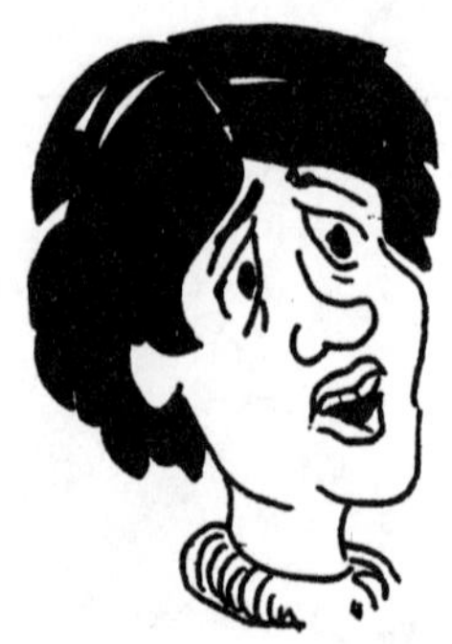

NAME ______________________________

Celia wants to go to Stanford University when she graduates from high school. She realizes that the admissions requirements are high and that many students with terrific grades apply and are not accepted. Celia wants to keep her grades up but realizes she will need to do more to stand out and be accepted by Stanford. She is worried that if she joins the band, plays in sports, holds a student government office, and tutors students in math she may become exhausted by trying too many things.

Goal: ______________________________

____

Problem: ______________________________

____

Suggestions for solutions: ______________________________

____

1. ______________________________

   Advantages: ______________________________

   Disadvantages: ______________________________

2. ______________________________

   Advantages: ______________________________

   Disadvantages: ______________________________

3. ______________________________

   Advantages: ______________________________

   Disadvantages: ______________________________

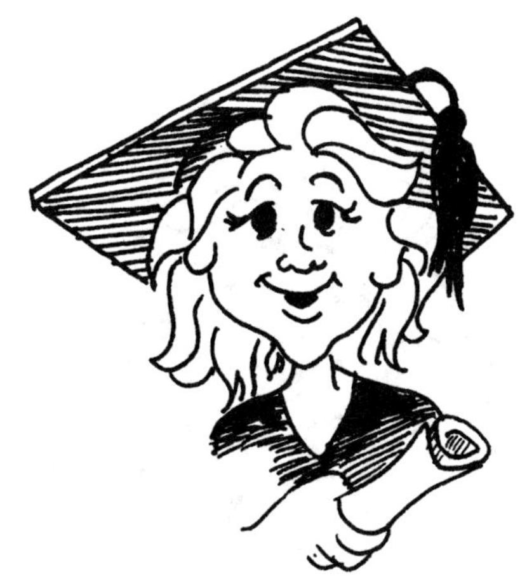

NAME ___________________________

Sadie is popular in school and has many friends. Her life has not been easy, however. Her father took off when Sadie was two years old and her mother struggles to keep the family surviving. Sadie takes pride in the fact that her mother is honest and hardworking, even though they do not have many things. Sadie has been voted Prom Queen by her class and does not have the money to get a new dress. The prom is two weeks away.

Goal: ___________________________

____

Problem: ___________________________

____

Suggestions for solutions: ___________________________

____

1. ___________________________

Advantages: ___________________________

Disadvantages: ___________________________

2. ___________________________

Advantages: ___________________________

Disadvantages: ___________________________

3. ___________________________

Advantages: ___________________________

Disadvantages: ___________________________

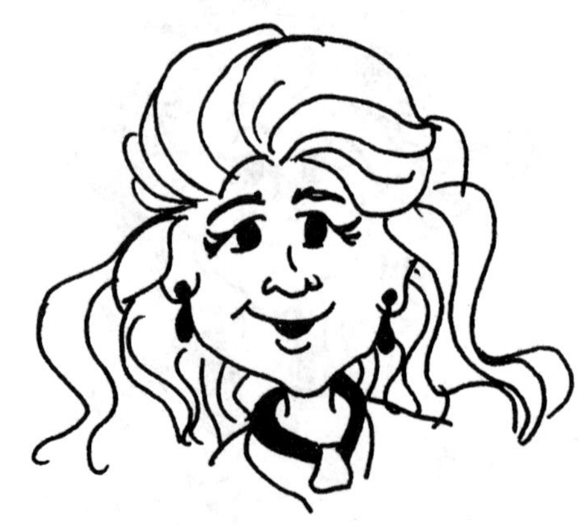

NAME ____________________

Long-Term Goals

Write one goal you would like to achieve in your lifetime:

____

____

List some of the obstacles that might prevent you from reaching this goal:

____

____

____

List three alternative suggestions to overcoming the obstacles:

① ____

② ____

③ ____

List any specific training, education, or skills you will need to reach your goal:

____

____

____

____

____

What resources do you already have at your disposal to achieve your goal?

____

____

____

____

NAME ______________________

Taking Risks

Think of risky situations similar to risks you have faced. Think of the worst thing that could happen in taking that risk. Think of the best thing that could happen in taking that risk. Then decide the best way to proceed in attempting the risky endeavor.

1. A risky situation: ______________________

   ____

   ____

   What is the worst thing that might happen?

   ____

   What is the best thing that might happen?

   ____

   This is how I would reduce the risk and achieve success: ______________________

   ____

   ____

   ____

2. A risky situation: ______________________

   ____

   ____

   What is the worst thing that might happen?

   ____

   What is the best thing that might happen?

   ____

   This is how I would reduce the risk and achieve success: ______________________

   ____

   ____

   ____

NAME ______________________________

3. A risky situation: ______________________________

____

____

What is the worst thing that might happen?

____

What is the best thing that might happen?

____

This is how I would reduce the risk and achieve success: ______________________________

____

____

____

4. A risky situation: ______________________________

____

____

What is the worst thing that might happen?

____

What is the best thing that might happen?

____

This is how I would reduce the risk and achieve success: ______________________________

____

____

____

NAME ____________________

S.T.A.R. Decisions

S -

T -

A -

R -

Problem: ____________________

Positive	Negative	Interesting

Solution: ____________________

Adapted with permission from *Prevention Skills for Youth,* ETR Associates Training Department. Santa Cruz, CA, 1987–1998.

NAME ____________________

What Would You Do?

Use the S.T.A.R. method of making decisions and solve the problems presented below. Work as a group in brainstorming ideas. Record all your ideas for each of the steps.

Situation 1:

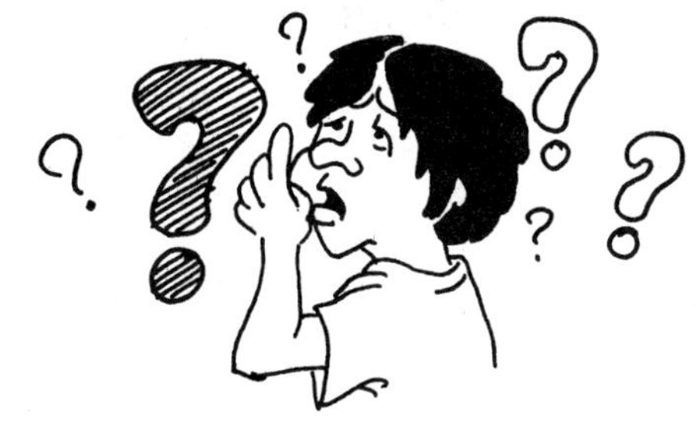

Lately there have been rumors around the school that the dress code will be changing. Many adults think that what people wear is reflected by their behavior. You and four other leaders from the student body have been called to the principal's office and told to decide whether the dress code should be changed and students required to wear uniforms.

STOP and identify the problem: ____________________

____

THINK:

Positive	Negative	Interesting

ACT (Your decision): ____________________

____

RE-ACT (Your method of evaluating your decision): ____________________

____

NAME ______________________

Situation 2:

Your parents are angry about the amount of time you spend on the telephone. They complain that none of their important calls can get through. They are considering limiting your time on the phone to fifteen minutes a day. They have asked you for your opinion.

STOP and identify the problem: ______________________

____

THINK:

Positive	Negative	Interesting

ACT (Your decision): ______________________

____

RE-ACT (Your method of evaluating your decision): ______________________

____

NAME ______________________

My Choices Have Consequences

Listed below are several situations. Think of three possible solutions for each of the situations. List at least three consequences for each of the solutions you present. Remember that consequences can be good and bad.

1. Your parents have dropped you off at the arcade for an hour while they go shopping. You meet some of your friends and they want to go to get something to eat but you will have to leave the arcade and walk about 1 mile. Your parents told you to stay at the arcade. What do you do?

______________________ ➔ ______________________
____
____

______________________ ➔ ______________________
____
____

______________________ ➔ ______________________
____
____

2. Your best friend is hooked on drugs. He cannot stop and is running out of money. He does not want to get help because he is afraid his parents will find out. What do you do?

______________________ ➔ ______________________
____
____

______________________ ➔ ______________________
____
____

______________________ ➔ ______________________
____
____

NAME ____________________

3. You and your boyfriend or girlfriend are at the movies. The movie was getting boring so your friend suggested that you go over to his or her house and "have a little fun." What do you do?

4. A person you are very good friends with and have known all your life asks you out. You do not know if you should date him or her because it might change your relationship and ruin your friendship. What do you do?

5. Your parents have gotten tickets for the whole family to go to a play and want you to attend with them, but your friends ask you to go with them to a party on the same night. You really want to go with your friends but your parents have tried hard to get these tickets and want this to be a family night. What do you do?

NAME ______________________

6. You are playing basketball during lunch at school. A very tough guy and his friends take the ball away and start harassing you. What do you do?

______________________ ➡ ______________________

____

____

______________________ ➡ ______________________

____

____

______________________ ➡ ______________________

____

____

7. You and a couple of friends are hanging out at the mall. To create some excitement, one of your friends suggests going into a store and shoplifting. What do you do?

______________________ ➡ ______________________

____

____

______________________ ➡ ______________________

____

____

______________________ ➡ ______________________

____

____

8. Your father and you argue all the time about almost everything. You are tired of all the fighting and want it to stop. What can you do?

______________________ ➡ ______________________

____

____

______________________ ➡ ______________________

____

____

______________________ ➡ ______________________

____

____

NAME ______________________________

Lifeboat

There are 100 people aboard a ship sailing around the world. They are having a lot of fun together and have become great friends. One night, they are singing and dancing during a party. Suddenly, a huge explosion occurs. The glass shatters, water pours in, and the people panic. Many people are killed in the initial explosion. Some people jump from the ship to save themselves from the fire that is spreading rapidly. People in the water are dying from the freezing temperatures. Those who survived the blast are running to the one lifeboat that is still intact. It has water, food, life jackets, and blankets for five people and no more. There are eight people at the boat who want to be saved. They know that only five of them can go into the lifeboat. Each one tells why he or she should be allowed to survive. It is up to you to decide who will board the lifeboat and who will be left behind to drown.

___ 1. *Mary, a small Hispanic woman.* "I am a few years older than the rest of the group and I am a teacher. People trust me and feel that I can take control of a situation and calm others. I have already calmed the people waiting at the lifeboat and have stopped them from fighting. Even though no one seems close to me and I am not very friendly, I feel I would be a valuable person because I can organize well and solve problems."

___ 2. *Hazel, a large black woman and a student in home economics.* "I know a lot about food and nutrition. I can ration food without waste. I am efficient to the point of being bossy."

___ 3. *Joe, a clean-cut, husky football player and star center of the basketball team.* "I am the only one strong enough to row and lift people, if necessary. I can physically stop fights between people because of my size and strength. I have already been scolded by Hazel for stealing a candy bar from the limited food supply."

___ 4. *Nancy, Bill's beautiful, blonde wife.* "I am a housewife and really nervous and upset by the explosion and the panic. I rely on Bill for everything. I am very scared because I am pregnant and expecting a baby in two months."

___ 5. *Bill, Nancy's husband.* "I am a Native American medical student nearing the end of my education. I have had experience in first aid and have worked during the summer as a medical director at a camp. I will not be saved unless Nancy is saved also. I have medical supplies with me. They include drugs like barbiturates, amphetamines, and marijuana—which I smoke regularly."

NAME ____________________

___ 6. *Don, an Asian businessman, a happy, playful person, very rich and very handsome.* "I can play the guitar and I have a great singing voice. I have a great sense of humor and know lots of jokes that will entertain us on the weary days ahead. I really want to be saved and will give each survivor $25,000 to let me get in the lifeboat."

___ 7. *Sam, a sailor and an angry bully who resents the guests on the ship.* "I know all there is to know about sailing on the ocean and I can repair anything on the lifeboat. I have practical skills although I have no formal education. I want to be saved but I don't want to have to talk to any of the ship's passengers."

___ 8. *Angelica, a member of the crew who is working as a waitress to earn her passage to the United States from Mexico.* "I am the oldest of seven children and I am very bright. My parents are sending me to the United States to go to school. I am 18 years old and have gotten in some trouble at home for hanging around with gangs, but I promise that I will improve my behavior if I am saved."

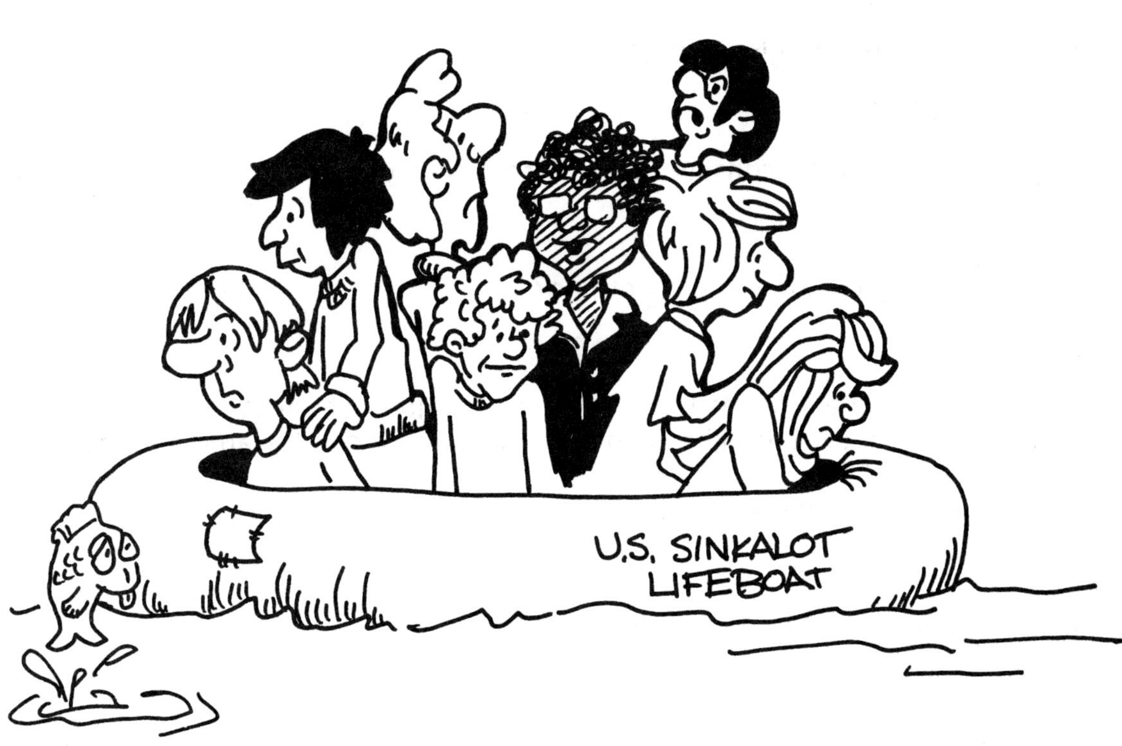

NAME ______________________________

Take My Advice

Practice making decisions by advising the people in each of the following situations. Use your experience in making decisions.

One of your best friends sits behind you in class and is not prepared for the test you are about to take. You are prepared and your friend wants you to allow them to cheat.

What advice can you give him or her?

What are some of the consequences of giving that advice?

What are some of the consequences of not helping him or her in any way?

Pattie's grades are falling and it is because she spends too much time on the telephone talking to her boyfriend.

What advice can you give Pattie?

What are some of the consequences of that advice?

What would happen if you did nothing?

Mike is a good friend and loves to read. He is also great at soccer. People at school want him to play soccer but Mike is shy and feels more comfortable reading.

What advice can you give Mike?

What are the consequences of that advice?

What would happen if you did nothing?

NAME ______________________

Angelica has been your friend since you were little kids. She is starting to wear heavy makeup and hang around a group of tough girls.

What advice can you give Angelica?

What are the consequences of that advice?

What would happen if you did nothing?

Your friend Tony is very smart and a good leader with many great ideas. Everyone wants him to run for class president at school, but Tony is shy and doesn't like to talk in front of groups of people.

What is your advice to Tony?

What are the consequences of your advice?

What would happen if you did nothing?

NAME ____________________

Commitment to Change

Using the steps for change discussed in class, identify a behavior that you would like to change and develop a plan to modify that behavior.

The behavior I want to change: ____________________

The behavior I would like instead—my "goal" behavior:

____

Obstacles that I may have to overcome: ____________________

____

____

____

Advice and information on changing the behavior: ____________________

____

____

____

____

Plan of action: ____________________

____

____

____

I will know I am successful when: ____________________

____

My reward for success will be: ____________________

NAME ____________________

This Is the Way I See It . . .

What would you think and feel in the following situations? Try to imagine the feelings of each of the people involved in the following situations. Describe how you think each person thinks and feels from their participation in the same incident.

You are waiting for tickets to a big game and the game sells out just before your turn to buy a ticket.

Viewpoint	Thought	Feeling
1. You		
2. Ticket sales person		
3 Owner of the stadium		
4. Player		

You are at school and a student pulls the fire alarm without reason.

Viewpoint	Thought	Feeling
1. Student in class		
2. Teacher		
3. Firefighter		
4. Janitor at the school		

NAME ______________________

A teen idol commits a serious crime.

Viewpoint	Thought	Feeling
1. The teen idol		
2. Teenagers		
3. Parents		
4. News reporters		

You see a person smoking in a public place designated "no smoking."

Viewpoint	Thought	Feeling
1. Person smoking		
2. Parent with new baby		
3. Tobacco company		
4. Person with lung cancer		

NAME ________________________

A teacher makes the whole class stay late into the lunch break because five students have been talking out of turn.

Viewpoint	Thought	Feeling
1. You		
2. The teacher		
3. Misbehaving students		
4. Cafeteria help		

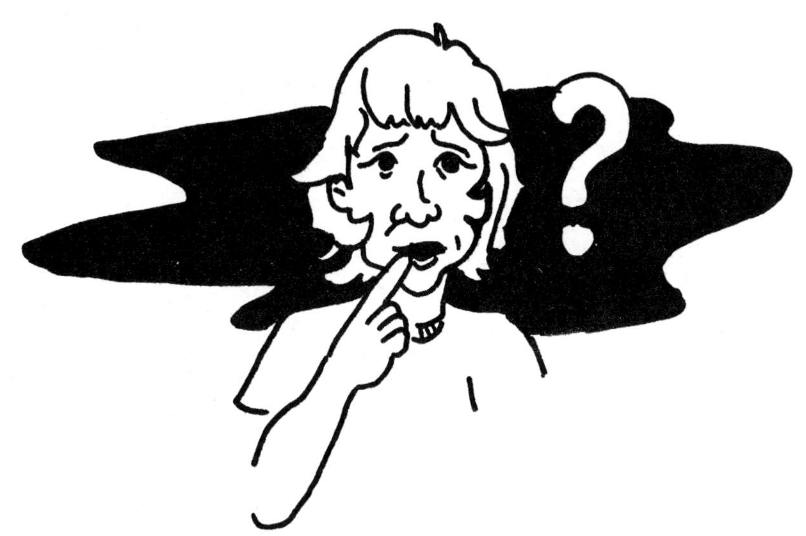

NAME ________________________________

Making Mistakes

Write down a negative thought you find yourself using a lot. Indicate the message that thought sends you. Choose a positive thought that you could use to replace the negative one.

Situation	Negative Thought	Message	Positive Thought
Bad hair day	"I really look ugly today."	"I don't look good enough to be around people."	"This is my chance to try a new hairstyle."

From Management Sciences for Health, Inc.

NAME ____________________

Identifying Stress

Read each event below. If that situation occurred in your life in the last 12 months, circle the number. When you have completed the list, add up the circled numbers.

EVENT	POINTS
Death of a parent or guardian	10
Caught using drugs	9
Going to detention at youth center/reform school/jail	9
Getting beaten by parents	9
Getting pregnant/becoming a father	9
Death of a close family member	9
Having a major illness/injury/car accident	8
Not getting promoted to the next grade	8
Getting attacked/raped/beaten	8
Parents getting a divorce or separation	8
Death of a close friend	8
Death of a pet	8
Getting a sexually transmitted disease	8
Starting to use drugs or alcohol	8
Fighting with parents	7
Caught cheating or lying repeatedly	7
Getting expelled or suspended from school	7
Going into serious debt	7
Being stereotyped by having bad rumors spread about you	7

NAME ______________________________

Moving to a different town/school and having to make new friends	7
Getting married	7
Pressure to take drugs or alcohol	7
Graduation	6
Getting pressure about having sex	6
Becoming religious or giving up religion	6
Suddenly having trouble getting a date	6
Developing problems with teachers or employers	6
Making career decisions (college/vocational)	6
Getting a traffic ticket or minor problems with the law	6
Breaking up with a boyfriend/girlfriend	6
Starting to perform (speeches/musical/drama)	6
Getting fired from a job	6
Taking finals or college entrance tests	6
Taking a driver's license test	6
Moving out of the house	6
Getting a bad haircut	6
Getting a bad report card	6
Being sent to the principal's office	5
Getting acne/warts	5
Starting to date	5
Arguing with peers/brothers/sisters	5
Trying to get a job or an interview	5

NAME ____________________

Getting an addition to the family	5
Getting braces	5
Losing or gaining weight	5
Getting glasses	5
Starting school	4
Starting to go to weekend concerts or parties	4
Being pressured to follow fads	4
Getting a car	4
Getting an award, honor, or office	4
Making a team (drill/athletic/debate)	4
Going to the dentist or doctor	4
Going on a diet	4
Getting a minor illness (cold/flu)	3
Changing exercise habits	2
Taking a test to identify stress levels	1

Total Points ____________

Compare your total points with the scale below.

0–40	No significant problem stress level
41–95	Stress levels are building
96–180	Moderate life crisis and feeling pressured
180–above	Severe pressure and going to blow!

The next question is—How can I get rid of the tension and stress in my life?

NAME ________________________________

Identify Your Feelings

Choose feelings from this list that best describe the way you would feel in the situations that follow the list. Write those feelings in the space provided.

Angry
Annoyed
Anxious
Bored
Brave
Calm
Cheerful
Confused
Cruel
Depressed
Disappointed
Disgusted
Disturbed
Embarrassed
Excited
Exhausted

Fearful
Foolish
Frightened
Frustrated
Free
Glad
Grumpy
Guilty
Happy
Hateful
Hurt
Jealous
Joyful
Kind
Lazy
Lonely

Lost
Mad
Mean
Naughty
Nervous
Overwhelmed
Panicked
Peaceful
Picked-on
Playful
Proud
Quiet
Rejected
Relaxed
Rested
Restless

Sad
Scared
Shocked
Shy
Silly
Sorrowful
Sorry
Special
Surprised
Tense
Thoughtful
Tired
Uncertain
Upset
Violent
Worried

Use the words listed above to explain how you feel in the following situations. Whatever you feel is okay. There is no *correct* feeling. You might be feeling several different emotions in one situation.

NAME ______________________________

Feelings | Situation

______________________ 1. Someone you care about says hello to you.

______________________ 2. You get an A on a difficult test in school.

______________________ 3. You help a friend mow the grass.

______________________ 4. You get punished for hitting your little brother.

______________________ 5. A popular person wants to copy your test in school.

______________________ 6. Your best friend wants to toilet paper your neighbor's house.

______________________ 7. Your date wants to go parking with you.

______________________ 8. Your parents are fighting.

______________________ 9. You have to choose between being with your friends and attending your father's birthday party.

______________________ 10. You get caught smoking cigarettes behind your house.

______________________ 11. You find $100 on the front seat of the school bus.

______________________ 12. Your older brother is drunk and wants you to help him not get caught.

______________________ 13. Someone breaks into your house.

______________________ 14. You help your grandmother clean her house.

______________________ 15. You find a baby bird that has fallen from its nest.

______________________ 16. You are held responsible for a fight that was not your fault.

______________________ 17. A popular girl or boy asks you to dance.

______________________ 18. You receive an award for getting good grades after working really hard during the semester.

______________________ 19. Your best friend moves to another state.

______________________ 20. Your mother brags about you on the phone to a relative.

NAME ______________________________

Reactions to Stress

People react in various ways to stressful situations. Circle the reactions you feel are healthy and are useful. Cross out the reactions you feel are detrimental or harmful.

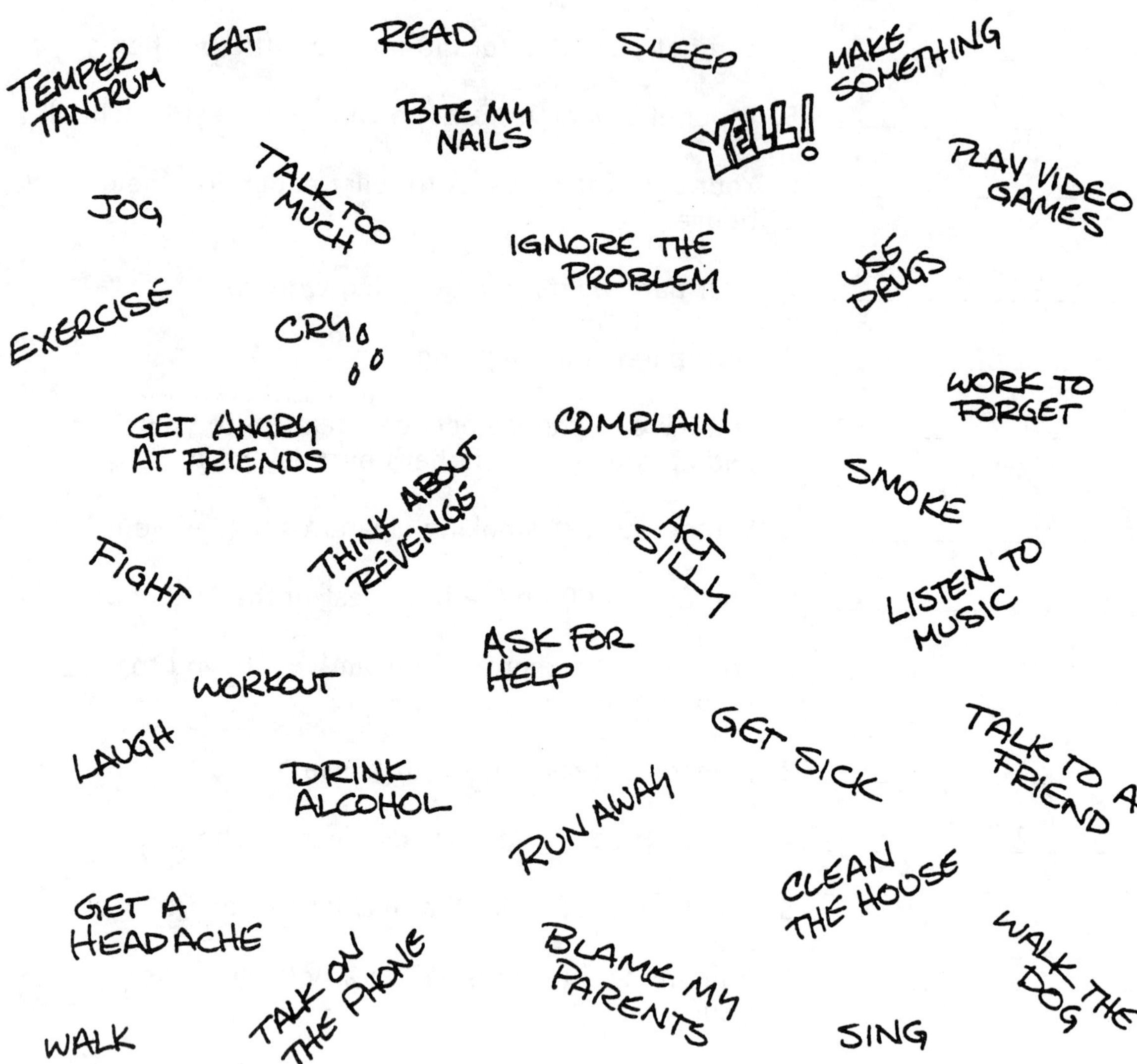

NAME ______________________

Stress Calendar

Keep a record of all the stressful situations you experience for a week. Briefly explain the stressful situation, the time it occurred, the people involved and your feeling caused by the stress.

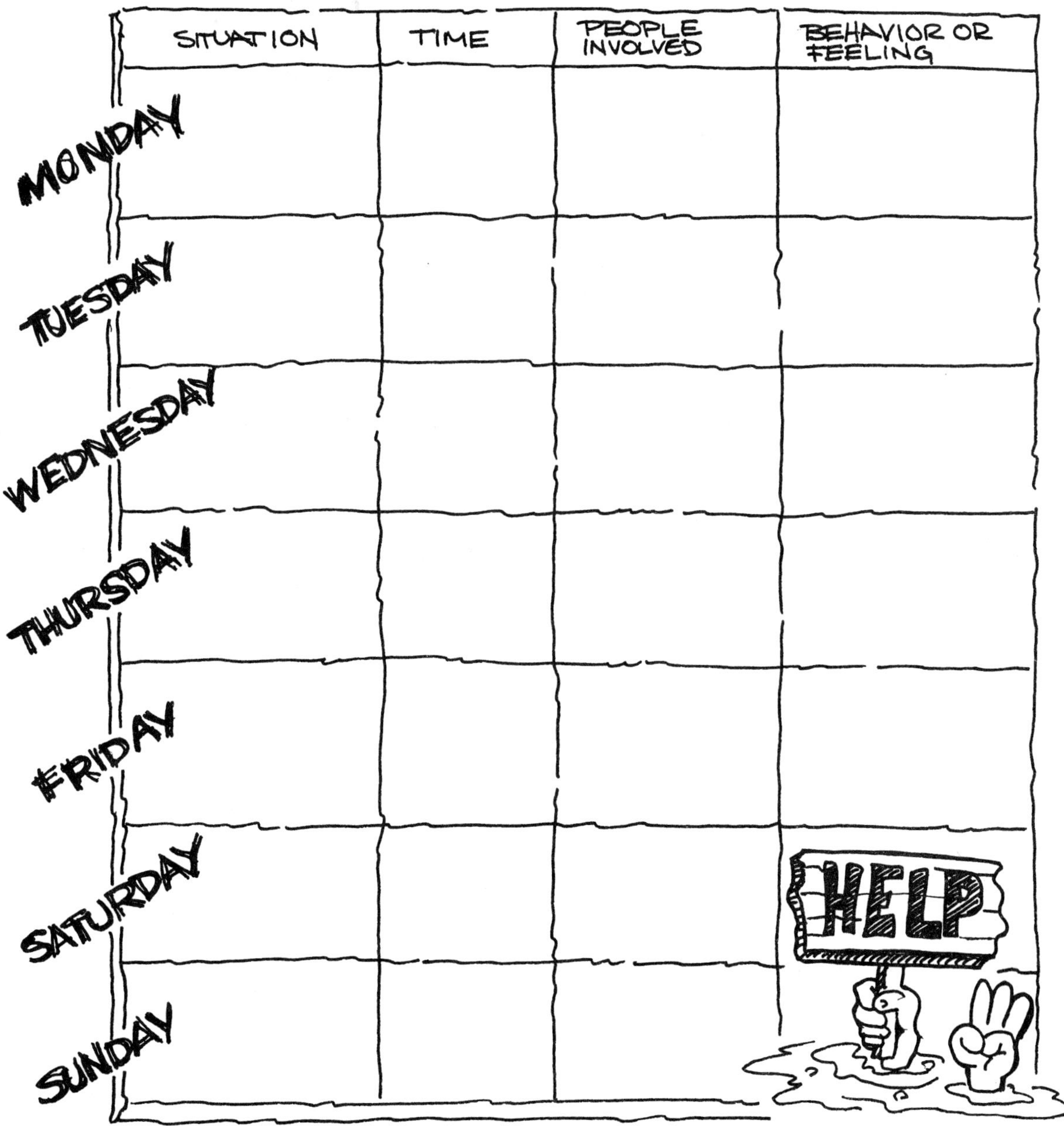

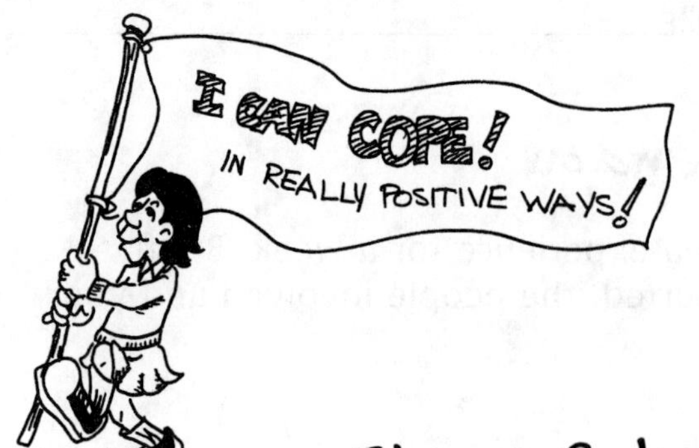

NAME ____________________

Stress Calendar Conclusions

Answer the following questions about your week and the stress you experienced.

1. Write your definition for *stress.*

2. What time of day seems to be the most stressful for you?

3. Who are the people who seem to be around when you are feeling stress?

4. What feelings occur most often when you are experiencing a stressful situation?

5. How do you react when you are experiencing stress?

6. Write an observation about you and your ability to deal with stress.

7. List some of the things you could change in your life to reduce the stress you feel.

8. How could you change your attitude to better deal with stress?

NAME ________________________________

Coping with Stress

Relaxation: You have the ability to calm your mind and body. You will restore a sense of well-being by allowing yourself to relax.

Relaxation takes many forms. Practice many forms of relaxation to find a style that works best for you.

Thoughtful and deliberate breathing is a good way to relax and can be performed almost anywhere at any time.

Conscious Breathing: Sit comfortably in a chair or lie down. Inhale deeply through your nose, allowing your stomach to push out as you take in air. Imagine each molecule of air entering your nose, filtering into your throat, passing down your bronchial tubes, and filling your lungs. When your lungs are filled, slowly release the air while allowing your stomach to relax naturally. Think about the air as it retraces its path from the lungs, back through the bronchial tubes to your throat, back through your nose, to the outside.

Try to make your breathing slow down as much as possible and concentrate on each breath. Closing your eyes will aide in relaxation.

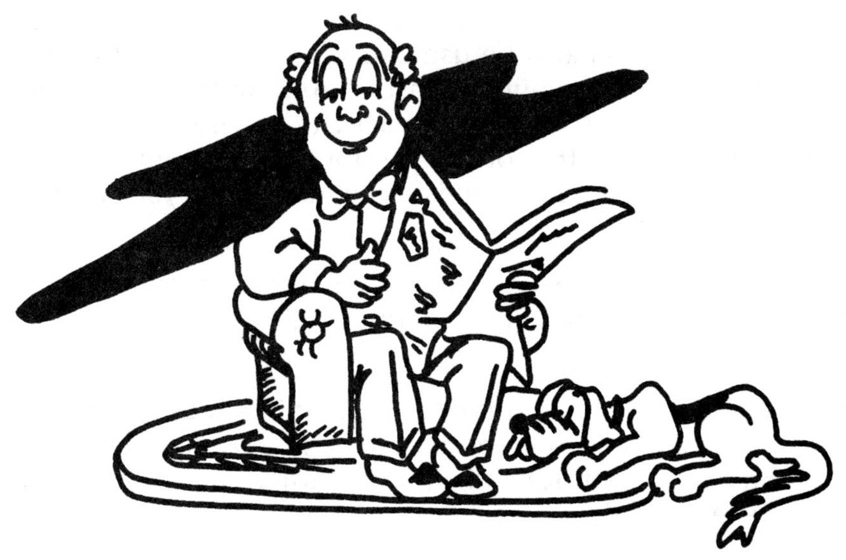

NAME ______________________________

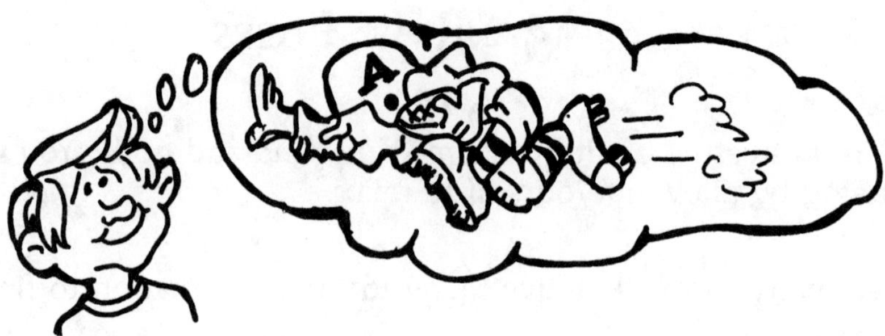

Visualization: Your mind will respond to what you are thinking as if it is really happening. Fool your mind into taking vacations or practicing for physical events without ever leaving your chair. This is almost like daydreaming, but you are in control of the dream.

Sit comfortably or lie down and practice controlled breathing. When you feel your body relaxing, picture yourself in a favorite place that brings you happiness or peace. Use all of your senses as you notice your surroundings. Look at the scene—notice every color and item. Feel the texture of the things that are touching you. If you are outside, notice the wind blowing your hair and feel the warmth of the sun or the cool dampness of the rain. Smell and taste the things around you.

Allow yourself to continue the visualization for several minutes. Enjoy the experience, then slowly open your eyes when you feel ready. Slowly start to move around and resume your activities.

Many athletes use visualization to relax and calm themselves before a game or competition. Visualization can also be used successfully as a form of practice for competition. Relax, and picture yourself participating in the activity you want to practice. Picture each and every step of the activity as you would perform it perfectly. Notice each detail in the form or performance. Picture yourself performing perfectly and feel your friends' acceptance and your own pride.

When you have completed the visualization, take a few controlled breaths and slowly open your eyes and resume your normal activities.

These methods of relieving stress are great for helping get rid of fear or anxiety before a big test. Try taking a few deep breaths and closing your eyes for a minute before you start your next test. It will help you gather your thoughts and be ready—you also have to study.

NAME ____________________________

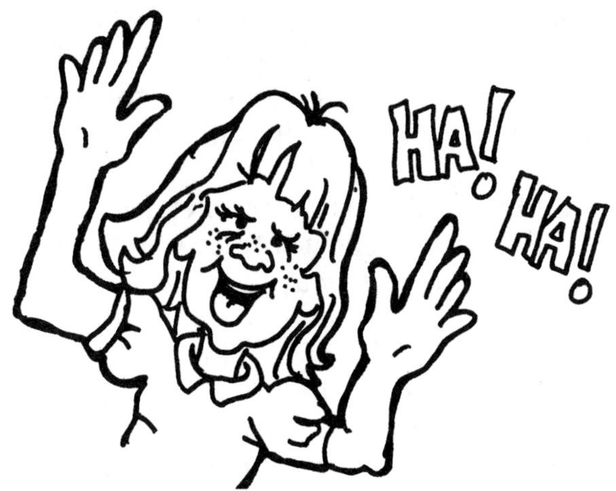

Look for a laugh: Humor or a good belly laugh is a great way to relieve tension. Laughing increases the amount of oxygen to the brain. The brain sends out chemicals called endorphins. These chemicals are used by the brain to reduce pain. That's what happens physically—what is important is that you feel better after a good laugh.

Take the opportunity to read jokes, call a friend who makes you laugh, watch a funny movie, or remember a good laugh you shared with a friend. Take the time to laugh.

Exercise: People tend to carry tension in muscles in various parts of their bodies. Some people carry tension in their neck, some in their back, some in their legs. Almost any physical activity will help to relieve the tension in muscles—swim, play basketball, run, lift weights, dance, walk to a friend's house, ride your bike, roller blade, go skiing—whatever.

Write a letter: A great way to relieve stress and reduce your anger at a particular person is to write that person a letter.

Write the letter to someone who has hurt your feelings or made you angry. It doesn't matter who that person is because they are not going to read the letter.

NAME ______________________________

In the letter, tell them exactly how you feel. Use whatever language you need to tell them off. Tell them why you feel that way. What did they do to hurt you or make you angry? Then tell them how they can make the situation better and what they need to do to improve their relationship with you. Sign the letter.

After making sure that you have told that person everything they need to know about the incident, rip up the letter. Tear it into a million pieces and then wad it up and throw the problem (and the letter) away.

This letter should *not* be given to the person. This letter is meant as a method of release for you. Get rid of your disappointment, anger, or hurt without showing the other person. Of course, it might be a good idea to talk rationally to that person about the problem when you have calmed down.

What a weapon!: You will need another person for this activity. If you are angry with someone, this is sometimes a fun way for both of you to release that frustration without getting hurt.

Get two *empty* paper grocery bags. Fill them with air and hold onto the open end, trapping the air inside. Each person has one bag. Hold the bag with one hand and stand about arm's length away from the other person. Say "go" and take thirty seconds to whack the daylights out of the other person using only the empty bag as a weapon. You may hit only below the waist, so aim carefully.

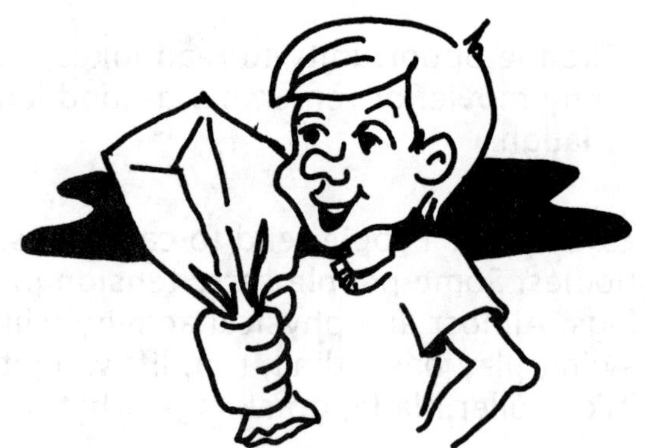

Punch a pillow: A variation of the bag activity is to punch a pillow. All you need is a good, soft pillow. Beat up the pillow instead of another person. Hit the pillow until all the anger and frustrations are gone and all you have left is exhaustion. No one will get hurt and you will have released all your anger in a very physical, but safe, manner.

NAME ____________________

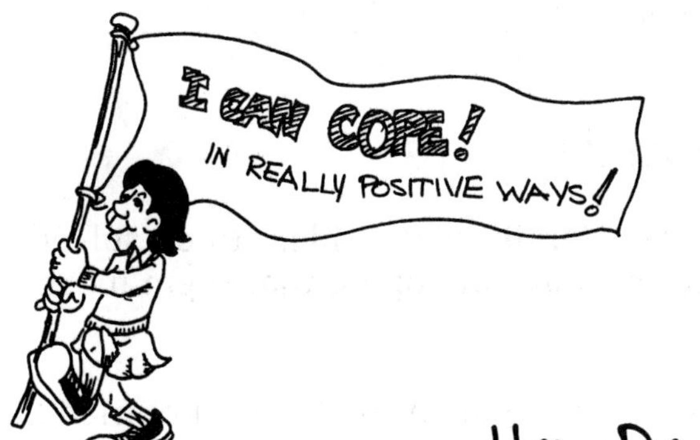

How Do You Cope?

Think of three adults who handle stress in a healthy manner. Ask each of those people to describe a stressful situation they often experience. Have them describe ways they cope with stress.

	STRESSFUL SITUATION	WAYS TO COPE
Name ______		
Name ______		
Name ______		

NAME ____________________

Take That!

Pretend that you are in the following situations. Identify the problem to be solved and list several possible ways to react. Circle the ways of coping that seem most appropriate.

1. You are in class but you have just had a terrible argument with your boyfriend or girlfriend. You are angry. Your feelings are hurt. You are afraid your relationship is over.

   What are you feeling?

   List several ways you could express your feelings. (Circle the most appropriate choice.)

2. You are in a restaurant with your parents. They have just told you that they are going to separate because they fight too much and want to have time alone. You had no suspicion that anything was wrong.

   What are you feeling?

   List several ways you could express your feelings. (Circle the most appropriate choice.)

3. You have just finished singing in a performance you have worked on for 6 months. This is the first time you have performed in public. You are standing in a group of adults that include your parents. Your parents are bragging about you to their friends.

   What are you feeling?

   List several ways you could express your feelings. (Circle the most appropriate choice.)

NAME ____________________

4. You are having a soda in a restaurant with your best friend. You are dying to tell him or her about the first kiss from your new boyfriend or girlfriend. You can't because your best friend broke up with that same person last week.

   What are you feeling?

   List several ways you could express your feelings. (Circle the most appropriate choice.)

5. You are at Disneyland on a crowded day. You reach for your wallet to pay for an ice cream cone and suddenly realize your wallet is missing. Your wallet contains all of the vacation money you have saved the entire year for. You race back to the last ride and as you approach the attendant, a little boy taps you on the arm. He has your wallet and tells you that he noticed it after you got off the ride. You check—all the money is still there.

   What are you feeling?

   List several ways you could express your feelings. (Circle the most appropriate choice.)

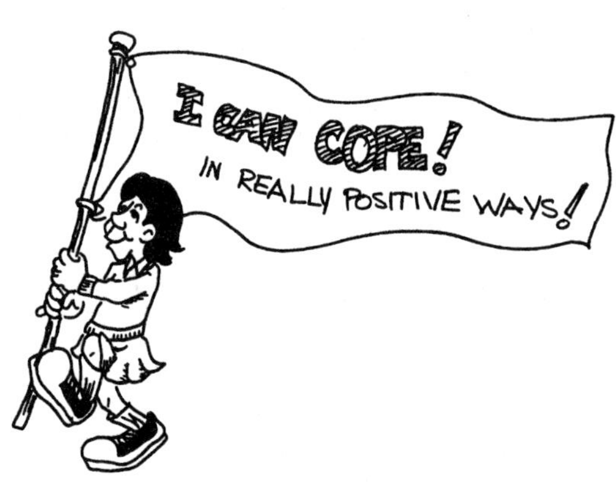

NAME ____________________

This Hurts Me

Draw a picture that represents a hurtful experience in your life. Write a sentence describing your feelings. Answer the questions at the bottom of the page. Look at this picture in the future and see how you feel as time passes.

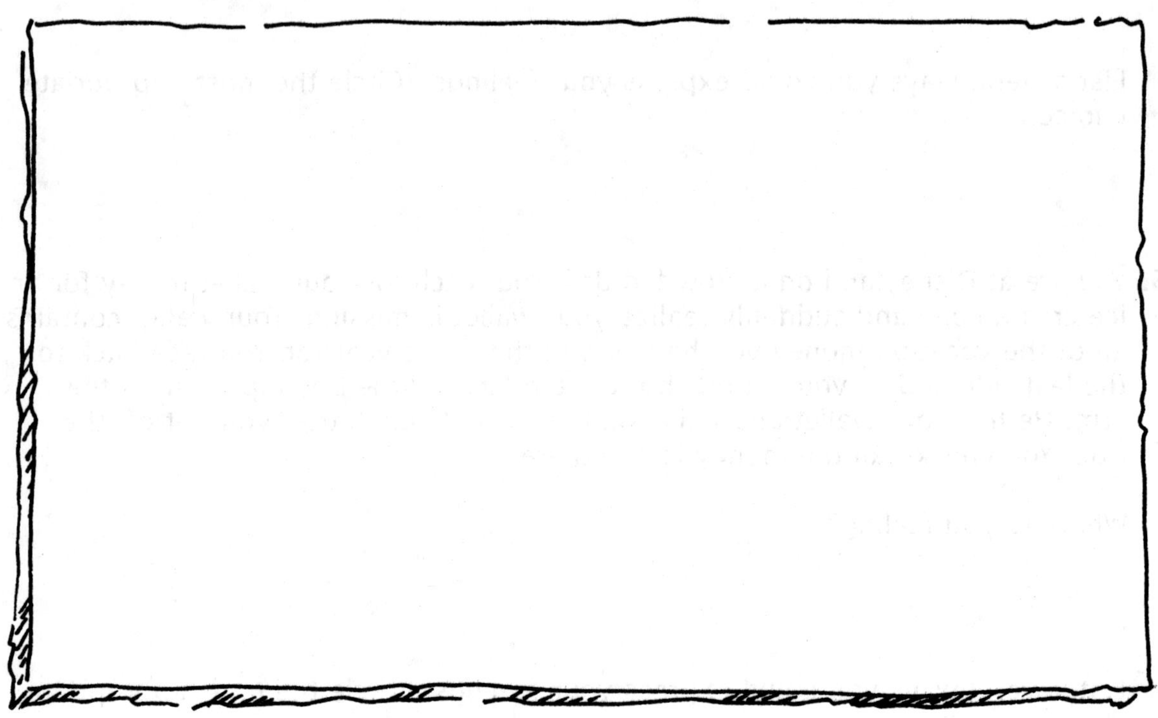

How could you have made the experience end differently?

What were your feelings immediately after the experience?

How have your feelings changed over time?

What did you learn from this painful experience?

NAME ____________________

Good Choices and Changes

List three situations you have experienced that upset you or made you feel uncomfortable. Describe your feelings in those situations, ideas to improve them, barriers to changing, and how you can break down those barriers.

☞ Uncomfortable situation: ____________________

____

____

My feelings at the time: ____________________

____

Ways I can improve the situation: ____________________

____

Barriers to improvement: ____________________

____

I can break down those barriers by: ____________________

____

☞ Uncomfortable situation: ____________________

____

____

My feelings at the time: ____________________

____

Ways I can improve the situation: ____________________

____

From Management Sciences for Health, Inc.

NAME ______________________

Barriers to improvement: ______________________

____

I can break down those barriers by: ______________________

____

☞ Uncomfortable situation: ______________________

____

____

My feelings at the time: ______________________

____

Ways I can improve the situation: ______________________

____

Barriers to improvement: ______________________

____

I can break down those barriers by: ______________________

____

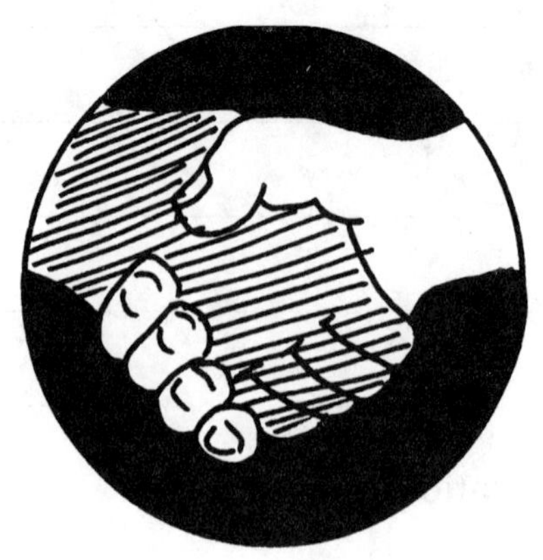

NAME ______________________

Emergency Plan

There may be times when you need an emergency plan. Record the names and phone numbers of people you can go to for help in emergencies.

Adults I can go to for advice and support: (list addresses and phone numbers)

______________ ______________ ______________

______________ ______________ ______________

______________ ______________ ______________

Adults I can stay with if I need to: (list addresses and phone numbers)

______________ ______________ ______________

______________ ______________ ______________

______________ ______________ ______________

Friends I can rely on for support: (List addresses and phone numbers)

______________ ______________ ______________

______________ ______________ ______________

______________ ______________ ______________

Phone numbers to remember:

Parent's work: ______________

Police: ______________

Fire Department: ______________

Home: ______________

Other: ______________

Doctor: ______________

Hospital: ______________

NAME ____________________

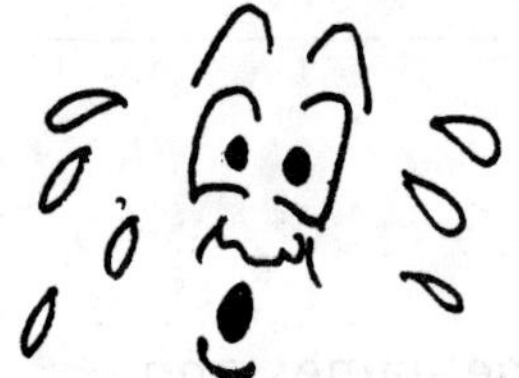

Body Language

Use the following examples to tell what the person is saying with body language. What message is being communicated?

1. "Your mother and I are very happy that you got an A on your test." (They are sitting, reading the newspaper. They don't even look up when you tell them the good news.) ____________________

2. "I don't care if I ever see him again!" (She is sitting slumped over, holding her chin in her hands. Her eyes are constantly darting around the room looking at people.) ____________________

3. "I'm *not* angry!" (You have just stomped into the house, slammed the door, and thrown your books across the room.) ____________________

4. "Stop kissing me. I don't think we should go any further on our first date." (You are tickling your boyfriend or girlfriend behind the ear and putting your arm around him or her as you snuggle up.) ____________________

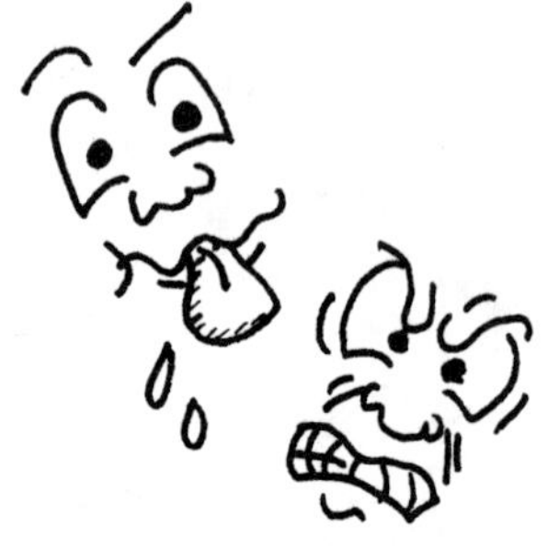

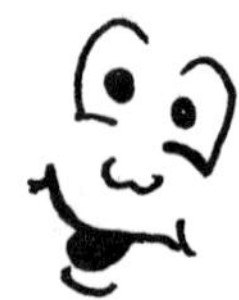

NAME ______________________

5 "Yes, teacher, I'm listening." (You are sitting slumped over your desk with your arms crossed under your head and your eyes are closed.) ______________________

____

____

6 "I feel fine." (You are sweating and pale. You are listless and barely move when answering.) ______________________

____

____

7. "Of course I love you. I want to spend as much time with you as possible." (You are sitting, leaning away from the person and avoiding eye contact.) ______________________

____

____

8. "I am really excited to hear more about your trip." (You are sitting, leaning forward toward the person. You have direct eye contact and are waiting for them to answer.) ______________________

____

____

NAME ____________________

Sending Clear Messages

One person will role-play one of the situations below. The listeners explain the message they received and give recommendations on how to improve communication. Take turns role-playing and listening.

1. You are about to leave a fun party. You have had a great time and want to tell the person giving the party how much you appreciated being asked.

   Listeners: What did you understand the message to be? ____________________

   Recommendations: ____________________

2. You are standing at the bus stop and see a new face. You realize that this person could be from the family that just moved in. You decide to show him or her that you are a friendly person and willing to help him or her get started at school.

   Listeners: What did you understand the message to be? ____________________

   Recommendations: ____________________

3. You are calling your boyfriend or girlfriend on the telephone. You want to clear up a fight you had at school. His or her father answers the phone and sounds angry after you identify yourself.

   Listeners: What did you understand the message to be? ____________________

NAME ______________________

Recommendations: ______________________

____

____

____

4. You are angry at your friends for spreading rumors about you. You see them standing by themselves after school so you walk up to them to straighten things out and try to salvage your friendship.

   Listeners: What did you understand the message to be? ______________________

   ____

   ____

   Recommendations: ______________________

   ____

   ____

   ____

5. You have always wanted to play in the school band. Tryouts are held after school in front of a large group of students. You are really embarrassed about performing alone in front of people and want to ask the band director to audition you last—when everyone has gone.

   Listeners: What did you understand the message to be? ______________________

   ____

   ____

   Recommendations: ______________________

   ____

   ____

   ____

NAME ____________________

Am I Clear?

Think about a common activity you do every day—making a peanut butter and jelly sandwich or brushing your teeth. Organize your thoughts clearly and explain each step in order. Pretend that you are telling a person from another planet how to do the activity—be clear!

The activity: ____________________

1. ____________________
2. ____________________
3. ____________________
4. ____________________
5. ____________________
6. ____________________
7. ____________________
8. ____________________
9. ____________________
10. ____________________
11. ____________________
12. ____________________
13. ____________________
14. ____________________
15. ____________________

Check your work by following your own directions as you act it out.

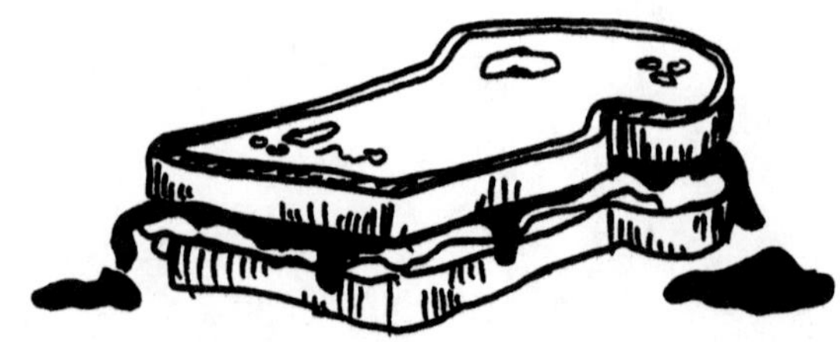

NAME ____________________

Explain a Puzzle

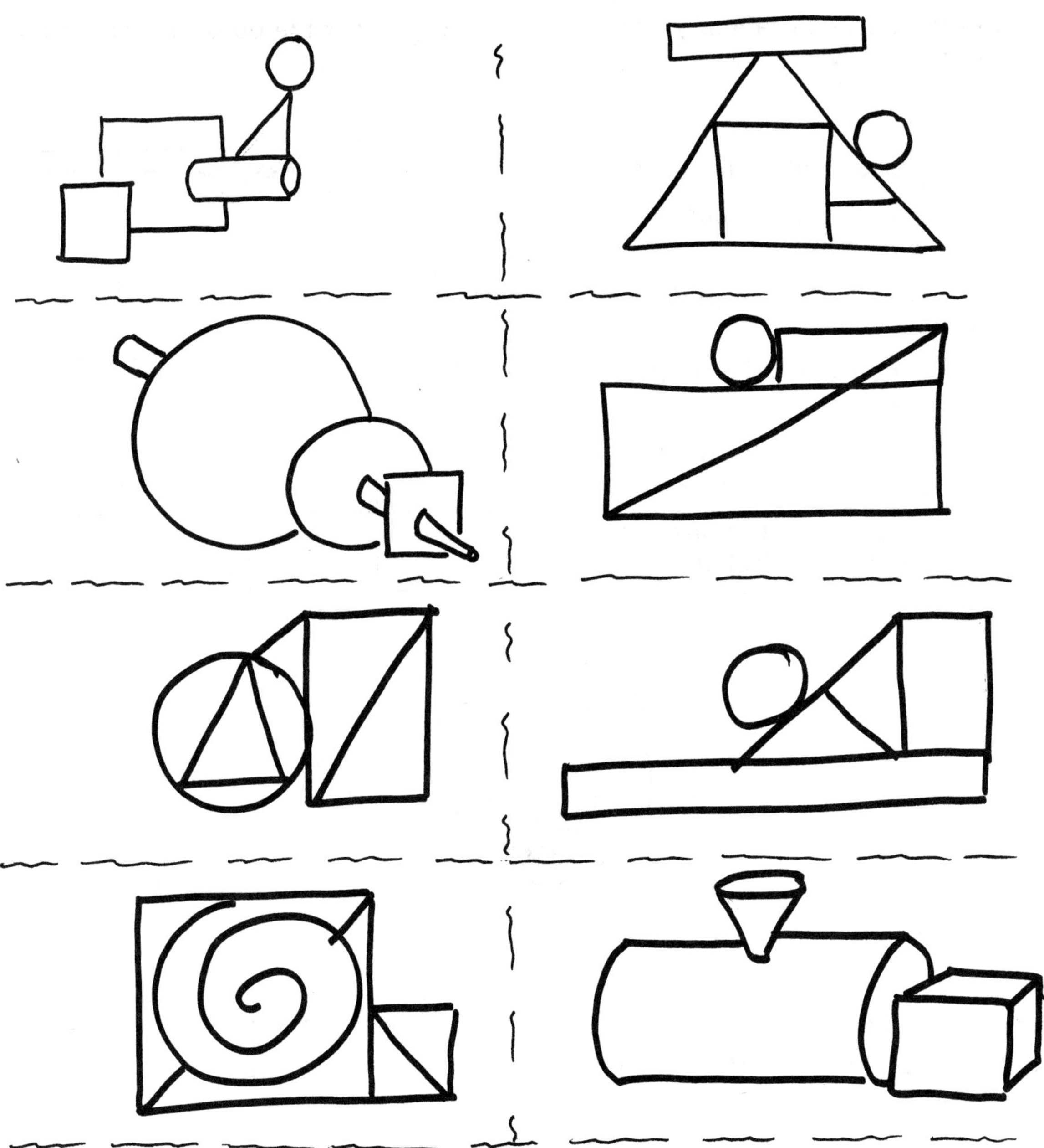

Make up some of your own—
Have students design
their own!

NAME ______________________

Listening Skills

Answer the questions about yourself in Part One. Answer the questions about the listener in Part Two.

Part One

Evaluate your own listening skills:

	Always	Sometimes	Seldom	Never
1. I retain eye contact throughout the conversation.				
2. I keep an open mind during the conversation.				
3. I do not interrupt when someone else is speaking.				
4. I use body language to show signs of understanding and interest.				
5. I ask the speaker questions or make comments for clarification.				

Part Two

Name of the person you are observing ______________________

Evaluate the listener's skills:

	Always	Sometimes	Seldom	Never
1. They retain eye contact throughout the conversation.				
2. They keep an open mind during the conversation.				
3. They do not interrupt when someone else is speaking.				
4. They use body language to show signs of understanding and interest.				
5. They ask the speaker questions or make comments for clarification.				

NAME ____________________

Recognizing Attitudes

There are three choices you can make when you react in a situation. You can choose to be passive, assertive, or aggressive. Below are examples of all three reactions to each situation. Label the behavior type for each answer.

1. You are watching your favorite television show. Your brother walks in and changes the channel.

   ____________ You yell, "Can't you see I was watching that show? Get out of here!"

   ____________ You get up and stomp out of the room.

   ____________ You say, "Please turn the channel back. I want to see the other program."

2. A group of people are gossiping about a friend of yours.

   ____________ You say, "I don't feel comfortable talking about my friend behind his back. Let's change the subject."

   ____________ You join in and tell some stories.

   ____________ You loyally defend your friend by correcting the others.

3. You are buying a notebook at the store and give the clerk a 10 dollar bill. The clerk gives you change for 5 dollars.

   ____________ You say, "Hey! I gave you 10 dollars. Don't rip me off!"

   ____________ You say nothing and leave the store feeling upset.

   ____________ You say, "Excuse me. I gave you 10 dollars. Please check my change."

4. You are waiting in line for tickets at the movies. Someone barges in front of you.

   ____________ You let him or her barge in without comment. After all, it's only one person.

   ____________ You say, "Excuse me. I'm waiting in line. The end of the line is behind me."

   ____________ You push the person and say, "I was here first. Wait your turn like everyone else."

NAME ______________________________

5. Your parents have grounded you for the weekend because you came in late from your last date.

   ______________ You stomp your feet and yell, "Everyone else stayed late. Why am I the only person who has to be home early?"

   ______________ You sneak out during the weekend without your parents knowing.

   ______________ You say, "I realize I was wrong by coming in late last weekend. Can I work off my punishment by mowing the lawn?"

6. You are with a group of friends at the mall and you are hungry. One friend asks where you would like to go eat.

   ______________ You say, "I feel like having pizza. Let's go get some pizza."

   ______________ You say, "I don't care. Wherever you want to go is fine."

   ______________ You say, "Hamburgers are disgusting! The only place that's any good at all is the pizza place."

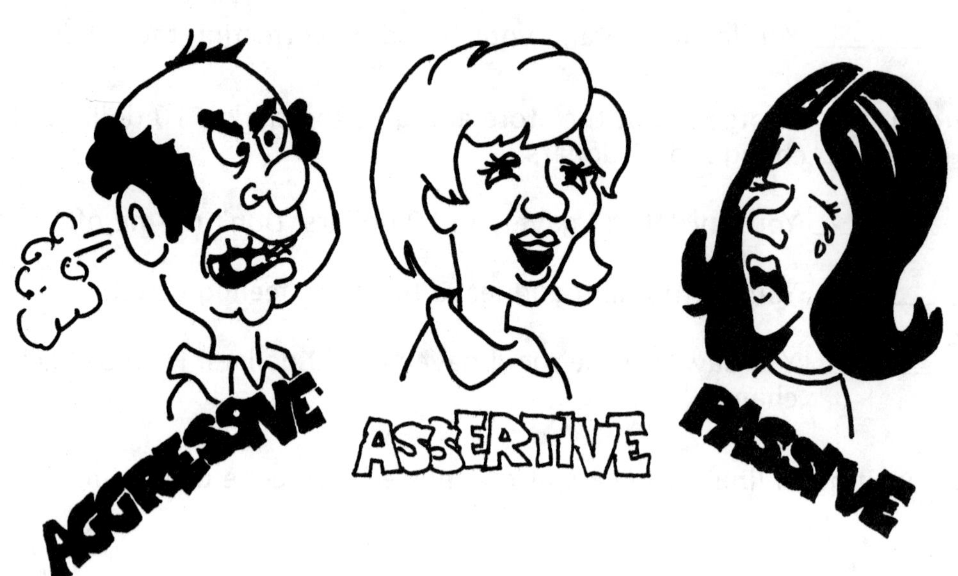

NAME ____________________

Practicing Assertive Behavior

Write an assertive response to the following situations.

➪ You feel your parents should increase your allowance.

Response:

➪ You asked your mother if you could go to the school dance with your friends and she has not given you an answer. The dance is tonight and you need to know now.

Response:

➪ A friend borrowed your in-line skates a week ago and you want them back.

Response:

➪ You get an important test back from the teacher and realize that she has made a mistake by marking your answer incorrect.

Response:

➪ You tried out for the basketball team but the coach says you did not make the team. You feel that you should be on the team because you made more points than some people who made the team.

Response:

➪ You have been sitting in a restaurant for 15 minutes without being waited on.

Response:

NAME ____________________

➪ Your teacher has already explained the homework to the class but you still do not understand it.

Response:

➪ You are with your friends at the theater and they ask which of the five movies playing you would like to see.

Response:

➪ You are on a long car trip and want to stop for something to eat. Your dad is driving and trying to reach the destination in record time.

Response:

➪ Your parents don't like the person you are dating. You think they are wrong about this person.

Response:

➪ Your parents are busy but you need help with your homework. You know they are good at this subject.

Response:

NAME ______________________________

Friendly Refusals

Include the steps for writing a friendly refusal in each of your responses to the situations presented.

Steps for a friendly refusal:

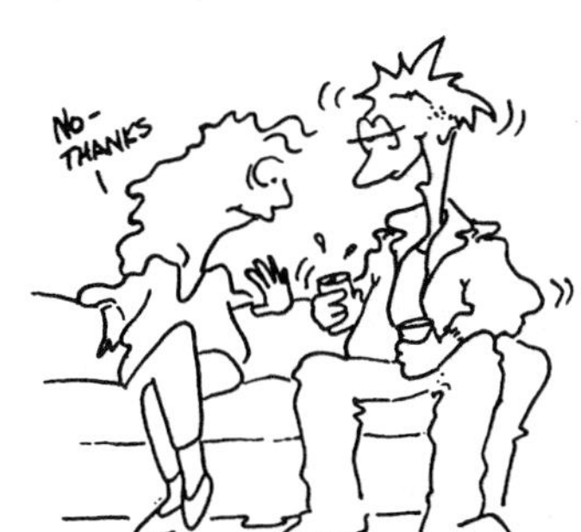

- Use the word "no" in your refusal.
- Emphasize your refusal by repeating the refusal and using body language.
- Give your reasons for refusing or list possible consequences.
- Suggest an alternative that includes your friend.
- Change the subject or walk away.

Practice writing refusals.

➪ Your friend asks you over to his or her house for the weekend. You don't want to go because you are tired and don't feel like going out this weekend.

Response:

➪ You are on a date with a special person who wants you to go parking with him or her. You really care for him or her and are afraid you might go further than you should.

Response:

➪ You are at a party and your friend offers you a beer. You don't want to drink.

Response:

NAME ___________________________

➪ You are at the mall with a group of friends. They are bored and decide to try shoplifting. You don't think it is a good idea.

Response:

➪ A friend sits beside you in math and wants to copy answers for the test that he or she didn't study for. You are afraid of getting caught.

Response:

➪ You are asked out by a friend. You are afraid that dating may ruin your friendship and don't want to go.

Response:

➪ A teacher asks you to stay after school to review information for a subject that you have been failing. You want to be with your friends that day.

Response:

NAME ____________________

Role-Play: Friendly Refusal

Ineffective Refusal

Charlie is the school's star athlete and is dating Meg. He is nervous about the big game tomorrow and feels pressure because the coach really depends on him to score points. Meg is trying to reassure him. They are standing at Meg's locker. Listen to Charlie's refusal.

Charlie: I'm really nervous about the game tomorrow. I haven't had a good practice all week.

Meg: Don't worry so much. Listen, if you're so nervous, I've got something to calm you down.

Charlie: What is that? Are those downers? Are you crazy? That stuff is dangerous!

Meg: Don't be a wussy. This will make you relax and get your head ready for the game.

Charlie: I just don't know if I want to do it, that's all.

Meg: There's nothing to be afraid of. I use them all the time before big tests and I get good grades.

Charlie: I don't know. I am afraid it will mess me up for the game.

Meg: It will help you for the game. You are the only kid in school *not* taking anything to help you. Here, put these pills in your pocket for later.

Charlie: Well, I'll hold them but I still may not take them. It doesn't seem right.

Meg: The thing that would seem right is winning the game, and we need you relaxed and loose. Take the pills and do the school a favor.

Charlie: I'll see. Oh! There's the bell for class. I'm late.

Meg: See you later. Be cool and be loose.

NAME ______________________________

Role-Play: Friendly Refusal

Effective Refusal

Charlie is the school's star athlete and dating Meg. He is nervous about the big game tomorrow and feels pressure because the coach really depends on him to score points. Meg is trying to reassure him. They are standing at Meg's locker. Listen to Charlie's refusal.

Charlie: I'm really nervous about the game tomorrow. I haven't had a good practice all week.

Meg: Don't worry so much. Listen, if you're so nervous, I've got something to calm you down.

Charlie: What is that? Those pills look like downers. They're dangerous.

Meg: Don't be a wussy. This will make you relax and get your head ready for the game.

Charlie: No. If I get caught with drugs, I could be suspended and kicked off the team.

Meg: There's nothing to be afraid of. I use them all the time before big tests and I get good grades.

Charlie: Taking drugs won't help. Drugs can have long-term effects and create more problems for both of us.

Meg: It will help you for the game. You are the only kid in school *not* taking anything to help you. Here, put these pills in your pocket for later.

Charlie: No. I don't want them. I don't feel it's right to take drugs.

Meg: The thing that would seem right is winning the game, and we need you relaxed and loose. Take the pills and do the school a favor.

Charlie: I'll do the school a favor by staying drug-free. Come watch me at the game tomorrow. I've got to go to class. See ya! (walks away)

Meg: See you later. Be cool and be loose.

NAME ___________________________

Role-Play: Friendly Refusal

You and a friend are at a party where there is a lot of alcohol and probably drugs. You feel a little nervous because many people have been going out to the backyard in small groups. These are the popular kids that you have been trying to impress. Your friend comes in from the backyard and is acting weird.

Person 1: You should go out back and see what's going on. There's lots of free stuff out there.

Person 2:

Person 1: Don't be shy! These people are our friends. They wouldn't do anything to hurt us.

Person 2:

Person 1: Let's just try some. It's free and everyone will think we're cool if we join them.

Person 2:

Person 1: I thought you would be a lot of fun. Don't wreck everything for us. This is our chance.

Person 2:

Person 1: You act like you're afraid. Grow up and experiment a little.

Person 2:

Person 1: Well, I just want to have a little fun. C'mon, let's go.

Person 2:

NAME ____________________

Am I Normal?

Adolescence is a time of change. You mature in many of the same ways your parents did. Ask one or both of your parents, or another significant adult, to answer the following questions. You do *not* need to write down the answers.

1. How did you feel about being a teenager?
2. Did you mature earlier or later than your friends?
3. How did you feel about your body as you matured?
4. Do you recall a significant event during adolescence that troubled you?
5. What significant events were occurring in society at this time?
6. What did you worry about most?
7. What ideas did you have at that time that were mistaken?
8. What did your parents tell you about sex?
9. What do you wish your parents had done to better prepare you for being an adult?
10. What do you think I need to know?

☞ The adult being interviewed should sign the form below, verifying that you talked to him or her and tell what relationship they are to you.

Signed ____________________ Relationship ____________________

NAME ______________________________

MALES ♂

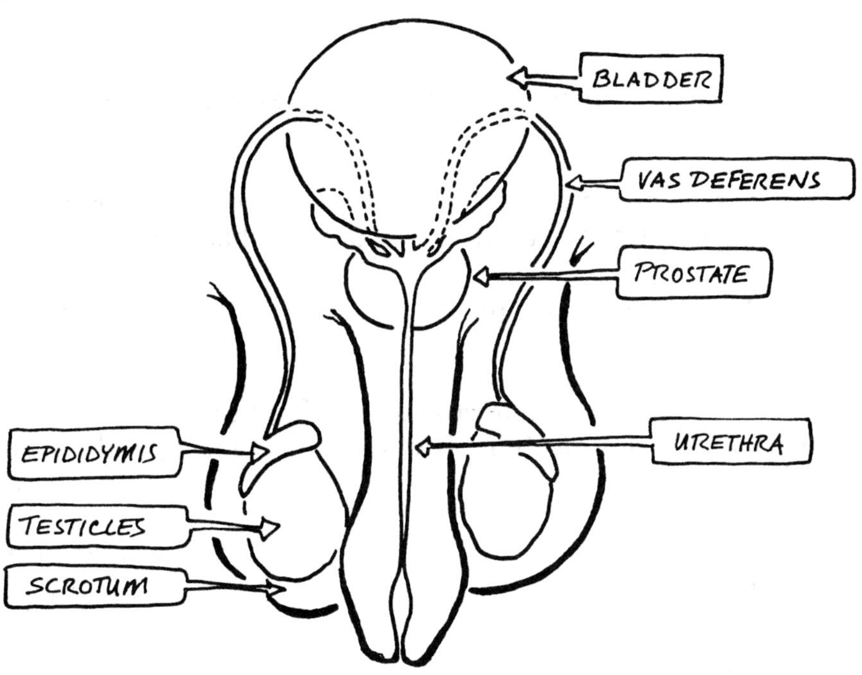

BLADDER
VAS DEFERENS
PROSTATE
EPIDIDYMIS
URETHRA
TESTICLES
SCROTUM

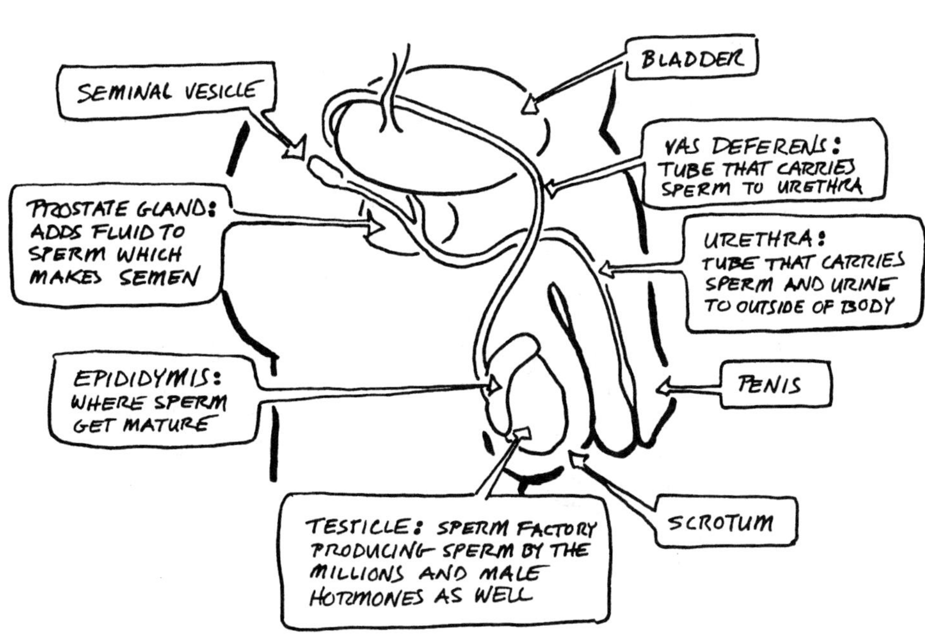

SEMINAL VESICLE
BLADDER
VAS DEFERENS: TUBE THAT CARRIES SPERM TO URETHRA
PROSTATE GLAND: ADDS FLUID TO SPERM WHICH MAKES SEMEN
URETHRA: TUBE THAT CARRIES SPERM AND URINE TO OUTSIDE OF BODY
EPIDIDYMIS: WHERE SPERM GET MATURE
PENIS
SCROTUM
TESTICLE: SPERM FACTORY PRODUCING SPERM BY THE MILLIONS AND MALE HORMONES AS WELL

NAME ____________________

See What You Have Learned: Male Reproductive System

Below is a picture of the male reproductive system that has not been labeled. See if you can follow the path of the sperm to the outside of the body. Choose a different color for each part of the system and color the square with that color.

- ❑ Find the *testes* (or testicles) and color them the same color. The testes produce sperm cells.
- ❑ On each testicle is an organ that stores the sperm while they mature. This is called the *epididymus.* Choose a different color to shade them in.
- ❑ Find the *vas deferens* that carry the sperm through the body. Choose a new color for these tiny tubes.
- ❑ Choose a color for the glands that provide the fluid that mixes with the sperm to give them mobility and nutrition. The names of these glands are the *seminal vesicles* and the *prostate.*
- ❑ The *urethra* is the tube that carries the semen through the penis. Choose a color for the urethra.

When you finish, check your work by looking at the labeled diagram of the male reproductive system.

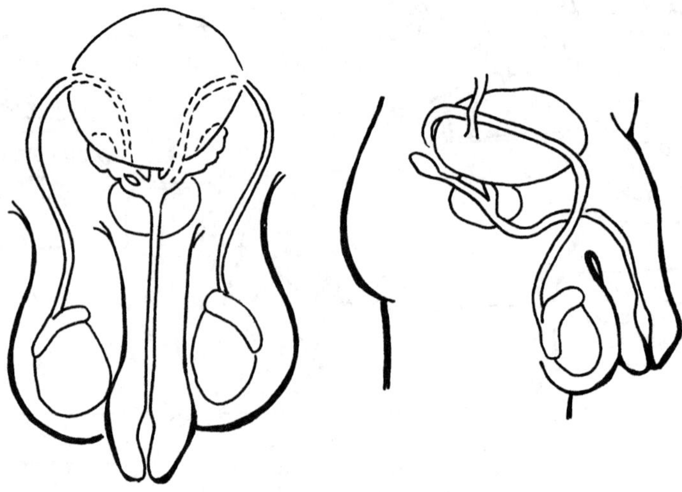

NAME ____________________

FEMALES ♀

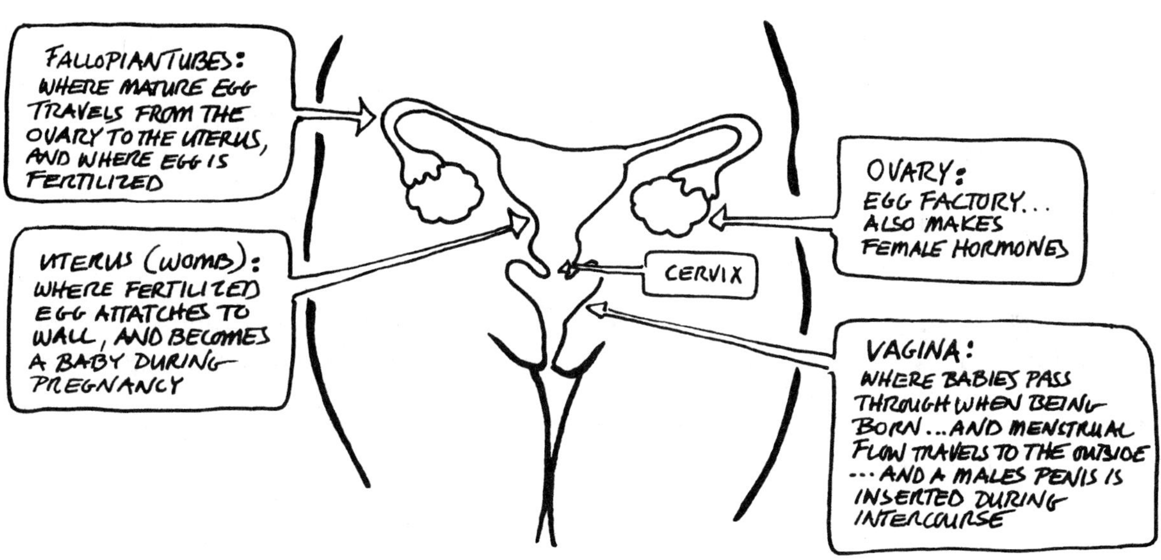

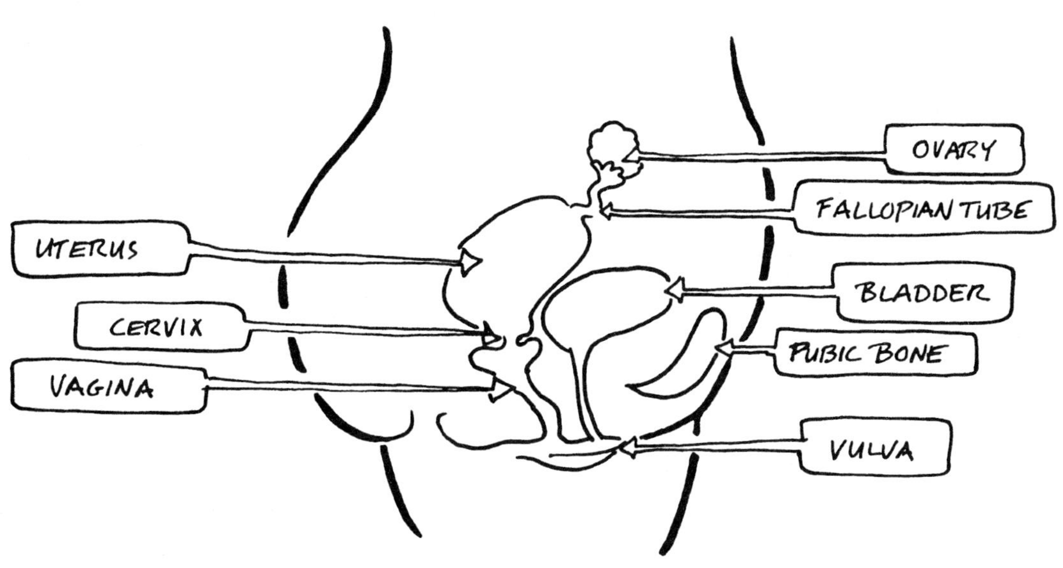

NAME ______________________

See What You Have Learned: Female Reproductive System

Follow the path of the ova through the female reproductive system. Choose a different color for each part of the system and color the square with that color.

- ❑ The *ovaries* are the glands that produce the ova. Color the ovaries and the square to the left the same color.
- ❑ The *Fallopian tubes* are the pathway to the uterus and the place where fertilization takes place if sperm are present. Choose a different color for these tubes.
- ❑ A spongy, thick lining is waiting for the ovum inside a muscular organ called the *uterus.* Choose a color for the uterus.
- ❑ The *cervix* is the opening at the bottom of the uterus and must dilate, or open, to allow a baby to be born. Choose a new color and shade in the cervix.
- ❑ The *vagina* is the passageway for menstrual blood to leave the body. Choose a color for this area.

When you finish, check your work by looking at the labeled diagram of the male reproductive system.

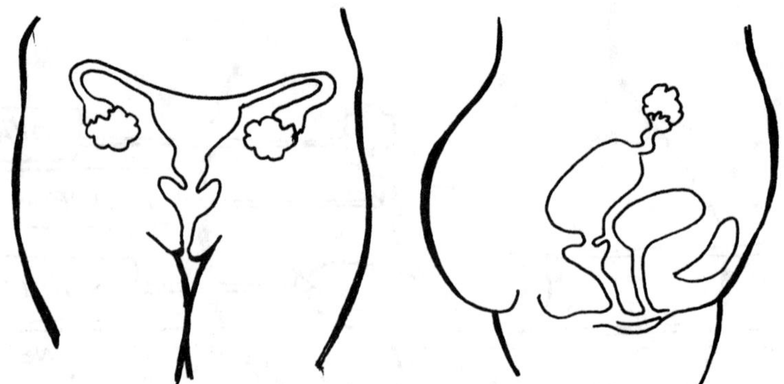

NAME ______________________________

MENSTRUATION

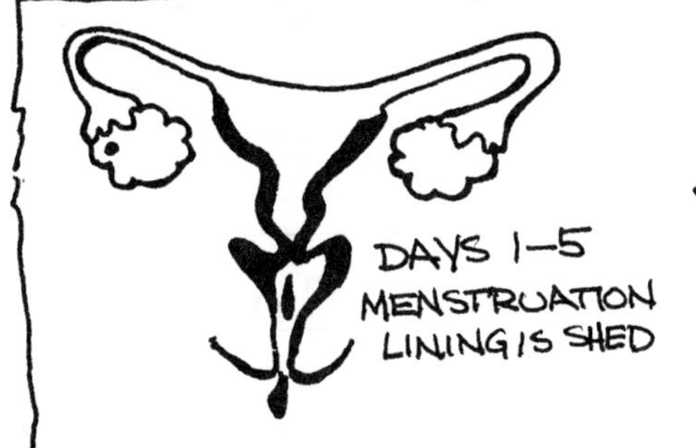

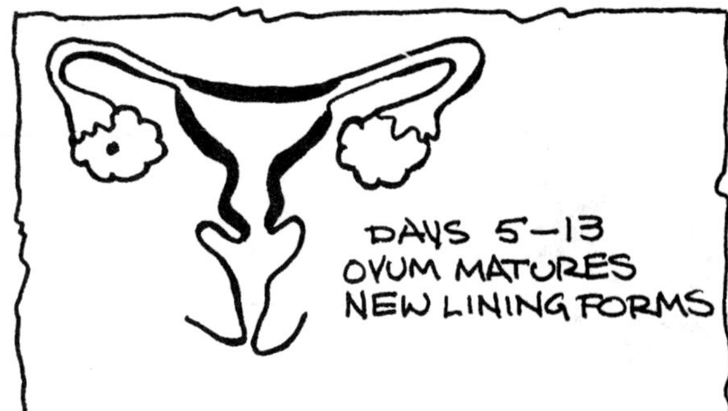

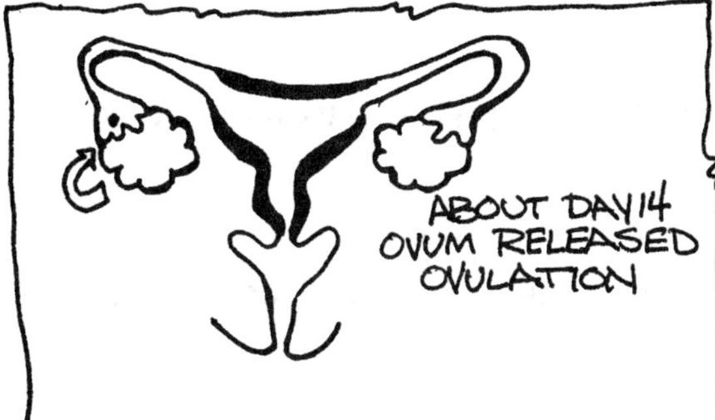

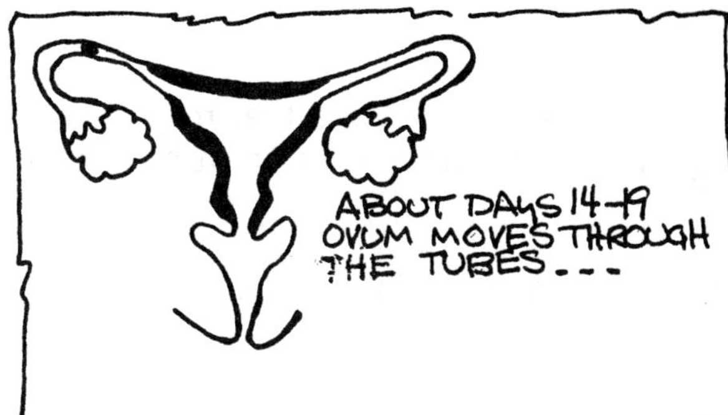

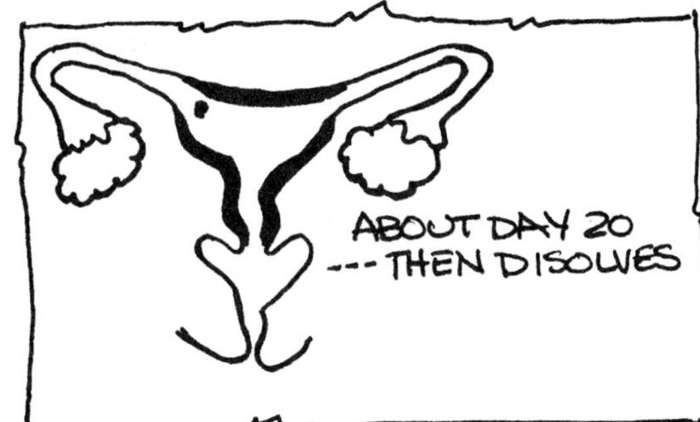

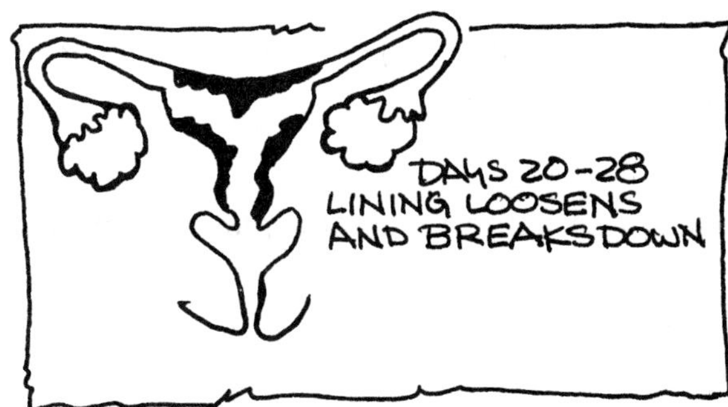

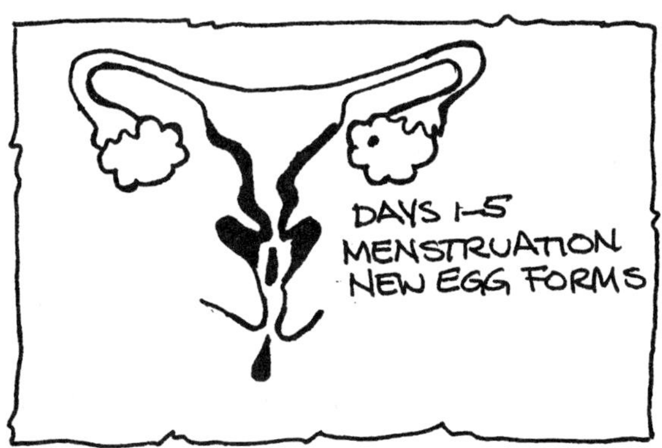

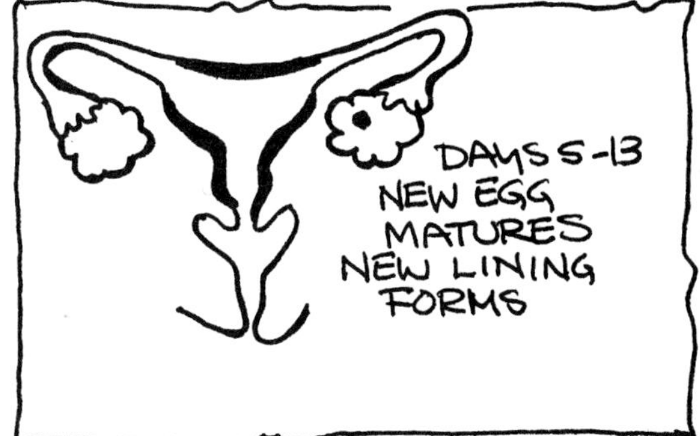

NAME ______________________

Recognize Affection

Think of ten ways that you can show how much you love someone *without* having sex.

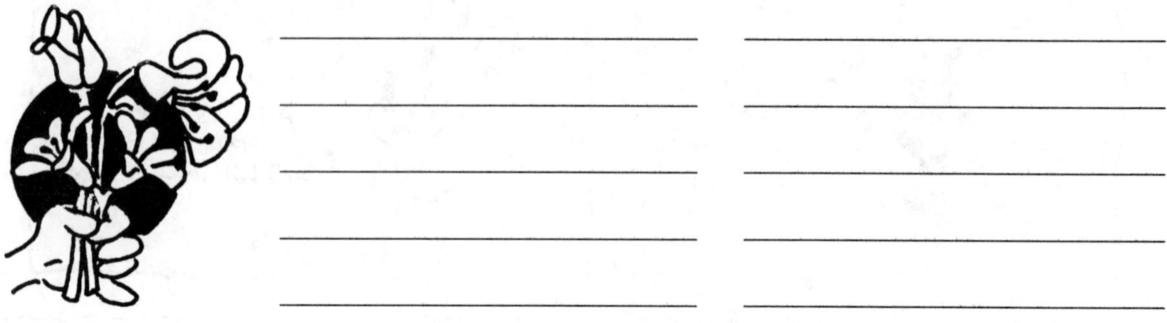

Circle any of those ideas that might be misinterpreted by your partner as a signal that you might be interested in having sex.

Using the ideas from your list, place them on the continuum from least romantic to most romantic.

Least Romantic ———————————— Most Romantic

Use those same ideas and place them on the continuum below from least risky to most risky.

Least Risky ———————————— Most Risky

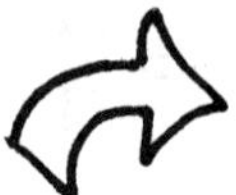

Compare the two continuums. What are your thoughts?

Adapted with permission from *Prevention Skills for Youth,* ETR Associates Training Department. Santa Cruz, CA, 1987–1998.

NAME ______________________________

Fetal Development during Pregnancy

When the sperm pushes into an egg in the Fallopian tube, the tail of the sperm drops off and the egg begins to divide into more cells. This is the moment of conception.

First Trimester

Weeks 1–12

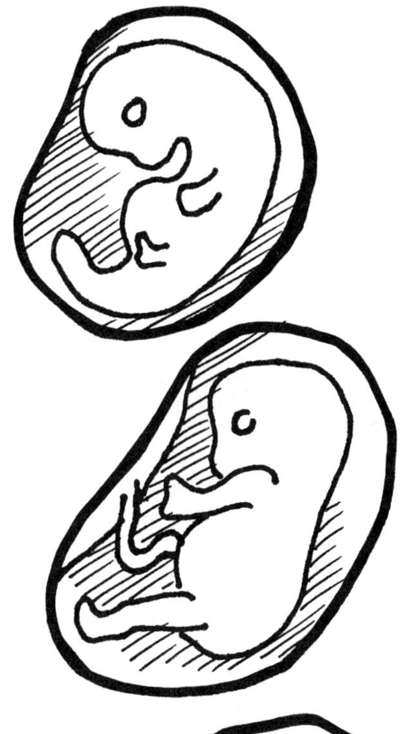

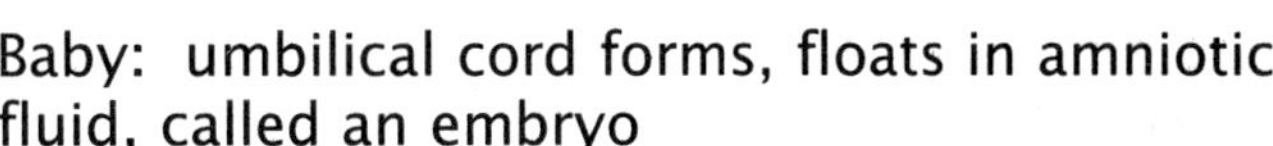

Baby: umbilical cord forms, floats in amniotic fluid, called an embryo

Mother: possible morning sickness, feels tired, skips her period.

Baby: umbilical cord and placenta form, organs develop, heart and brain active

Mother: feels very tired, urinates more, is sick all day

Baby: mouth, nose, and ears show, testicles or ovaries grow, fingers and toes appear, called a fetus

Mother: breasts grow larger and may produce fluid from nipples, may have back pain

FETUS

NAME ____________________________

Second Trimester

Weeks 13–26

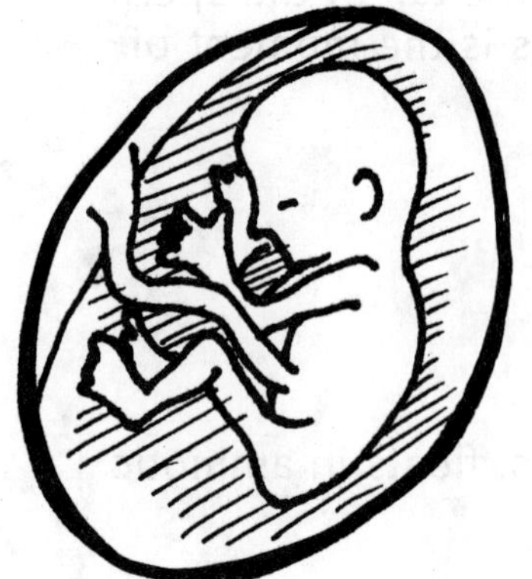

Baby: growth rate increases, starts moving, sucks thumb, hair appears

Mother: gains 3–4 pounds a month, clothes get tight, increase in hormones causes feeling of fullness and blotches on skin

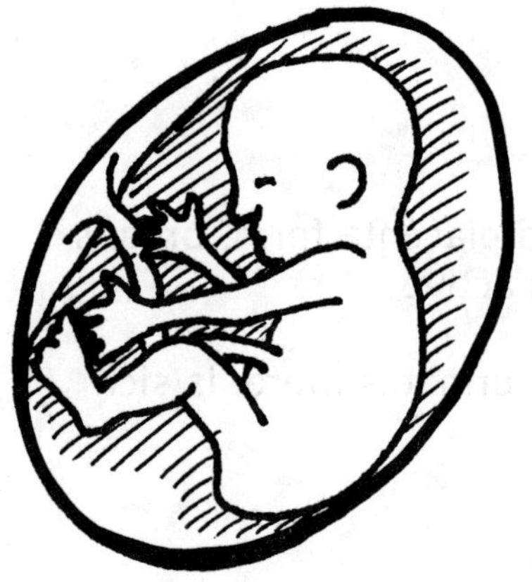

Baby: heartbeat can be heard, arms and legs move, bones begin to grow

Mother: feels baby moving, pressure on rectum can cause constipation, varicose veins can appear

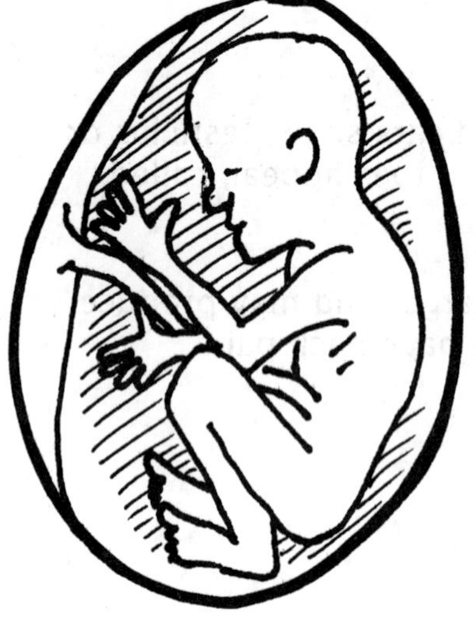

Baby: starts kicking hard, nails and hair grow, increase in size and weight

Mother: time of greatest weight gain, stretched ligaments cause pain in groin, increased need to urinate

NAME ____________________

Third Trimester

Weeks 27–40

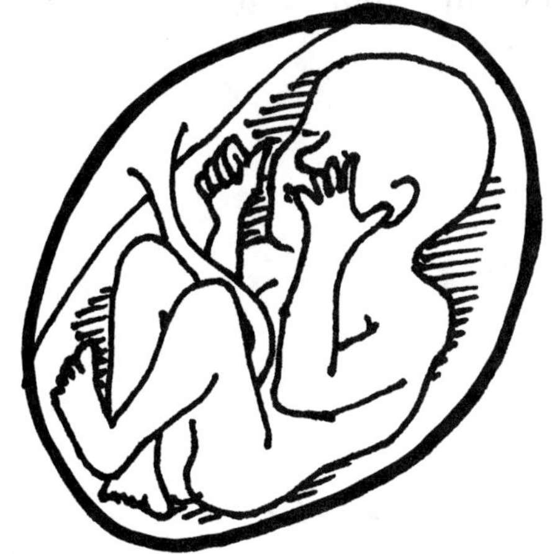

Baby: about 12 inches long, weighs 1¼ pounds, moves vigorously, responds to sound, able to survive if born

Mother: backache common, still gaining weight, stretch marks can occur

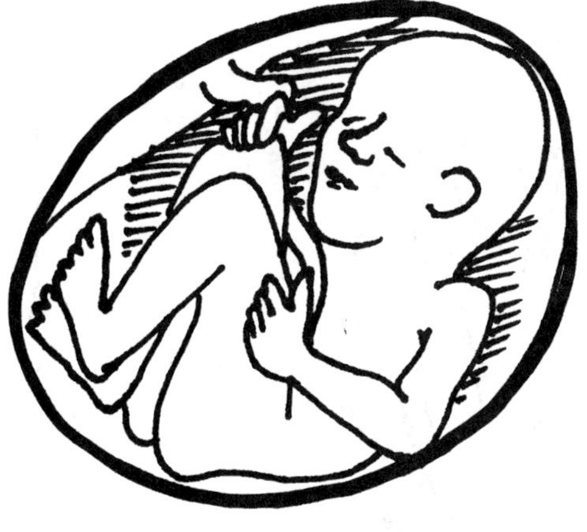

Baby: most rapid weight gain, organs ready to work on their own, reproductive organs in place, brain cells developed

Mother: inner organs crowded as baby takes up more room, joints ache, sleep interrupted by baby movement

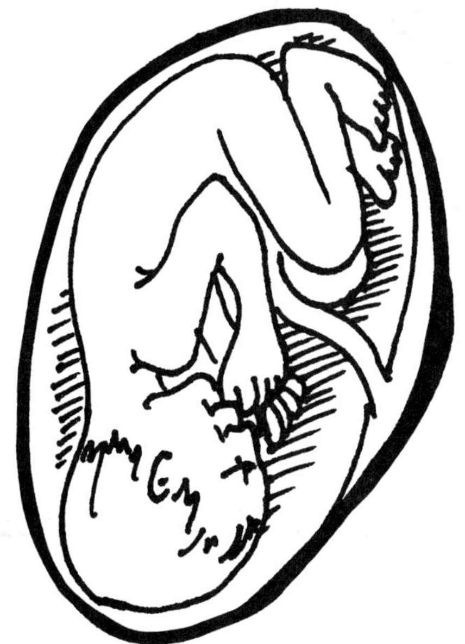

Baby: brain waves same as newborn, moves into birth position with head down

Mother: size of baby causes increased pressure and shortness of breath, has difficulty eating and sleeping, uncomfortable most of the time

NAME ______________________

Fetal Development

Look at the illustration of the developing fetus in the ninth month of pregnancy. Find and label the following things on the illustration:

Placenta	Umbilical cord
Uterus	Cervix
Fetus	Amniotic sac
Amniotic fluid	Vagina

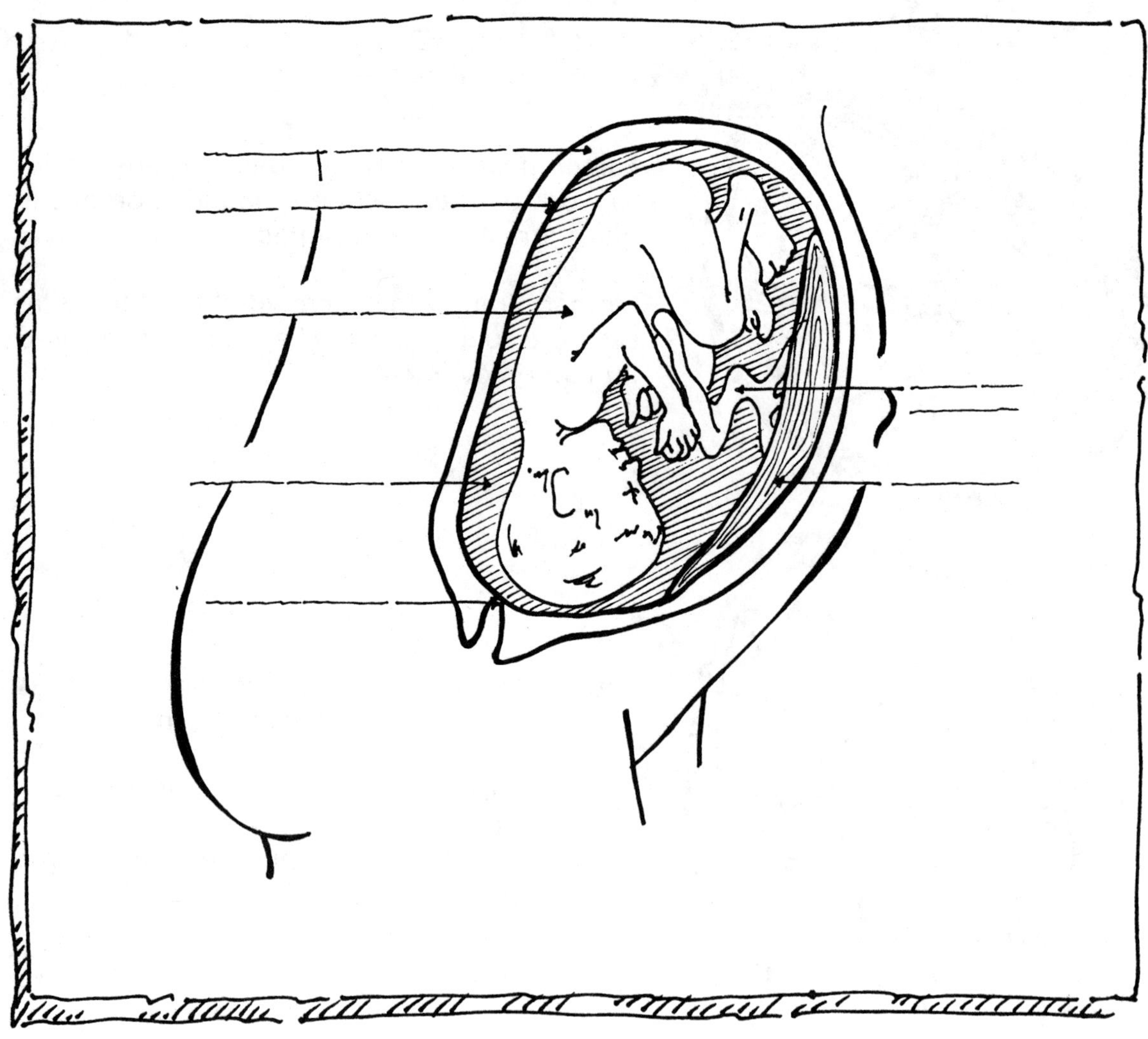

NAME ____________________

Stages of Labor

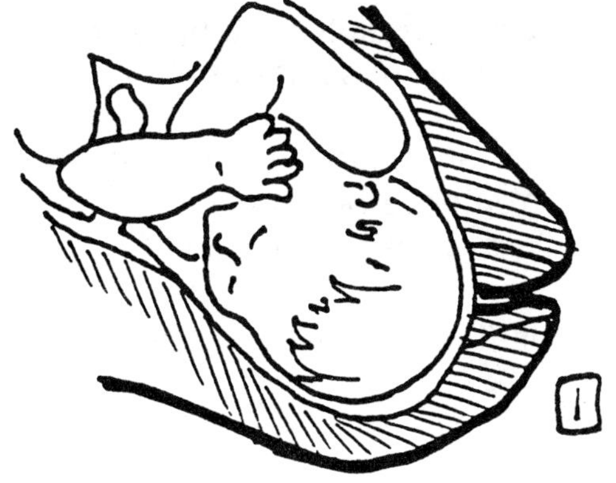

Stage 1

Baby: moves down in the uterus and pushes against the cervix

Mother: experiences mild contractions of the uterus spaced far apart, uncomfortable

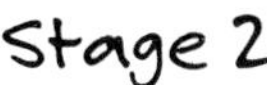

Stage 2

Baby: still pressing against cervix

Mother: bag of waters may break, contractions stronger and closer

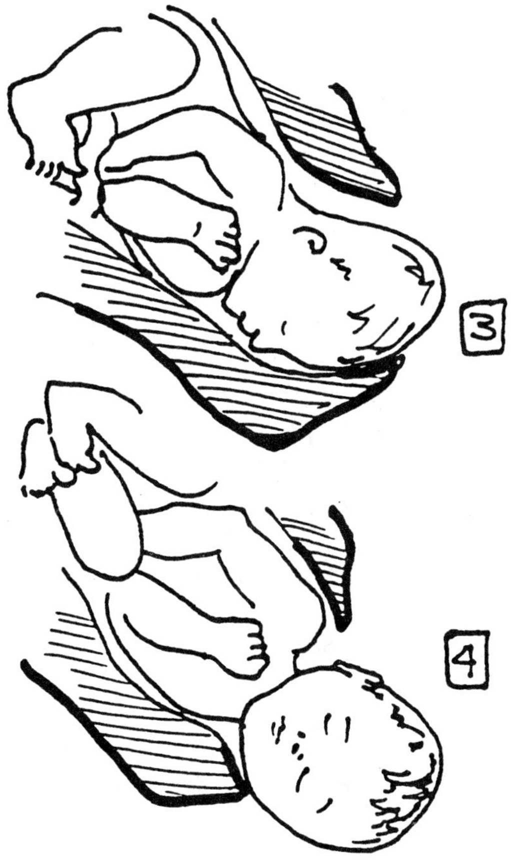

Stage 3

Baby: crowning occurs—when the top of the head can be seen outside the vagina

Mother: has strong contractions close together, wants to push

Stage 4

Baby: head out, turns to get shoulders out

Mother: continues pushing two or three times to release baby

Stage 5

Baby: umbilical cord cut and tied, separated from mother

Mother: rests

Stage 6

Mother: has contractions to push out afterbirth

NAME ______________________________

Responsible Choices

Read each situation and decide what you see as the main problem. Work together as a group to solve the problem in two different ways. Then use the check sheet to evaluate those solutions.

You are on a date and your boyfriend or girlfriend starts pressuring you to have sex. You have both been drinking and you are tired of saying no. Your date just won't take no for an answer.

Problem: ______________________________

____

Solution #1: ______________________________

____

Solution #2: ______________________________

____

Evaluation:

Criteria	#1	#2
Is the solution safe?		
Is the solution legal?		
Does the solution help me achieve my goals?		
Does the solution show respect for all involved?		

You are at a party. Groups of kids are going into the back rooms and whispering. They look really loaded or high when they return. Your friends want you to join them as they go to the rooms to check it out.

Problem: ______________________________

____

Solution #1: ______________________________

____

NAME ____________________

Solution #2: ____________________

____

Evaluation:

Criteria	#1	#2
Is the solution safe?		
Is the solution legal?		
Does the solution help me achieve my goals?		
Does the solution show respect for all involved?		

Your girlfriend looks really beautiful and is your date to the big school dance. You think you are in love with her and want to share sex with her. You brought condoms with you but she does not want to have sex.

Problem: ____________________

____

Solution #1: ____________________

____

Solution #2: ____________________

____

Evaluation:

Criteria	#1	#2
Is the solution safe?		
Is the solution legal?		
Does the solution help me achieve my goals?		
Does the solution show respect for all involved?		

NAME ______________________

You have recently started dating a girl who you really like. There are rumors around school suggesting that you are sexually active and are a real stud. You know if your girlfriend hears these rumors she will be offended and think you only want her for sex.

Problem: ______________________

____

Solution #1: ______________________

____

Solution #2: ______________________

____

Evaluation:

Criteria	#1	#2
Is the solution safe?		
Is the solution legal?		
Does the solution help me achieve my goals?		
Does the solution show respect for all involved?		

NAME ______________________

Sexually Transmitted Diseases

Symptoms, Treatment, and Consequences

STD	SYMPTOMS	CONSEQUENCES
AIDS/HIV Treatment: see a doctor. Even though there is no cure, there are ways to fight the disease that give hope.	Unexplained weight loss Night sweats Diarrhea White spots in the mouth Unexplained fatigue Swollen lymph glands Symptoms may appear months or years after infection	You can infect another person through sexual activity or by sharing an IV drug needle. AIDS cannot be cured. You will die from it. AIDS/HIV can be spread from a pregnant woman to her child.
Syphilis Treatment: early treatment with antibiotics can stop the disease.	1st stage Painless sore or blister on the mouth or sex organ 2nd stage Flu-like symptoms may occur 1–6 months after sore appears 3rd stage Occurs years later and causes heart and brain damage Death	You can pass syphilis to your sexual partner. Heart disease, brain damage, blindness and death. Passed from pregnant woman to unborn child.
Herpes Treatment: cannot be cured but sores can be treated with a drug called acyclovir. Keep sores clean and dry.	Sores may come and go but the virus remains Fluid-filled blisters in the mouth or on sex organs Swollen glands Flu-like symptoms	You can pass herpes to your sexual partner. Herpes sores will recur. Herpes cannot be cured. Passed from pregnant woman to child during childbirth.
Genital Warts Treatment: removal of warts clinically. Reduce stress and keep area dry around warts.	Small bumpy warts on or around the sex organs Flat or cauliflower shaped Painless but can cause itching or burning in the area affected	You can pass genital warts to your sexual partner. More warts will grow. May lead to cancer. Passed from mother to child during childbirth.

NAME ______________________

Gonorrhea Treatment: a doctor can treat gonorrhea with antibiotics. Avoid sexual activity until cured.	Discharge from the sex organs Pain in the pelvic area Painful urination Pain possible during menstruation	Passed to sexual partner during sexual activity. Can lead to Pelvic Inflammatory Disease in women. Sterility may result. Heart trouble, arthritis, skin disease. Passed from mother to child during childbirth.
Chlamydia Treatment: a doctor can cure Chlamydia with the right medicine. Avoid sexual activity until cured.	Discharge from the sex organs Painful urination Unusual bleeding from the vagina. Pain in the pelvic area	Passed to sexual partner. Can lead to Pelvic Inflammatory Disease in women. Sterility may result. Damage to reproductive organs. Passed from mother to child during childbirth.

Other diseases passed from one partner to another by sexual activity include:

Vaginitis—symptoms include a whitish or clear discharge from the vagina that can be accompanied by pain, itching, and unpleasant odor. Treatment with over-the-counter medications is available.

Hepatitis B—can be spread through sexual activity or by sharing drug needles. This disease can cause serious illness and damage to the liver. There is no cure but it can be prevented with a series of shots.

General Statements True of All Sexually Transmitted Diseases

Eliminate the risk by abstaining from sexual intercourse and not using intravenous drugs. Have only one sexual partner for life.

Reduce the risks by using latex condoms with spermicidal foam, avoid multiple sex partners, and avoid drugs and alcohol.

Responsibility of a Person Infected with an STD

- Go to a doctor or medical clinic for treatment.
- Tell your sexual partner so he or she can get checked and treated if necessary.
- Avoid sexual activity until you are cured or no longer infectious.

NAME ____________________

Information Guide for Reporters

Name of newspaper group: ____________________

Reporter: ____________________

This guide will help you collect facts needed for your story.

Name of the disease:

How common is this disease?

How does a person get this sexually transmitted disease?

Is there a cure for this STD?

What are the signs or symptoms of this disease?

What is the treatment for this STD?

Where would a person go to get help if they noticed some of the symptoms for this disease?

NAME ______________________________

What behaviors increase the risks of catching this disease?

What three things would a responsible person do if they notice symptoms of this disease?

How can a person avoid catching this sexually transmitted disease?

Additional information pertaining to this STD:

NAME ____________________

Newsflash!

Sexually Transmitted Diseases

Name of newspaper group: ____________________

Editor: ____________________

Reporters and the topic researched:

____

____

____

____

____

____

____

____

Reports are in! Sexually transmitted diseases, also known as STDs, are a continuing problem among sexually active people. The numbers of people with STDs are surprising. Some of these diseases are so common that the following numbers of people might be infected:

____

A person can catch one of these diseases in the following ways:

____

____

____

____

Some of these diseases have no cure. The diseases that can be cured are:

____

____

____

NAME ______________________________

The STDs that cannot be cured are:

____

____

Some of these diseases can kill if left untreated. The STDs that are deadly are:

____

The STDs that can cause permanent scarring and damage to the reproductive organs are:

____

Some sexually transmitted diseases can cause sterility when left untreated. Sterility is defined as:

____

____

Each of the sexually transmitted diseases has definite symptoms or signs of that disease. List the diseases reported on and the major symptoms for each disease.

____

____

____

____

____

____

____

____

____

____

____

____

____

NAME ______________________________

Each disease has some kind of treatment available. List each disease reported on and the treatment or cure for that disease.

____

____

____

____

____

____

____

____

____

The best way to avoid getting any of these diseases is:

____

____

If a person must be sexually active, which increases his or her risk of getting a sexually transmitted disease, he or she can protect himself or herself to some degree by using a specific method of contraceptive. The only form of birth control that places a barrier between you and your partner is:

____

There are several ways of lowering the risks of catching a sexually transmitted disease if a person is sexually active. The methods of lowering the risks are:

____

____

____

____

____

____

NAME ____________________

The three things a responsible person can do if they notice signs or symptoms of any of these diseases are:

____

____

____

____

____

There are places in the community where a person suffering these symptoms can go to for help and treatment. Below is a list of some of those places available in our community:

____

____

____

____

____

____

____

____

____

Some additional information concerning specific diseases:

____

____

____

____

____

____

NAME ____________________

AIDS/HIV Puppet Show Puppets

COLOR: BLUE

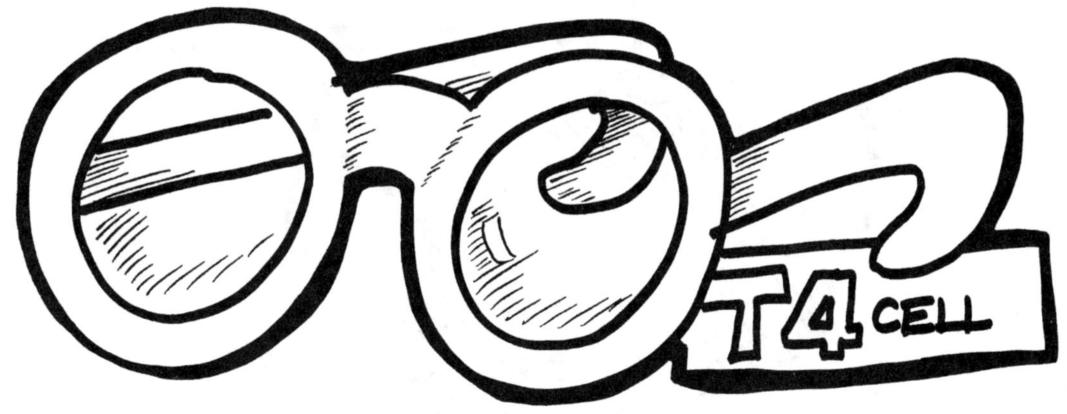

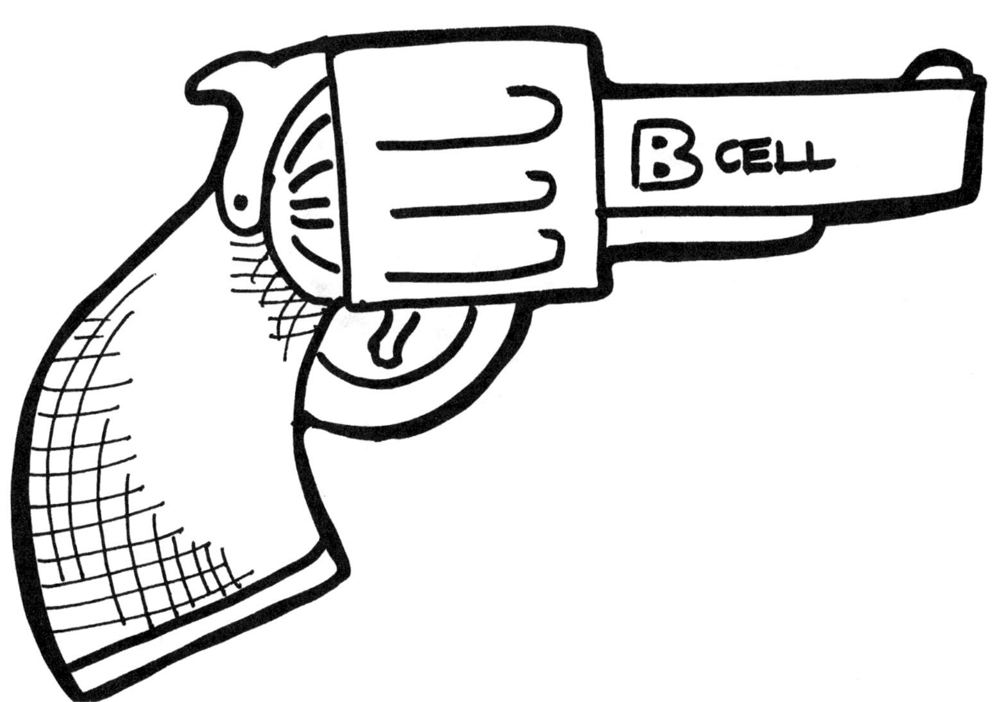

Directions: Cut figures out on the heavy black line, color with bright colors, glue to 3 × 5 cards and glue to tongue depressor. Stick the tongue depressor into the cup bottom. See illustration on following page.

NAME ____________________

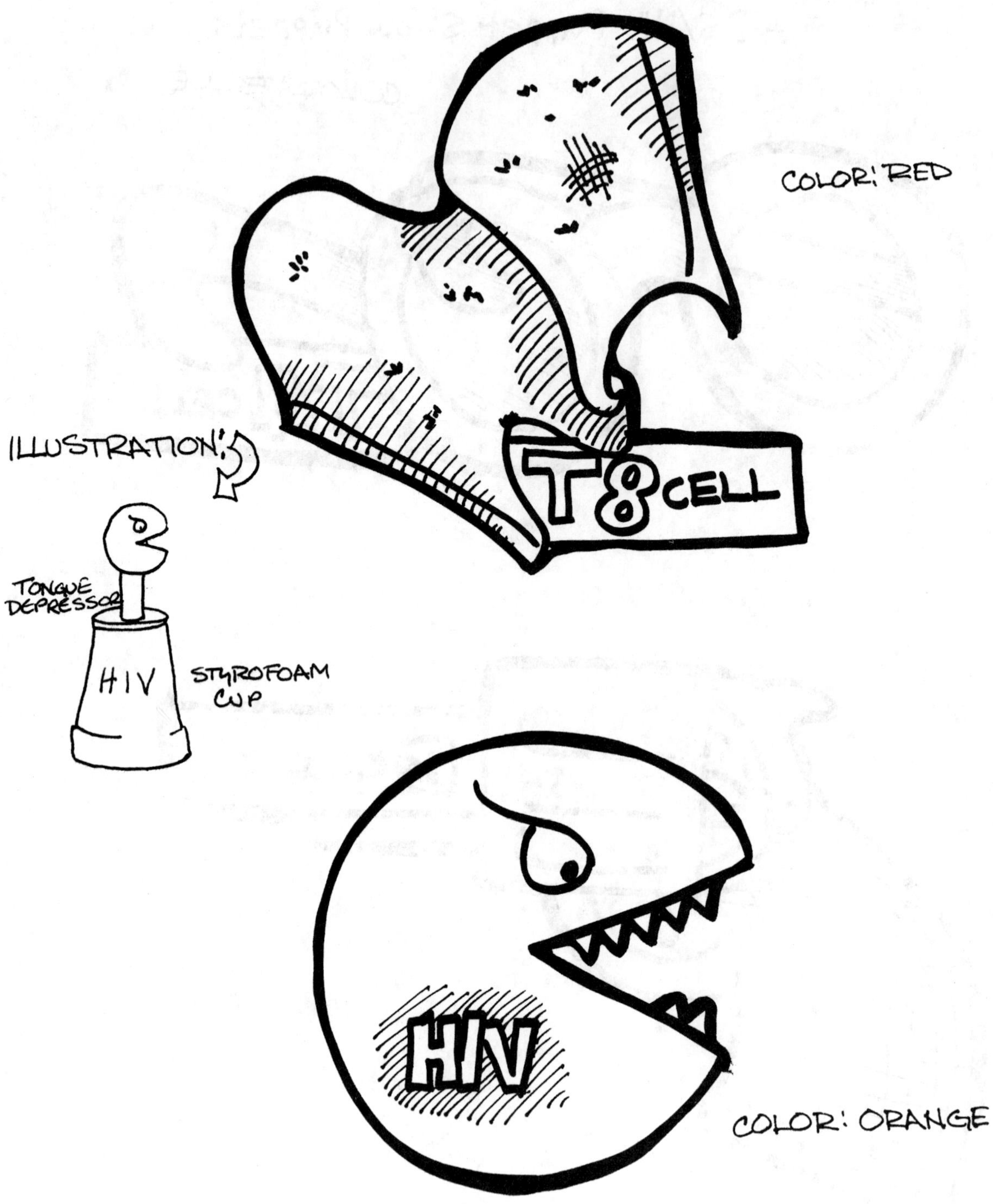
COLOR: RED
T8 CELL
ILLUSTRATION:
TONGUE DEPRESSOR
HIV
STYROFOAM CUP
HIV
COLOR: ORANGE

NAME ______________________

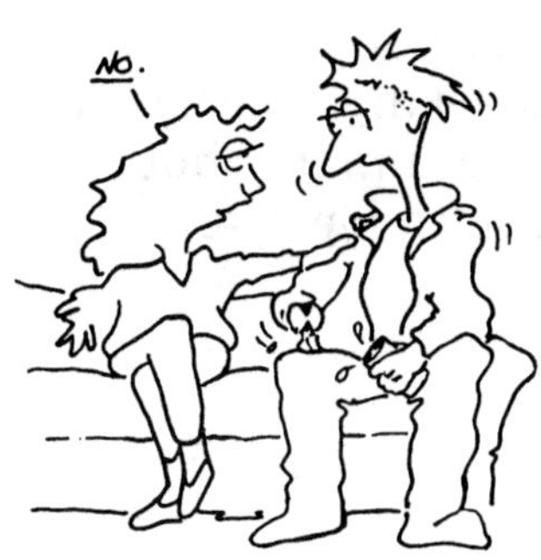

How Do You Feel?

You have just received a lot of information about sexually transmitted diseases including AIDS. Go through some of the situations below and ask yourself how you would react, keeping in mind the information you have learned about these diseases.

1. You are with a group of friends and have just decided to make this an exclusive club. Proof of membership is to become blood brothers and sisters by cutting your thumb and placing all the cut thumbs together in a pledge of loyalty.

   What are you going to do?

2. You are at camp sharing a cabin with five other teenagers. You just found out that one of your bunkmates shoots up drugs. You all share the same bathroom.

   What are you going to do?

NAME ___________________________

3. You have been dating the most popular guy in school for 3 months. Every girl has been envious of you and asking if all the rumors about his sexual abilities are true. You are not sure if the rumors about him sleeping with many girls are true. He has not pressured you to have sex . . . until tonight.

   What do you do?

4. Your uncle is dying of AIDS. You are seeing him probably for the last time. He reaches out to hug you and say good-bye.

   What should you do?

5. Your best friend tells you how much she loves her boyfriend. She and her boyfriend have thought it over and decided to have intercourse. She tells you that her boyfriend refuses to use a condom.

   What do you do?

6. There is a new girl in your room at school. She sits next to you and she confides that she had to leave her other school because people were afraid of her. She is HIV positive.

   What do you do?

NAME ______________________

Test Your Knowledge of AIDS

This is it! See if you really understand the important facts about AIDS. Just answer whether the question is true or false in the space provided.

Don't worry—you are not going to get a grade. This is for you to see if you have all the facts.

1. ____________ A person can be HIV positive and look perfectly healthy.
2. ____________ Only adults get AIDS.
3. ____________ You can catch AIDS by donating blood.
4. ____________ The HIV virus destroys the immune system in a person.
5. ____________ There is a cure for AIDS.
6. ____________ Using a condom is a sure way of preventing AIDS.
7. ____________ All types of condoms will offer some protection against AIDS.
8. ____________ Abstinence is a good way to avoid becoming infected with AIDS.
9. ____________ AIDS is caused by the human immunodeficiency virus called HIV.
10. ____________ Kissing a person with AIDS is dangerous.
11. ____________ Only people with full blown AIDS can infect other people.
12. ____________ Only homosexuals get AIDS.
13. ____________ I can take action to prevent getting AIDS.
14. ____________ People usually recover from AIDS after being very ill.
15 ____________ Only adults can get tested for AIDS.
16. ____________ HIV can be spread by using someone's personal belongings, such as a hairbrush or lipstick.
17. ____________ Most people who become infected with HIV will usually develop AIDS in the future.
18. ____________ I can avoid becoming infected with HIV by exercising regularly.
19. ____________ HIV infection is not as big a problem as the media makes it out to be.
20. ____________ I need to be aware of and knowledgeable about HIV infections and AIDS.

NAME ______________________________

An Innocent Date

Read the following story about a teenager preparing for a date with her boyfriend. Underline all the preparations that seem to be risky. Circle those preparations that may be dangerous.

Julie is so excited to be going out with Jake! She has been trying to get his attention for several weeks. She realizes tonight is the perfect night for this date because she doesn't have her period and she feels great.

Jake is going to pick her up at 7:00 p.m. so Julie jumps into the shower at 5:00 p.m. to start getting ready. She washes her hair and shaves her legs, making sure she shaves up to the top of her thighs even though she doesn't usually shave that high. She puts extra rinse on her hair to make sure it smells really good.

After showering, she picks out her sexiest pair of black lace panties and bra. She puts on the panties and discards the bra, deciding that she looks too uptight with a bra. She chooses a clean blouse and skirt her friends helped pick out just for tonight. Before putting them on, she sprays perfume behind her knees and on her neck. She goes to the bathroom, brushes her hair, brushes her teeth, rinses her mouth with mouthwash, and puts on her makeup. She grabs her brush, makeup, and two condoms and stuffs them all into her purse.

She checks with her parents to make sure they are still going out for the evening and reassures herself that they won't be back until 3:00 a.m. Julie sneaks a pint of rum out of the liquor cabinet in case the evening gets dull and hides it in her purse. She sits down to wait for Jake and giggles at how she got her little brother to spend the night at Grandma's. She is all set for this date. She is eager to make a good impression.

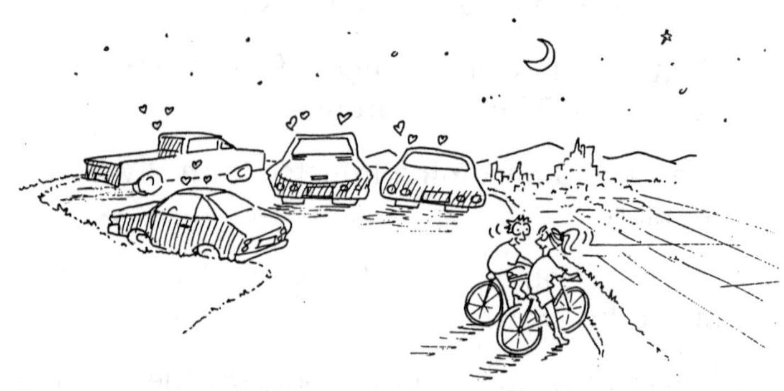

NAME ______________________

That was how Julie prepared for the evening. Let's see what Jake was doing to get ready. Underline the preparations he makes that might lead to trouble later. Circle the preparations that seem dangerous.

Jake is really excited to go out with Julie. He has had his eye on her for quite a while but had to get his courage up to ask her out. He was surprised when she said yes. He made arrangements to go to dinner with Joe and Diane so they can all feel relaxed but told Joe that he is ditching them later. He is planning on taking Julie to the drive-in movie . . . alone.

Jake washes and dries his car. He gets the vacuum out for the big job of getting the inside of the car presentable. He checks the mechanism on the front seat that lowers the seat back and decides it needs oil. He makes sure the seat pushes up and back easily. Jake checks the glove compartment to make sure he has a box of condoms available and that they are not too old. He stashes a fifth of good vodka under the seat in case Julie wants a drink during the date. He wants everything to be just right.

Jake is a little behind schedule so he rushes into the shower, towels off, and brushes his teeth. He checks his face for stubble and decides to leave the few whiskers because it makes him look more mature. He puts on his sexiest shirt that is cut low enough to show the hair that is sprouting on his chest. Jake tears through the pile of clothes at the bottom of his closet to find his favorite black jeans that hang just right on his hips and make his butt look so tight—or at least that's what his last girlfriend, Mary, said.

Jake combs his hair and grabs the keys to his car and starts out the door. He runs back to his room to pick up the clutter and straighten his bed in case Julie wants to see his room later. He checks his pocket for the house key. He congratulates himself again on not having to spend the weekend with his family at the cabin—he has the house all to himself.

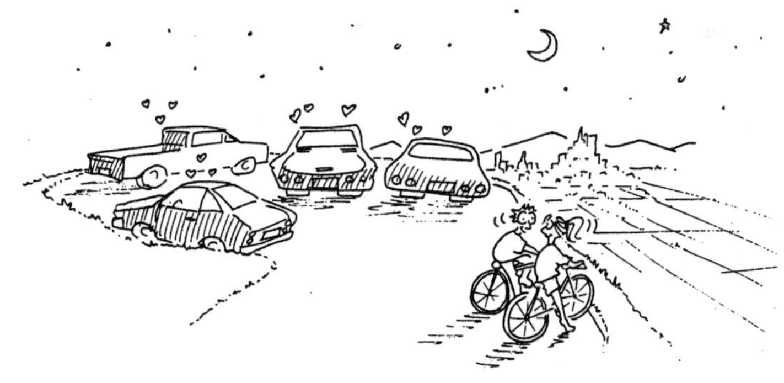

NAME ______________________________

Why Choose Abstinence?

Abstinence is choosing not to have sexual intercourse. Choosing to be abstinent can be a sign of emotional maturity and integrity. It takes maturity and honesty to resist the pressure imposed by someone you love and make a decision that will be consistent with your own values and needs.

Think of some reasons why it would be better for you to delay sexual intercourse in a relationship during adolescence.

Personal reasons: ______________________________

____

____

Financial reasons: ______________________________

____

____

Relationship reasons: ______________________________

____

____

Social reasons: ______________________________

____

____

How could abstinence affect your future and your goals? ______________________________

____

____

____

NAME ______________________________

Last Saturday

Write down everything you did last Saturday. Start at 1:00 a.m.—in the middle of the night. Be as specific as you can. Write down how you felt as you went through the activities of the day.

Last Saturday:

Time	I was doing . . .	I was feeling . . .
1:00 a.m.		
2:00 a.m.		
3:00 a.m.		
4:00 a.m.		
5:00 a.m.		
6:00 a.m.		
7:00 a.m.		
8:00 a.m.		
9:00 a.m.		
10:00 a.m.		
11:00 a.m.		
12:00 noon		

NAME ______________________________

1:00 p.m.		
2:00 p.m.		
3:00 p.m.		
4:00 p.m.		
5:00 p.m.		
6:00 p.m.		
7:00 p.m.		
8:00 p.m.		
9:00 p.m.		
10:00 p.m.		
11:00 p.m.		
12:00 midnight		

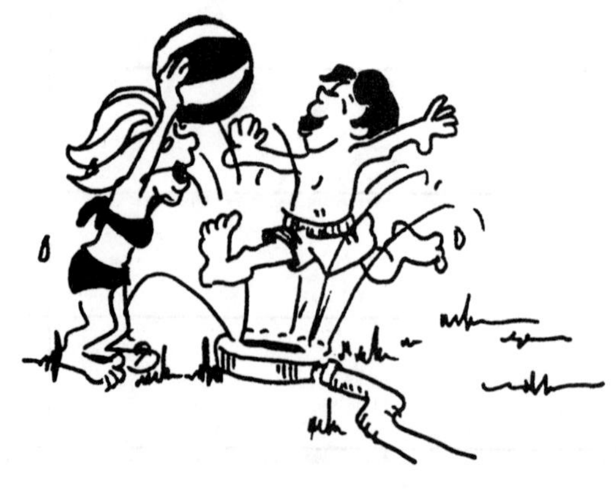

NAME ____________________

Last Saturday with a Baby

How would your life be different if you had a baby? Assume that the child is your responsibility and you alone must tend the baby. Remember to feed the baby, change diapers, comfort the baby, and take the baby outside for a while. Remember to take care of your needs but you will have to fit them in around those of the baby.

Last Saturday with a baby:

Time	I was doing . . .	I was feeling . . .
1:00 a.m.		
2:00 a.m.		
3:00 a.m.		
4:00 a.m.		
5:00 a.m.		
6:00 a.m.		
7:00 a.m.		
8:00 a.m.		
9:00 a.m.		
10:00 a.m.		
11:00 a.m.		
12:00 noon		

NAME ______________________________

1:00 p.m.		
2:00 p.m.		
3:00 p.m.		
4:00 p.m.		
5:00 p.m.		
6:00 p.m.		
7:00 p.m.		
8:00 p.m.		
9:00 p.m.		
10:00 p.m.		
11:00 p.m.		
12:00 midnight		

How do you feel after comparing the two views of last Saturday?

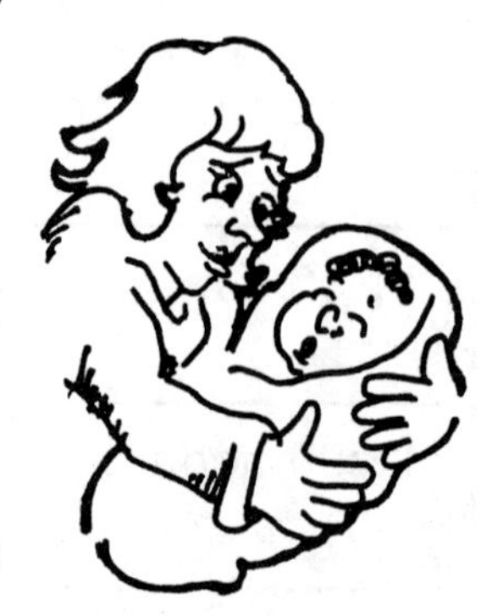

NAME ______________________

Baby Journal

Opinion before Parenting

______________ What is your age now?

______________ Do you plan to have children?

______________ If you answered yes, how many do you want? At what age do you want to have your first child? ______________

Why is it recommended that two adults raise children? ______________________

____

____

____

How do you think having a baby affects a couple's relationship? ______________

____

____

____

How does an extended family (relatives, friends) affect the baby? ______________

____

____

____

How many hours a day (on average) do you think are required to care for a new baby? ______________

Note any profound thoughts and comments on parenting before the actual experience.

____

____

____

NAME ______________________________

Parenting Contract

I, ______________________________, agree to accept full responsibility for my child, and promise to do the following:

1. I will take care of my baby as if he or she was a real, live baby and my own child.
2. I will carry my baby and all of the items needed to care for him or her with me wherever I go.
3. I will never abuse or neglect my baby. I will treat him or her gently and patiently.
4. I will protect my baby from other people who may do harm to my baby.
5. I will keep a daily log of the feeding and diaper changes required for my baby.
6. I promise to do my best to be a responsible parent.

Signed ______________________________

Witness ______________________________ Date ______________________________

NAME ____________________

Birth Certificate

This certifies that ____________________
was born on __________ *the* __________ *day*
of ______________, *in the year* ________.

This baby was born in ______________ *county at*
____
while in attendance in the ______________
class at said institution.

The parent's name is ____________________

The baby's weight at birth is ________ *lb.* ________ *oz.*
The baby's length at birth is ________ *inches.*

NAME ______________________

Baby Journal

Daily Log

Day number:

Feeding Times

____

____

____

Diaper Change Times

____

____

____

Daily Activities

____

____

____

____

____

Expenditures

____

____

____

Items Purchased

____

____

____

Important Addresses and Phone Numbers

____

____

____

Emergency Phone Numbers

____

____

____

NAME ______________________________

Incident Report
Child Protective Services

Date of the incident: ____________ Person reporting the incident: ____________________

Name of parent being cited: ____

Name of the baby: ____

Description of the incident in question:

____

____

____

____

____

Witnesses to the incident in question:

______________________ ______________________

______________________ ______________________

Official Use Only

Recommendations:

Signature of official:

____

NAME ______________________________

Interview an Exceptional Parent

Conduct an interview with a real parent who demonstrates exceptional parenting skills. Ask them the following questions and record their answers.

How would you describe the job of parenting?

What are some of the benefits of being a parent?

What is the optimal age to begin parenting?

What are the benefits of having two people parent a child?

What are some of the difficulties involved in parenting?

What special skills are necessary to be a good parent?

What advice would you give to young people about parenting?

NAME ______________________________

How Much Do Children Cost?

Find the prices for each of the items listed below. Check stores, talk to new parents, and look at newspaper ads for prices.

Product	**Price**	**Product**	**Price**
Formula for one month		Crib	
Bottles (10)		Mattress	
Baby vitamins		Plastic mattress cover	
Infant cereal		Sheets	
Bibs (6)		Blanket	
Bathtub for baby		Bumper pads	
Baby oil		Cloth diapers (12)	
Baby powder		Disposable diapers	
Desitin		Diaper service (1 month)	
Q-Tips (cotton swabs)		Baby wipes	
Receiving blanket		Diaper pail	
Undershirts (10)		Changing table	
Sleepers (5)		Stroller	
Booties		Car seat	
Hat		Washer	
Sweater or jacket		Dryer	
Socks		Doctor examination	
Nail clippers		Cost of delivery	
Tweezers		Hospital expenses	

NAME ____________________

Baby Journal

Opinion after Parenting

Answer the questions below after taking care of your baby for 5 days. See if your thoughts about parenting have changed.

__________ Do you plan to have children?

__________ If you answered yes, how many do you want? At what age do you want to have your first child? __________.

Why is it recommended that two adults raise children? ____________________

____

____

____

How do you think having a baby affects a couple's relationship? ____________________

____

____

____

How does an extended family (relatives, friends) affect the baby? ____________________

____

____

____

How many hours a day (on average) do you think are required to care for a new baby? __________

How is tending your pretend baby like caring for a real baby? ____________________

____

____

____

NAME ____________________

Explain how caring for your pretend baby is different than caring for a real baby?

Note any profound thoughts and comments on parenting *after* the actual experience.

List some of the benefits of being a parent.

List some of the disadvantages of parenting.

List some of the benefits of waiting until you are really ready to accept the responsibilities of being a parent.

When is the *best* time to have a baby? Why?

Thank you for your courage and enthusiasm in participating in this simulation.

In order to get a more beneficial experience from this simulation, compare your parenting to that of your own parents. Ask them how their experience with you as a baby was the same or different. Were they scared or embarrassed at times? How did they cope?

NAME ______________________________

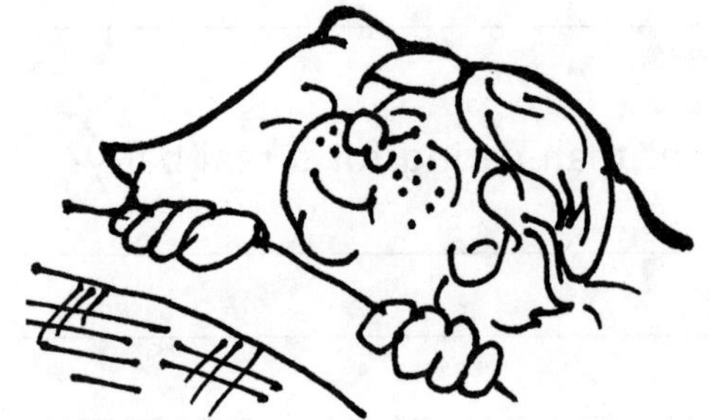

Am I Healthy?

Answer the questions below about the choices you make concerning your health. Check how often you do each of the things listed below.

	ALWAYS	SOMETIMES	NEVER
1. I get seven to eight hours of sleep every night.			
2. I eat breakfast before school.			
3. I try to stay away from fatty foods.			
4. I limit the amount of fast foods as I make food choices throughout the week.			
5. I eat something from each of the food groups every day.			
6. I get adequate exercise every day.			
7. I stay away from cigarettes and other tobacco products.			

NAME ____________________

	ALWAYS	SOMETIMES	NEVER
8. I stay away from alcohol and drugs.			
9. I make sure that my body and clothes are clean.			
10. I brush my teeth every day.			
11. I limit the amount of television I watch and balance that time with exercise.			
12. I wear a helmet when riding my bike.			
13. I wear a seat belt when riding in the car.			
14. I make decisions based on my own needs and not the pressure of friends.			
15. I evaluate dangerous situations for my safety before taking risks.			

NAME ____________________

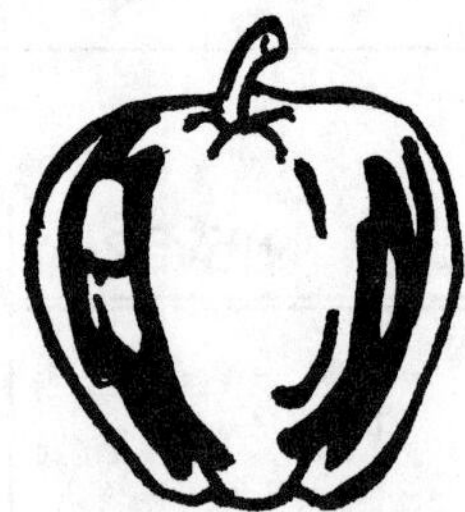

A Pound of Fat

In order to gain 1 pound, you must take in 3,500 calories. If you want to lose 1 pound, you must use up 3,500 more calories than you take into your body. A calorie is a measure of body heat produced when you consume a certain amount of food. One calorie is the amount of food necessary to raise the temperature of 1 square inch of water 1 degree.

Figure out the answers to the following problems concerning weight loss and weight gain.

Assumption: 3,500 calories equals 1 pound of body weight.

Fact: To maintain good health, lose no more than 2 pounds a week.

1. You normally consume 2,500 calories a day. You normally use about 2,500 calories a day but have increased your physical activity recently and use 3,000 calories a day. How many days will it take to lose 1 pound?

   ____

2. If you continued exercising and burning 3,000 calories, how could you lose one more pound in a week?

   ____

3. How many pounds will you lose in a week if you increase the number of calories you use each day by 500, and you decrease the amount of calories you consume by 500?

   ____

4. Following the weight loss plan above, how many pounds will you lose in 4 weeks? In a year? (52 weeks)

   ____

5. Write a general description of a safe and healthy plan to lose 10 pounds and tell how long it will take to accomplish the goal.

NAME ___________________________

Food Diary

Write down all the food that you consumed yesterday from the moment you woke up in the morning until you went to bed at night. List every cookie, candy bar, French fry, and soda. Place a check mark in the box for the groups that each food item satisfies.

Foods consumed	Grain	Veggies	Fruits	Dairy	Meat	Extra
Totals						

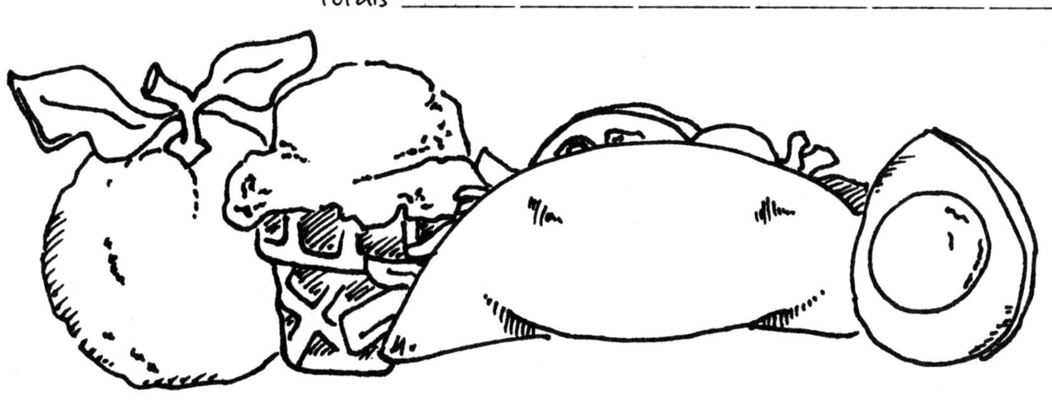

NAME ________________________________

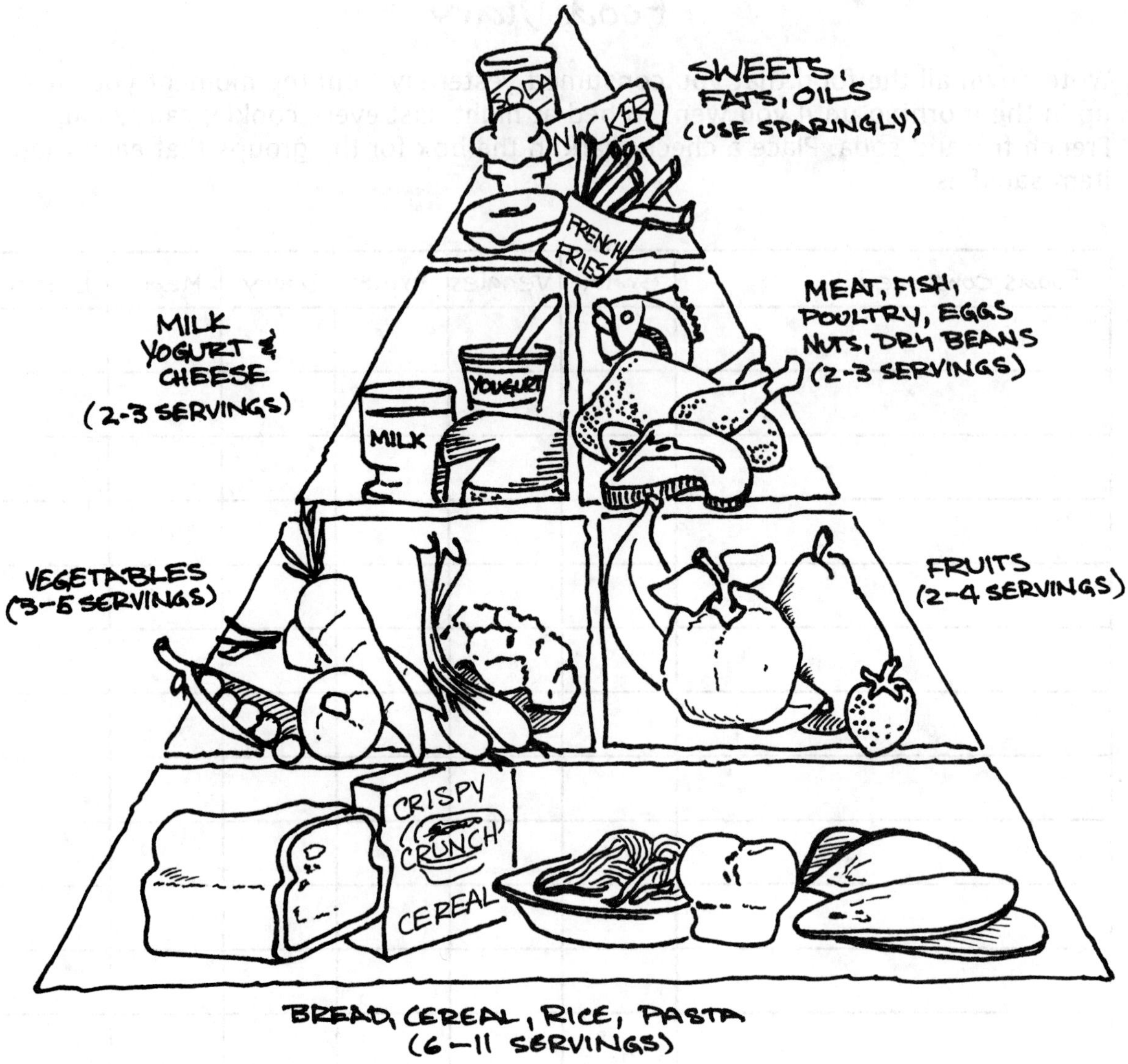

SWEETS, FATS, OILS (USE SPARINGLY)
SODA
SNICKERS
FRENCH FRIES
MILK YOGURT & CHEESE (2-3 SERVINGS)
YOGURT
MILK
MEAT, FISH, POULTRY, EGGS NUTS, DRY BEANS (2-3 SERVINGS)
VEGETABLES (3-5 SERVINGS)
FRUITS (2-4 SERVINGS)
CRISPY CRUNCH CEREAL
BREAD, CEREAL, RICE, PASTA (6-11 SERVINGS)

FOOD PYRAMID GUIDE

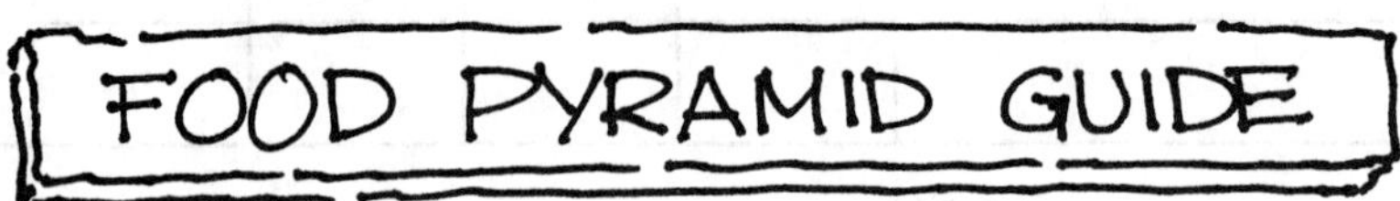

NAME ______________________________

Foods and the Uses to the Body

FOOD GROUP	PROVIDES	USE IN BODY	FOODS
Bread, Cereal, Pasta 6-11 servings	Complex Carbohydrate	Good source of energy	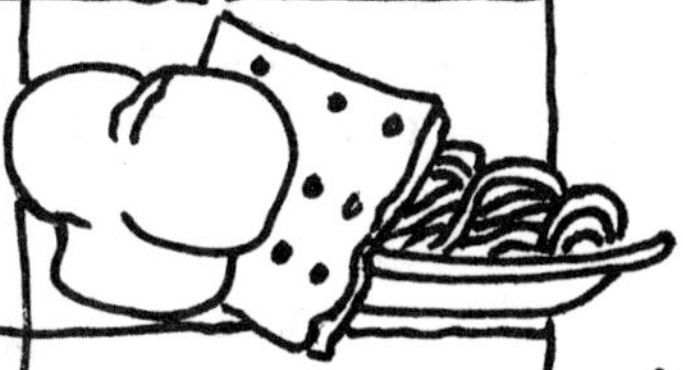
Vegetables 3-5 servings	Water, roughage vitamins, minerals	Cleans digestive system, helps body function normally	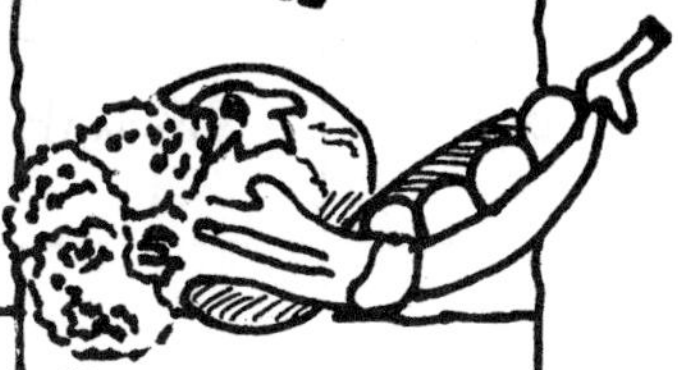
Fruits 2-4 servings	Water, roughage vitamins, minerals	Cleans digestive system, helps body function normally	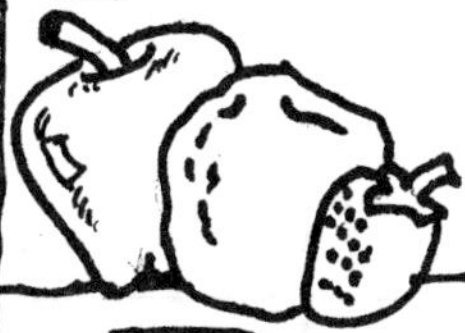
Milk, Cheese, Yogurt 2-3 servings	Calcium, Vitamin B2	Builds strong bones , B2 converts food to energy	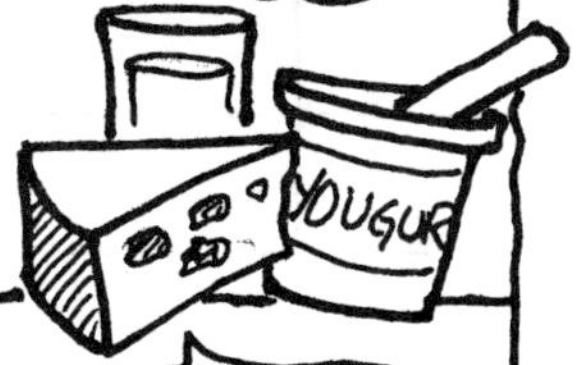 YOUGUR
Meat, Fish, Dry Beans, Nuts, Eggs 2-3 servings	Protein, Amino Acids	Growth and repair of muscle tissue	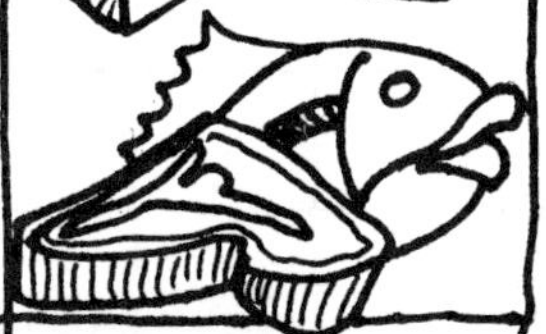
Fat use sparingly	Lipids	Part of every cell, aid in getting vitamins into body	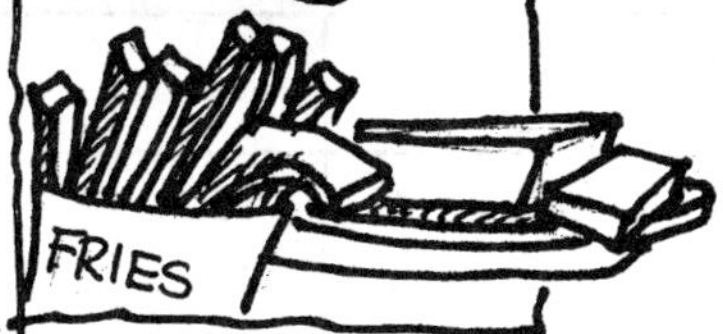 FRIES
Water 6 8oz servings	Essential Liquid	Part of every cell, aids in digestion, transport nutrients	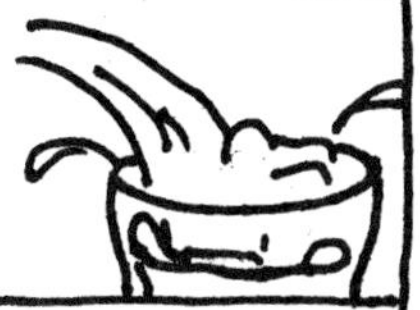
Extra Foods use sparingly	Sugars and Fats	Empty calories, cause high cholesterol	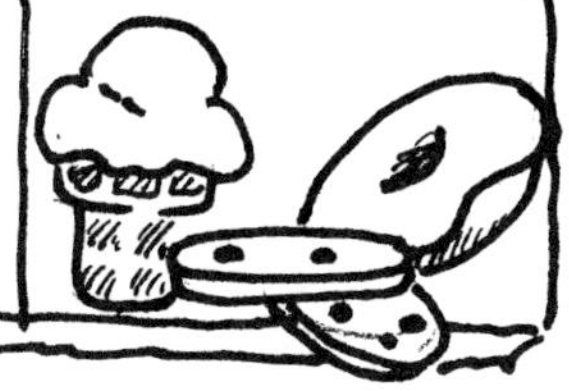

NAME ____________________

My Activity Level

Using the chart below, write down everything you eat for one day on the left-hand side of the chart. Write down all the activities you do during the day on the right-hand side of the chart. Use the "Sample Calorie Chart" and "Caloric Output for Exercise" handouts to determine the number of calories consumed and burned. Total both columns and circle the higher total.

Calories Consumed			Calories Used		
Food	Amount	Number Calories	Activity	Time	Calories Used

Total ____________ Total ____________

Have you maintained your weight? Or did you gain or lose weight? ____________

NAME ____________________

Sample Calorie Chart

Breakfast:	
Bagel	163
Bagel with cream cheese	263
Cereal with milk	180
English muffin with butter	189
Pancakes with butter and syrup	519
Eggs, 2 scrambled	200

Sandwiches:	
Cheeseburger	320
Cheeseburger with bacon	608
Chicken filet	515
Fish filet	431
Hamburger	279
Ham and cheese	350
Hot dog	242
Hot dog with chili	324
The following sandwiches are on whole wheat bread	
BLT	290
Bologna	305
Chicken salad	255
Corned beef	296
Cream cheese and jelly	370
Peanut butter and jelly	385
Roast beef with gravy	421
Tunafish	275

Condiments:	
Butter	100
Catsup	3
Mayonnaise	81
Mustard	4
Sugar	25

Mexican Foods:	
Burritos	
Bean	448
Bean and meat	508
Beef	523
Chimichanga with beef	425
Enchilada with cheese and beef	324
Nachos with cheese	345
Taco with beef	425

Other:	
Chicken nuggets	290
Pizza with cheese (1 slice)	110
Shrimp (breaded and fried)	454

Desserts:	
Brownie	243
Pies	266
Ice cream cone	230
Vanilla shake	350

Side Orders:	
Chili	268
Coleslaw	147
Corn on the cob with butter	155
Potato, baked with sour cream	394
Potatoes, French fried	325
Potato chips	148

NAME ______________________________

Caloric Output for Exercise

This chart is based on calories used by a 160 pound adult. The bigger and more vigorous you are, the more calories you will use for an activity.

Activity:	Calories/Hr.	Average Calories Used
Sleeping	65	520 (for 8 hours)
Watching television	80	80 (for 1 hour)
Shopping	165	165 (for 1 hour)
Bowling	190	190 (for 1 hour)
Dancing (slow)	250	105 (for 5 dances)
Dancing (fast)	445	222 (for ½ hour)
Walking, 25 min./mile	255	127 (for ½ hour)
Walking, 15 min./mile	345	172 (for ½ hour)
Baseball (not pitching or catching)	280	560 (for 2 hours)
Weight training	300	150 (for ½ hour)
Swimming, moderate	300	150 (for ½ hour)
Swimming, vigorous	600	300 (for ½ hour)
Bicycling, 6 min./mile	415	207 (for ½ hour)
Tennis	425	425 (for 1 hour)
Downhill skiing	595	1,190 (for 2 hours)
Touch football	600	300 (for ½ hour)
Soccer	600	600 (for 1 hour)
Jogging, 11 min./mile	655	327 (for ½ hour)
Basketball, full court	750	750 (for 1 hour)
Martial arts (judo, karate)	790	395 (for ½ hour)
Running, 7.5 min./mile	800	400 (for ½ hour)
Ice hockey	900	900 (for 1 hour)
Lacrosse	900	900 (for 1 hour)

NAME ______________________________

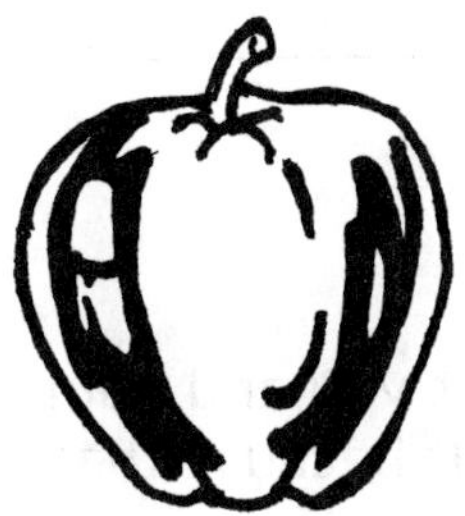

Design a Diet

Design a menu for one day that will provide all the necessary nutrients a teenage will need. Make the choices on the menu attractive so that a teenager would want to eat the food suggested.

Meal	Grains 6–11 servings	Veggies 2–5 servings	Fruits 2–4 servings	Dairy 2–4 servings	Proteins 2–3 servings
BREAKFAST					
LUNCH					
DINNER					
SNACK					

NAME ______________________

I'm the Cook

Now you can really test your skills. Design a menu for one meal that you and your family can share. You need to choose items you can prepare yourself because that is the challenge—and surprise—for your family. You are going to plan, prepare, and clean up after a meal.

Choose foods that will fill all the food groups in the pyramid so that you have a well-rounded meal. Be aware of the color of the food you choose. Try to make the meal attractive by selecting food with a variety of colors and textures. You also need to be aware of preparation and cooking time. Will everything be ready on time?

Planning Chart

Food Choices	Food Group	Color	Prep Time	Cooking Time

NAME ____________________

Target Heart Rate

Instructions	Sample for a 15-year-old	Figure yours here
Everyone starts here	220	220
Subtract your age	– 15	–
This is your maximum heart rate—the fastest your heart should beat at your age	205	
Subtract your resting heart rate	– 72	
(Answer)	133	
Choose your level of fitness. Beginning exercisers use 60% Regular exercisers use 70% Competitive athletes use 80% Multiply by the % you choose	× .70	×
(Answer)	89.13	
Add your resting heart rate in again	+ 72	+
This is your Target Heart Rate	161(.13)	
(Divide your Target Heart Rate by 6 so that you can take your pulse in 10 seconds when exercising)	÷ 6	÷ 6
This is your 10 second Target Heart Rate		☐

NAME ______________________________

Investigate Food

Watch your favorite television channel on Saturday morning and count the number of food commercials. Record the type of food promoted.

TV Channel ____________________ Time: From ________ To ________

Number of Commercials: ______________________________

Types of Foods

Food Groups	Name and Type of Food
Bread, cereal, rice, pasta	
Vegetables	
Fruits	
Dairy—milk, yogurt, cheese	
Meat, poultry, fish, dried beans, eggs	
Extras—snack food with lots of sugar, salt or fats	

Which types of foods are advertised the most?

____

____

Why do you think this happens?

____

NAME ____________________

Go to the supermarket and determine which types of foods are at eye level for kids. Record your findings below:

____

____

____

____

Generally, which products and food items are in the most convenient locations and easily reached? Record your findings below:

____

____

____

____

Why do you think the products are displayed in this way?

____

____

____

____

____

What age group do you think is targeted the most for snack foods?

1–5 years   6–10 years   11–16 years   17–25 years   26–36 years   37+

Why do you think that age group is targeted?

____

____

____

____

NAME ______________________

Become a Smart Consumer

Below is a copy of the Nutrition Facts label from a box of cereal. Answer the questions concerning that cereal.

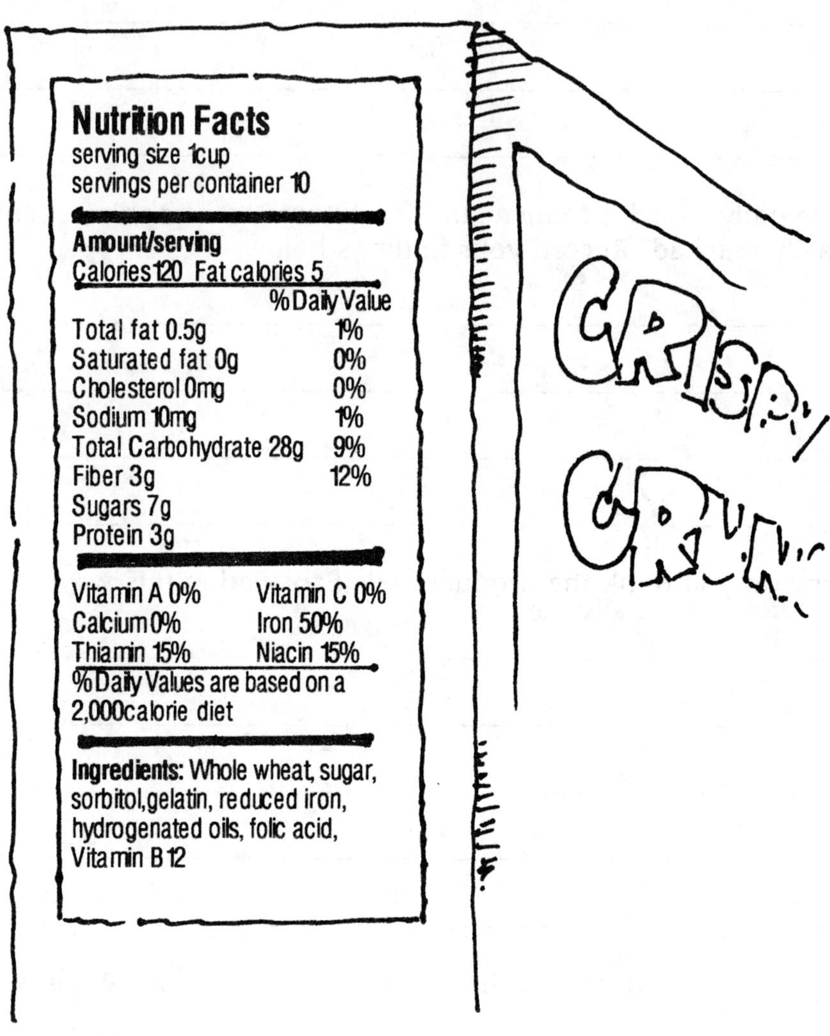

1. How many calories is each serving of cereal? ______________________
2. What is the size of one serving of cereal? ______________________
3. Is the serving size less than what you would normally eat? ______________________
4. How much sugar is in each serving? ______________________
5. How much fat is in each serving? ______________________
6. What is the major ingredient in this cereal? ______________________
7. If less than 30 percent fat is ideal for your day's total calories, is this cereal above the recommended amount of fat? ______________________

NAME ______________________________

Look at the Nutrition Facts label on five different foods. Answer the following questions concerning the information on the Nutrition Facts label.

1. Of the five foods, which has the highest number of calories per serving? ______

   ____

2. Which product has the most fat? ______________________________

3. What is the major ingredient in each of the five foods?

   a. ____

   b. ____

   c. ____

   d. ____

   e. ____

4. Which product has a serving size that seems appropriate to the amount you would normally consume?

   ____

   ____

5. Saturated fats are fats that come from animal sources such as lard, butter, and fatty meats. Partially hydrogenated sources of fat are found in coconut oil and palm oil. These fats should all be avoided. Which food is the highest in saturated fats?

   ____

6. Of the five food you are investigating, which food seems to provide the most nutrition with the least amount of harmful products? Why?

   ____

   ____

   ____

   ____

NAME ____________________

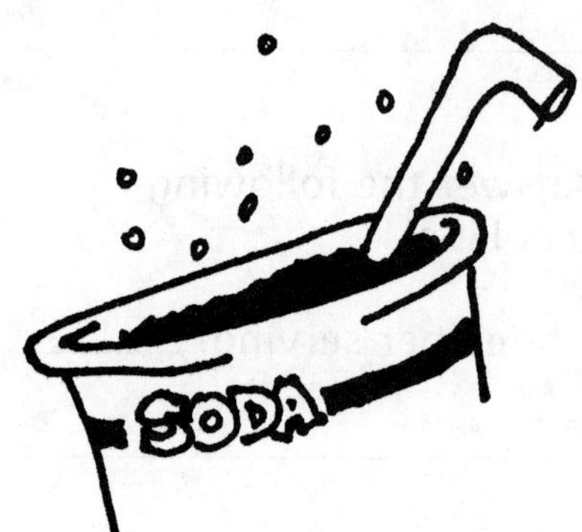

Fast Food Fun

Use the "Fast Food Guide" handout to answer the following questions:

1. Using the "Fast Food Guide," design a menu for lunch that would be under 1,000 calories and within the limits for fat and sugar. Individuals should limit fat intake to 15 teaspoons a day and sugar which contains wasted calories, to as little as possible.

2. A stick of butter (¼ lb.) contains 92 grams of fat and 810 calories. Design a common fast food meal that would equal or surpass the amount of fat and calories in a stick of butter.

3. Design a fast food dinner that would include foods from all the important categories in the food pyramid.

4. Here's a challenge for you. Assume you are on a diet and trying to lose weight. Design a tasty menu for one day—breakfast, lunch and dinner—providing fewer than 5 grams of fat and fewer that 2,200 calories *and* try to provide adequate servings of food from the food pyramid categories.

NAME ____________________

Fast Food Guide

NOTE: For a healthy diet, it is recommended that teenagers consume between 2,100–2,600 calories per day. They should have between 16–21 grams of fat and 2,000 mg of sodium. Of course, keep sugar to a minimum.

Company/Product	**Calories**	**Fat** (tsp.)	**Sugar/ Sodium**
Arby's Roast Beef, regular	353	3	0/590
Roy Roger's Roast Beef, regular	317	2	0/785
Arby's Bac'n Cheddar Deluxe Beef	561	8	0/1385
Long John Silver's Ocean Chef's Salad	229	2	0/986
Burger King Whaler Sandwich	488	6	0/592
McDonald's Filet-o-Fish	435	6	0/799
Kentucy Fried Chicken crispy drumstick	173	3	0/346
Arby's Chicken Breast, roasted	254	2	0/930
Wendy's Chicken Sandwich, multi-grain bun	320	2	0/500
Carl's Jr. Charbroiler Chicken Sandwich	450	3	0/1380
Wendy's Kid's Meal Hamburger	200	2	0/265
McDonald's Hamburger	263	3	0/506
McDonald's Quarter Pounder with Cheese	525	7	0/1220
Wendy's Triple Cheeseburger	1040	15	0/1848
Arby's French Fries	211	2	0/30
Long John Silver's Fries (no salt added)	247	3	0/6
McDonald's Fries	220	3	0/109
McDonald's Hash Brown Potatoes	144	9	0/325
Kentucky Fried Chicken Mashed Potatoes	59	1	0/228
Arby's Baked Potato, plain	290	1	0/12

NAME ______________________

Burger King Onion Rings, regular	274	16	0/655
Jack in the Box Club Pita	284	8	0/953
Jack in the Box Taco, regular	191	11	0/406
Jack in the Box Taco Salad	377	24	0/1436
Kentucky Fried Chicken Coleslaw	105	6	0/171
Roy Rogers' Breakfast Crescent Sandwich	401	27	0/867
Roy Rogers' Egg and Biscuit Platter	394	27	0/734
Wendy's French Toast (no syrup)	400	19	0/850
Wendy's Omelet with Ham and Chesse	250	21	0/570
McDonald's Sausage McMuffin with Egg	517	33	0/1045
McDonald's Hotcakes with syrup and butter	500	10	40/1070
Arby's Coke, medium, 16 fl. oz.	128	0	32/0
McDonald's Vanilla Shake, 10.2 fl. oz.	352	8	32/201
Roy Rogers' Chocolate Shake, 11.25 fl. oz.	358	10	39/290
Roy Rogers' Milk, 8 fl. oz.	150	8	0/120
Wendy's Orange Juice, 6 fl. oz.	80	0	0/0
Long John Silver's Cherry Pie	294	11	15/251
Dairy Queen Banana Split	540	11	30/150
Dairy Queen Mr. Misty, regular	250	0	63/trace
Dairy Queen Soft Ice Cream Cone, regular	240	7	30/80
Carl's Jr. Carrot Cake	50	18	14/375

NAME ______________________________

Fast Food Survey

Approach family members, relatives, friends, and teachers to survey their preferences in fast food. Record the names of five fast food restaurants in your community at the top of each column. Write in the items on the menus that are favorites. Survey at least fifteen different people.

← Restaurants →

Food ↕

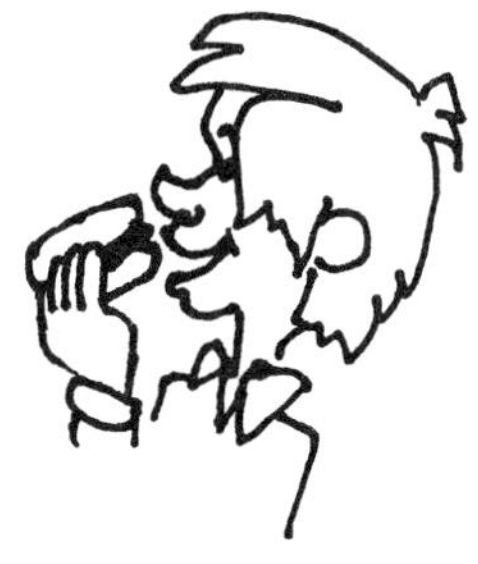

NAME ______________________________

Workout!

ACTIVITY	TIME	EQUIPMENT	SAFETY	REWARD
Monday				
Tuesday				
Wednesday				
Thursday				
Friday				
Saturday				
Sunday				

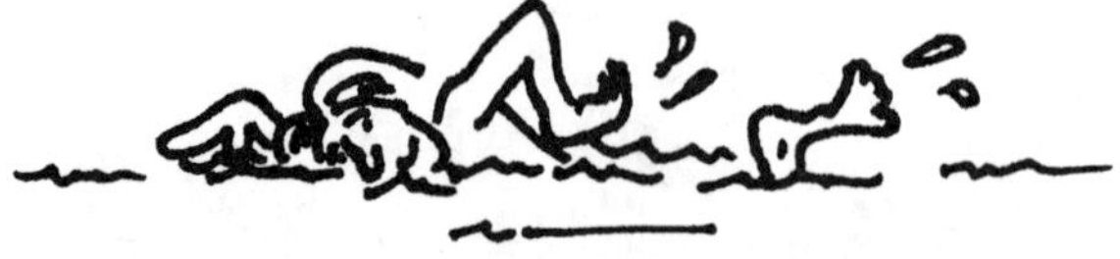

NAME ____________________

"Rube Goldberg" Gym Equipment

Pretend that you do not have the super chrome plated, advertised on television type gym equipment but still want to participate in a sport. Use your imagination and improvise the equipment you need from household products. Remember, If you want it bad enough, you will think of a way. Use the worksheet to illustrate your design:

NAME ______________________

The Ultimate Me!

Use the space below to form an image of yourself as you would like to be. Draw or use cut out pictures from magazines to create an image of yourself in peak condition. Use this image as a goal. Remember that in setting goals, your choices need to be realistic and achievable.

My goal for a healthy body:

My realistic methods for achieving my goal: ______________________

NAME ____________________

What's Available?

Make a list of all the activities that are available to you in your community. Check out the clubs available at school; look into the YMCA or YWCA; check the phone book for private dance or gymnastics clubs; look in your community for ice skating or roller skating rinks. Use the space below to form your activity list.

Name & Address	Type of Activity	Phone Number	Hours & Cost

NAME ______________________________

Good Grooming Habits

Listed below are things that you should do each day to practice good personal grooming habits. Use the list to check your own habits each day.

Personal Hygiene and Good Grooming Practices

	Mon.	Tues.	Wed.	Thurs.	Fri.	Sat.	Sun.
Clean hair							
Brush or comb hair							
Brush teeth (after each meal)							
Shower or bathe							
Use deodorant							
Scrub face							
Clean hands and fingernails							
Clean clothes							
Get proper nutrition							
Use good posture							
Have positive attitude							

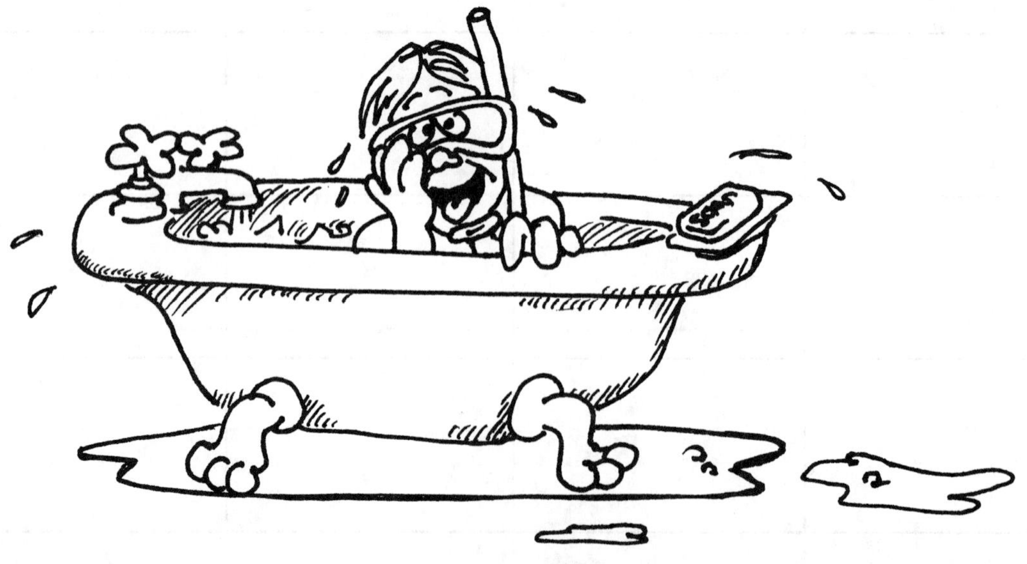

NAME ______________________

Preparation for a Date

What efforts would you make to look your best if you had the date of your dreams? On the list below, explain what you would do to prepare for that special date.

Hair care	
Skin	
Fingernails and hands	
Whole body	
Teeth	
Posture	
Nutrition	
Clothing	
General appearance	
Anything extra	

You made all those preparations for your dream date. What type of impression would you make on people if you did all those things every day?

NAME ____________________

I Can Improve

Follow the steps listed below for acquiring new personal grooming habits. Keep a log each day for a week in each of the categories.

Identify the new skill or habit to be learned:

Efforts toward achieving the new skill or practice:
People to go to for information and support:
Helpful reminders:
Reward for success:
Thoughts and feelings:

NAME ______________________________

Friends and Family Diagram

Friends:

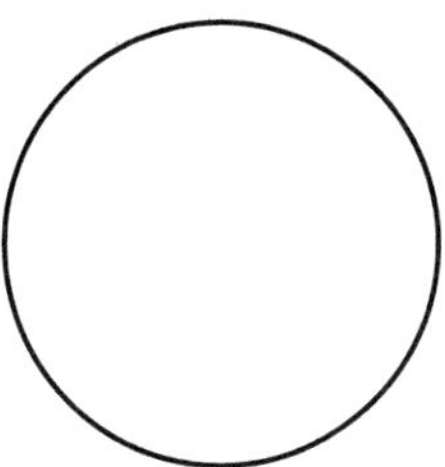

Family:

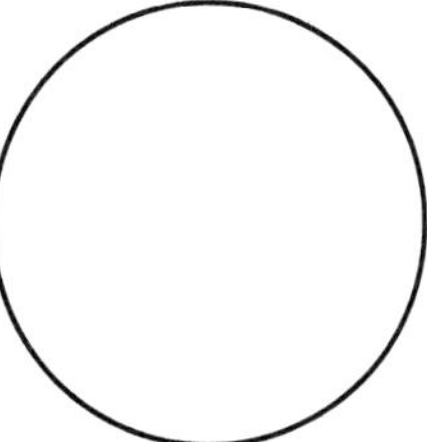

Adapted from *Can I Handle Alcohol/Drugs? A Self-Assessment Guide for Youth,* 1987, Johnson Institute, Minneapolis, MN.

NAME ______________________

Your Risks

Think about the phases of substance use. Write a brief description of the behavior of a person at each stage of substance abuse:

Experimentation:

Misuse:

Abuse:

Addiction:

Use a phone book or talk to adults to make a list of people or agencies available in your community for support and help if you need it. Some common agencies are listed. Look up the phone numbers for those.

Alcoholics Anonymous

Alateen

Al-Anon

Mothers Against Drunk Driving (MADD)

Students Against Drunk Driving (SADD)

D.A.R.E.

Make your own list, including adults such as teachers, counselors, or clergy who might be helpful.

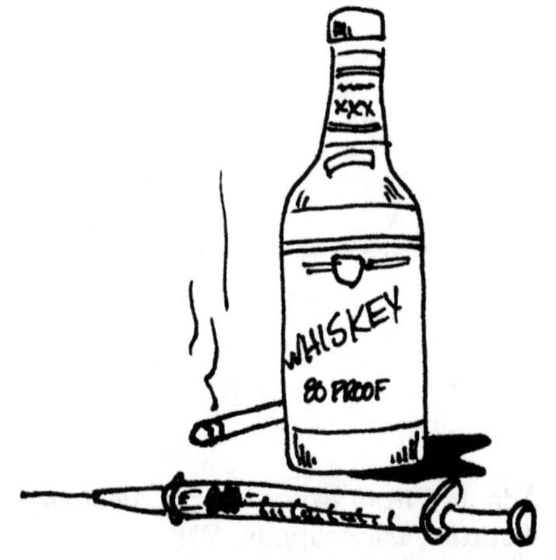

NAME ______________________________

Feelings Continuum

There are no right or wrong answers to this activity. Think about how you feel in each of the situations listed below. Record those feelings on the continuum below by writing the letter of the situation on the continuum in the appropriate place for you.

A. receiving your report card

B. your birthday

C. first day of a new year at school

D. a regular day at school

E. last day of school in the year

F. getting ready for a party

G. attending a family dinner

H. New Year's day

I. an evening with your family

J. a night at the movies with friends

K. being picked for a team at school

L. getting up in the morning

M. doing homework

N. watching television in the evening

O. after school just before dinner

P. going to bed at night

Q. doing daily chores at home

R. walking with friends

S. a family vacation

T. asked out on a date

U. receiving recognition or an award

V. lunch time at school

Place the letter of each of the experiences along the continuum where you feel it belongs between painful to joyful.

PAINFUL ———————————————————— JOYFUL

Explain how you deal with painful experiences.

Think about how you could better deal with those painful experiences. List five ways that you could feel better after experiencing something painful.

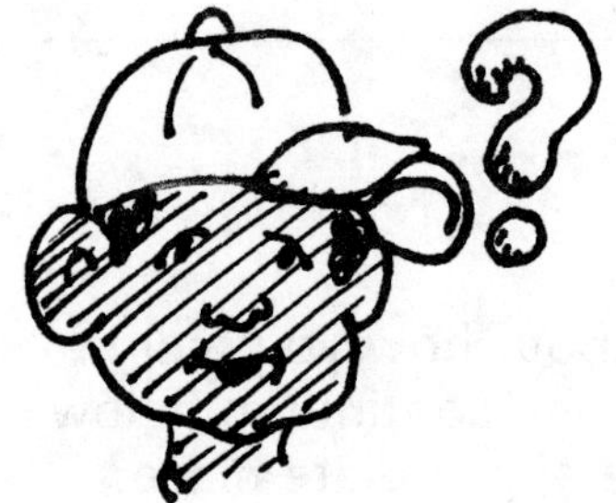

NAME ______________________________

Checklist of Traits

Below is a list of traits dealing with how you view yourself. Check only the traits that apply to you.

- ❑ Loyal
- ❑ Responsible
- ❑ Honest
- ❑ Unlikable
- ❑ Ambitious
- ❑ Shy
- ❑ Weak
- ❑ Sexy
- ❑ Poor student
- ❑ Bad temper
- ❑ Lots of interests
- ❑ Flexible
- ❑ Confident
- ❑ Out of control
- ❑ Hard worker
- ❑ Creative
- ❑ Attractive
- ❑ Likable
- ❑ Reliable
- ❑ Friendly
- ❑ Stubborn
- ❑ Boring
- ❑ Dumb
- ❑ Smart
- ❑ Ugly
- ❑ Outgoing
- ❑ Powerful
- ❑ Insecure
- ❑ Good sense of humor
- ❑ Controlling
- ❑ Imaginative
- ❑ Loving

What general opinion do you have of yourself?

____

____

____

NAME ______________________

Ad-Lib

Below is a list of techniques used by advertisers to promote their products. Use this list in evaluating commercials and advertisements you see every day.

1. Bandwagon. This method tries to convince you that everyone is buying the product and you need to hurry so you won't be left out.

   Examples: ______________________

2. Fantasy. You imagine yourself in the surroundings or using the product.

   Examples: ______________________

3. Humor. The more you laugh at or with the commercial, the more you will remember it.

   Examples: ______________________

4. Nostalgia. Helps you to remember or relive the good old days. This is often very back-to-nature or country oriented.

   Examples: ______________________

5. Sense appeal. You feel, smell, taste, hear, and generally experience the product.

   Examples: ______________________

6. Special effects. Fantastic technical effects are used to make the product memorable and appealing.

   Examples: ______________________

7. Statistics and comparisons. Statements of results from studies "proving" the validity and merit of a product. Uses a lot of numbers to sound impressive. Many times only a portion of the complete information is used so it can be misleading. One product says that their brand is better than Brand X.

   Examples: ______________________

8. Symbols. The ad emphasizes a brand logo or a catchy saying.

   Examples: ______________________

9. Testimonial. An important or famous person says they use the product and so should you.

   Examples: ______________________

10. Transfer and sex appeal. Handsome men and women, or rich and powerful people, are used to make you feel that if you use the product you, too, will be beautiful, rich, or powerful.

    Examples: ______________________

NAME ________________

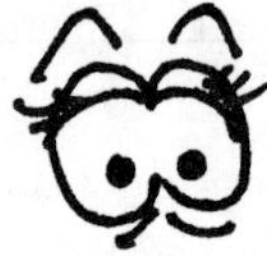

Consumer Awareness

Make a list of popular advertisements and commercials and tell what technique has been used to sell the product.

Advertisement/Commercial	Sales Technique

Use the guide below as you watch three commercials on television and analyze the technique used to sell the product.

☞ Name the product ________________

Briefly describe the ad or commercial ________________

____

What is the age group and population being targeted? ________________

____

Is the ad or commercial a realistic portrayal of life? Why? ________________

Why? ________________

The ad or commercial appeals to what basic need or desire? Why? ________________

____

Do you think the ad or commercial will be successful? Why? ________________

Why? ________________

NAME ______________________________

☞ Name the product ______________________________

Briefly describe the ad or commercial ______________________________

____

What is the age group and population being targeted? ______________________________

____

Is the ad or commercial a realistic portrayal of life? Why? ______________________________

Why? ______________________________

The ad or commercial appeals to what basic need or desire? Why? ______________________________

____

Do you think the ad or commercial will be successful? Why? ______________________________

Why? ______________________________

☞ Name the product ______________________________

Briefly describe the ad or commercial ______________________________

____

What is the age group and population being targeted? ______________________________

____

Is the ad or commercial a realistic portrayal of life? Why? ______________________________

Why? ______________________________

The ad or commercial appeals to what basic need or desire? Why? ______________________________

____

Do you think the ad or commercial will be successful? Why? ______________________________

Why? ______________________________

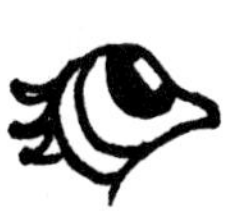

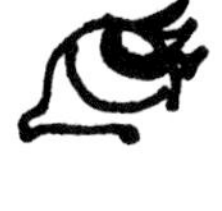

NAME ______________________________

Commercial Guide

Use this paper as a guide to plan your commercial.

Name and description of the product and its use: ______________________________

____

____

____

____

Story board of the action in the commercial:

NAME ____________________

Age group of the target group: ____________________

____

Population targeted: ____________________

____

____

Advertising technique used in promotion of the product:

____

____

Materials needed for production:

____

____

NAME ____________________

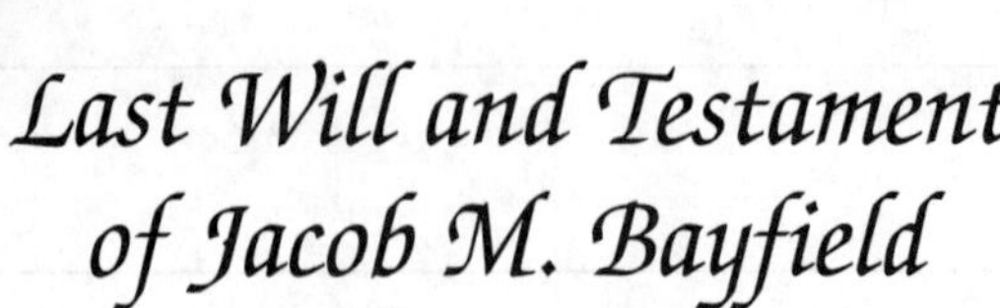

Last Will and Testament of Jacob M. Bayfield

I, Jacob M. Bayfield, being of sound mind but unhealthy body, do hereby declare that my entire estate be left to but one of my four children. This one child will be my sole heir and benefactor. All property and holdings will be left to this person.

A person's life is often best remembered by the deeds he or she has done and the lifestyle in which he or she has lived. While my business has prospered, and I have gained power beyond most, I have not set health and fitness as a personal goal. As a young boy, I started smoking. At that time we had no knowledge of the harm that smoking could cause. Rather than listen to medical experts and my own family, I continued to smoke for the rest of my life. And now I am sure, according to medical statistics, that this habit will lead to my premature death.

Therefore, I set before this court the task of determining which of my four children is the healthiest and least likely to become a smoker, being able to resist the influences to smoke which I could not. His or her life should be an example of good health and represent positive influences on the communities in which he or she lives. My entire estate will then be given to that child so that my wealth can be used for good health.

Signed: Jacob M. Bayfield

Adapted from *A Smoke-Free Generation*, "The Will to Be Healthy," Minnesota Coalition for a Smoke-Free Society 2000.

NAME ________________________

Biographical Sketch

Abby Bayfield

Abby is the second of the Bayfield children. She is the owner and operator of Bayfield Health Clubs, Inc. Abby started her business with one private health club that was frequented by athletes, weight lifters, and body builders and transformed it into a community facility. The health club now offers a wide variety of activities, from aerobics to intramural basketball teams and general fitness awareness classes. Because of her keen interest in community welfare, Abby has recently funded service projects for disadvantaged adolescents.

The success of the Bayfield Health Clubs is a reflection of Abby's views of the importance of physical fitness. She participates in many sports, particularly swimming, which she does faithfully every day. She also organized and coaches a city-wide girls' basketball league.

Abby is also the manager, financial officer, and chief administrator of the health clubs and the community help programs that she actively supports. In addition, she sits on a number of social action committees and boards of directors. After three hours of sleep, Abby goes nonstop in her neverending series of meetings. She has high blood pressure but says that is essential to keep her energy up. She often takes on more responsibility than time permits and becomes overly stressed when she cannot carry out her responsibilities to her satisfaction.

Because of Abby's busy schedule, she is always eating on the run, usually skipping breakfast, grabbing a quick burger and fries or a taco for lunch and then again for dinner. After a long day of work and meetings, it is typical of Abby to go home, grab a bowl of dip, a bag of chips, and a bottle of beer and turn on the television until the wee hours of the morning. These 4 or 5 hours of television are Abby's way of unwinding from her hectic day.

Although Abby is very confident in handling the pressures that go along with the business world, she is insecure about her social life. She has few close friends, is often alone, and has rarely gone out with the same guy more than once. As Abby would say, "I'm a great team manager, but I'm no good at playing the field." Recently, she has been dating her state senator, a heavy smoker. She accompanies him to cocktail parties and social gatherings. Abby is often uncomfortable at these parties because she doesn't think she fits in. Her boyfriend has noticed that when she feels uncomfortable, she tends to eat half the buffet table. This has made Abby even more self-conscious, though at the last party she noticed that the two people that she was talking to were smoking while she was pigging out on caviar and cheese chunks. Abby thought it was unfortunate that these attractive people reeked of smoke and had dragon breath.

Over the past 5 years, Abby has had six major car crashes. Luckily, she has not been injured; although others have been. Before his death, Jacob expressed his concern over Abby's fast-paced lifestyle and bad driving habits.

NAME ______________________

Biographical Sketch

Mollie Bayfield

Mollie is the youngest of the Bayfield children. Her father spoiled her as a child and Mollie has had a hard time growing up. When she was in junior high school, Mollie hung around with kids her parents strongly disapproved of. Her friends took drugs and drank alcohol on the weekends. At the age of fourteen, she ran away, started smoking, and lived on the streets. She continued this way of life for two years until she met an astrologer (a fortune teller) named Madame Crystal, who advised her to return home and begin a healthy lifestyle. Ever since, Mollie has been devoted to astrology and regularly consults Madame Crystal to have her fortune told and for guidance. Many of her personal and business decisions are based on the positions of the stars and planets according to the readings of Madame Crystal.

Proud of his daughter's recovery, 5 years ago Mollie's father gave her a restaurant for her birthday, which she has turned into a huge success. Upon the advice of her astrologer, she later purchased four more restaurants. Bayfield's Brunchola has become a chain of popular cafes where young professionals and athletes go for gourmet health food.

Mollie's expertise and creativity with gourmet health foods has been written up in several magazines. Although the overall business is a success, the employees often take advantage of Mollie's generous nature by borrowing money from her without paying it back and using her good nature to take extra days off work.

Mollie is an avid runner. She runs 20 miles a day and has won four marathons—one race away from a national record. She actually might have won her fifth marathon, but the local television station obtained pictures of her getting in a car halfway through the race and claimed she didn't run the whole way. Mollie denies this. She encourages her friends and family, as well as her restaurant customers, to exercise. For the last 5 years, she has sponsored statewide 10-kilometer races, with hundreds of thousands of dollars worth of proceeds going to charities.

The foods that Mollie eats are very healthy, but not enough for someone so active. Mollie is extremely conscious of her weight and is very thin. Her doctor is concerned about possible anorexic behavior and says that she needs to gain 20 pounds. Mollie's father was very worried about her weight. Mollie thinks she is slim but healthy, even though she has fainted twice this month.

Mollie has compassion for others and demonstrates that through her creation of "Meals on Heels"—a program to bring leftover restaurant food to poor, elderly people who are unable to cook for themselves. She has organized high school track teams throughout the city to deliver the meals. The hungry people she helps refer to her as Saint Mollie and the runners think of her as an important role model.

When Mollie's father died, she was devastated. The night before her father's sudden death, he asked her to come over for dinner. Although she had no special plans, she made up an excuse so that she could squeeze in an extra run. She never saw her father alive again. On hearing the news of her father's death, she was overcome with guilt. She sank into a deep depression, and was often unable to get up in the mornings or to make even the simplest decision. She stopped running and became nervous and jittery. Mollie consulted her astrologer who said, "The answer to your problems lies in the patterns of past smoke rings."

NAME ____________________

Biographical Sketch

Nick Bayfield

Nick is the oldest of the Bayfield children and was very upset by his father's death. Nick is the owner and president of the local semipro baseball team and in three years has turned the team from losers into world champs. Nick is a natural leader. He happily shakes hands and gives autographs to the people who seek him out. Most people in the community think of Nick as a local hero of sorts and some have even suggested that he run for Congress.

To his business partners, however, Nick is considered a "smoke-filled back room wheeler dealer," comparing him to the gangsters in the movies who make their deals in smoky rooms at the back of bars. Several times he has used his influence to take over smaller businesses, showing little compassion for those people whose lives and savings he has destroyed. It is rumored that he is under criminal investigation by the federal government for bribery and smuggling. Nick has been able to keep the investigation out of the news—along with the fact that he has had his driver's license revoked for drunken driving.

Nick's skills in negotiating business deals and his international connections have been recognized worldwide. He has been a chief negotiator in major peace treaties all over the world. Nick has not only helped end localized wars, but he has also helped fund rebuilding by providing aid to the victims of war-torn nations. These efforts have won him a Nobel Peace Prize nomination.

Nick has trouble keeping his weight down. He works out at Abby's health club three days a week and his major interest there is weight lifting and body building. He loves to swim and takes brisk walks. The family has a baseball-shaped swimming pool in the backyard which Jacob had built for them before his death. Nick makes good use of the pool.

Last week, a group of community leaders visited Nick to inquire about the unhealthy foods available at his ball park and the advertising of alcohol and tobacco products there. They claimed the hot dogs were full of fat and sugar, the popcorn was covered with salt, the Polish sausages were nothing but fat, and the ice cream was full of empty calories. They said that the advertising of alcohol and tobacco products was not good for impressionable youth. The group suggested some healthy alternatives that could be served in place of the unhealthy food items and mentioned other products that could be advertised. Nick refused to listen to their arguments and had the group removed from his office.

Because of Nick's high visibility and his celebrity status in the community, a new tobacco company has approached him to become its spokesperson and endorse its new low tar cigarettes. Nick agreed, provided he doesn't have to inhale in the ads. However, during the photo session of the commercial he became anxious after many takes had to be reshot. The director, a woman whom Nick finds extremely attractive (and vice versa), suggested that the real Nick will come out if he just inhales and relaxes, just as she does.

NAME ________________________________

Biographical Sketch

Ross Bayfield

Ross is the next to youngest of the Bayfield children. He owns and manages seven movie theaters and several apartment buildings. Though a confirmed family man, he shows little understanding or compassion for his low-income renters. Last winter he tried to cut off the heat and electricity of late-paying renters. He has been ticketed several times by the health department for violating city health codes.

Ross and his wife have four children. Because of the death of one of his small children, Ross is a major contributor to the children's wing of the hospital, of which he is chairman of the board. He has recently denied a board decision designating the hospital as a smoke-free space.

The loss of his infant child moved Ross to devote every waking hour to the invention of a new type of incubator that has already saved thousands of babies' lives but was too late to save his own daughter. Each night after a stressful day of decision-making, he leaves the family estate, working alone until dawn to improve the incubator to save even more lives. He is obsessed with preventing other families from suffering the loss as his did.

When his youngest child was a baby, Ross, a former state swimming and diving champion, had a serious diving accident which left him paralyzed from the waist down. He felt insecure and inferior because of his confinement to a wheelchair. Because of this, he looked for ways to seem more sophisticated and powerful. He often told people that he pictured himself as the "macho Marlboro man on wheels." Since the accident, he has become overprotective of his children. Because he is afraid that they might have an accident also, he does not allow them to get involved in many athletic sports. Ross's wife, however, does try to get the children out and active, against their father's wishes.

Despite his disability, Ross is an enthusiastic pilot. He owns a specially equipped Lear jet that he uses to transport dying infants from all over the world to his infant care facilities. He also flies medical teams to remote villages around the world to train local doctors in infant care and the lifesaving use of the incubators.

Ross is a great fan of the movies, especially those about fighter pilots. As he soars high above the clouds he likes to picture himself as a top gun fighter pilot, off on a daring adventure, cigarette dangling from his lips, courage in his heart, and romance in his eyes.

Lately Ross has been spending a great deal of time at the state capitol lobbying for a bill which would allow smoking in movie theaters. This sudden interest coincides with his recent investment in a large tobacco company.

NAME ___________________________

Recovery Rate from Quitting Smoking

Within 20 minutes of your last cigarette:
- you stop polluting the air
- blood pressure drops to normal
- pulse rate drops to a normal rate
- temperature of the hands and feet increases to normal

8 hours:
- carbon monoxide level in the blood drops to normal
- oxygen level in the blood increases to normal

24 hours:
- chance of heart attack decreases

48 hours:
- nerve endings adjust to the absence of nicotine
- ability to smell and taste is enhanced

72 hours:
- bronchial tubes relax, making breathing easier
- lung capacity increases

2 weeks to 3 months:
- circulation improves
- walking becomes easier
- lung function increases up to 30 percent

1–9 months:
- coughing, sinus congestion, fatigue, and shortness of breath all decrease
- cilia regrow in lungs, increasing ability to handle mucus, clean the lungs, and reduce infection
- body's overall energy increases

1 year:
- heart disease death rate is halfway back to that of a nonsmoker

5 years:
- heart disease death rate drops to the rate for nonsmokers
- lung cancer death rate decreases halfway back to that of nonsmokers

10 years:
- lung cancer death rate drops almost to the rate for nonsmokers
- precancerous cells are replaced
- incidence of other cancers—mouth, larynx, esophagus, bladder, kidney, and pancreas—decreases

NAME ______________________

What's in Cigarette Smoke

There are over 4,000 chemicals, including:

Over 12 cancer causing agents

Over 10 different metals

Acetone

nail polish remover

Acetic acid

vinegar

Ammonia

floor/toilet cleaner

Arsenic

poison

Butane

lighter fluid

Cadmium

rechargeable batteries

Carbon monoxide

car exhaust fumes

DDT/Dieldrin

insecticides

Ethanol

alcohol

Formaldehyde

preserver of body tissue

Hexamine

barbecue lighter fluid

Hydrogen cyanide

gas chamber poison

Methane

swamp gas

Methanol

rocket fuel

Napthalene

mothballs

Nicotine

insecticide/addictive drug

Nitrobenzene

gasoline additive

Nitrous oxide phenols

disinfectant

Stearic acid

candle wax

NAME ______________________

Important Facts about Tobacco

1. Smoking is the number one preventable cause of death in the nation.

2. Every thirteen seconds, someone in the world dies from a tobacco-related illness.

3. More people die from cigarette smoking and related illnesses than from AIDS, alcohol, traffic accidents, illicit drugs, murder, and suicide combined.

4. Cigarette smoking is responsible for one of every five deaths in the United States.

5. Tobacco kills nearly 435,000 Americans each year; cocaine kills no more than 1,000 annually.

6. Of the 3,000 children who smoke their first cigarette, 23 will be murdered, 30 will die in traffic accidents, and nearly 750 will be killed by smoking-related illnesses.

7. Short-term effects of smoking are rapid heart beat, increased pulse rate, bad breath, stained teeth, shortness of breath, smelly clothes and hair, reduced circulation, increased coughing and wheezing, allergy flare-ups, more colds and pneumonia, and decreased sense of taste and smell.

8. Smoking cigarettes can cause premature facial wrinkles and impotence.

9. Smokeless tobacco stains teeth an ugly, yellowish-brown color. It wears off the enamel on teeth and causes bad breath. After using smokeless tobacco for a few weeks, the user's lips and gums can begin to crack, bleed, and wrinkle and may develop sores and white spots that can lead to cancer.

NAME ____________________

The Addictive Aspect of Using Tobacco

1. The earlier people start smoking, the harder it is to quit when they are older. People who start smoking in their teenage years run the risk of becoming lifelong smokers.

2. Eighty-five percent of teenagers who smoke two or more cigarettes completely—and overcome the initial discomfort of smoking—will become regular smokers.

3. Most adolescents believe they can stop smoking whenever they wish.

4. Only 5 percent of high school seniors believed they would still be smoking years after graduation. In fact, 75 percent were still smoking 8 years later.

5. Nicotine, which is found in tobacco products, is more addictive than crack cocaine or alcohol. One out of six who experiment with crack will become addicted and one out of ten who experiment with alcohol will become addicted, *nine out of ten* who experiment with tobacco will become addicted.

6. Tobacco is a gateway drug. Those people who use tobacco are 14 times more likely to abuse alcohol, 100 times more likely to use marijuana, and 32 times more likely to use cocaine.

7. Forty percent of all movie tickets are purchased by individuals under the age of 21. Teenagers frequent movies three times more than adults. Movies have become the avenue for tobacco promotion through subliminal techniques such as having heroes, movie stars, and actors of all kinds smoke.

NAME ______________________

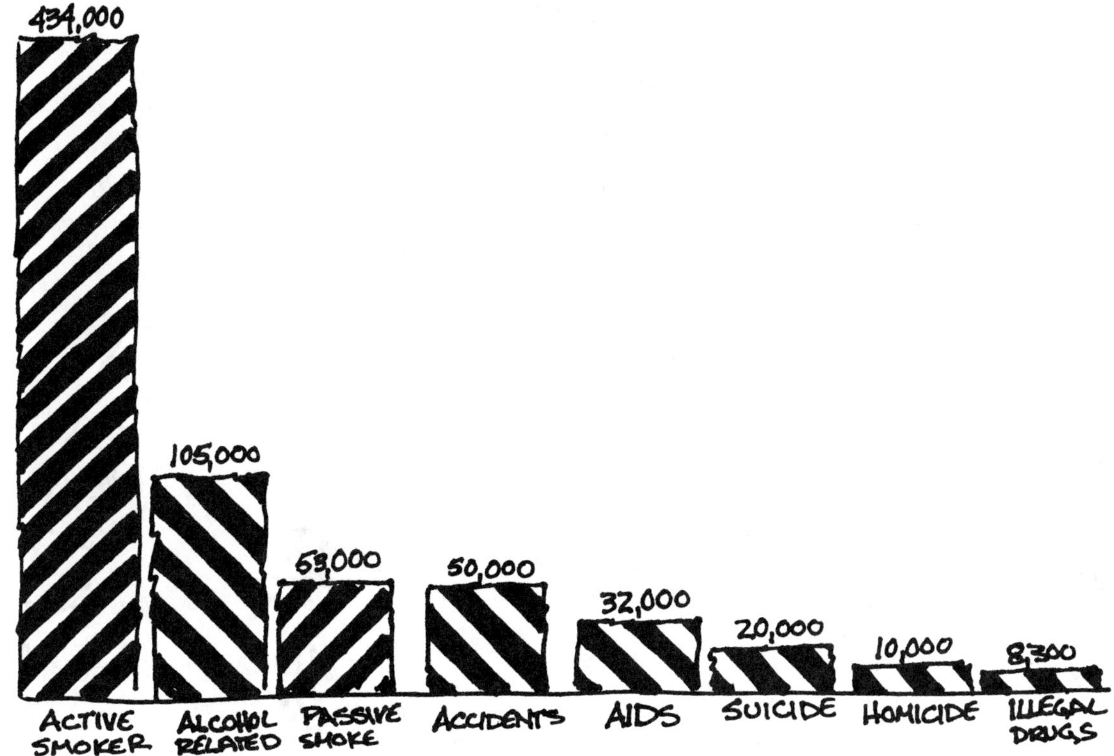

U.S. Deaths in 1989
434,000
105,000
53,000
50,000
32,000
20,000
10,000
8,300
ACTIVE SMOKER
ALCOHOL RELATED
PASSIVE SMOKE
ACCIDENTS
AIDS
SUICIDE
HOMICIDE
ILLEGAL DRUGS

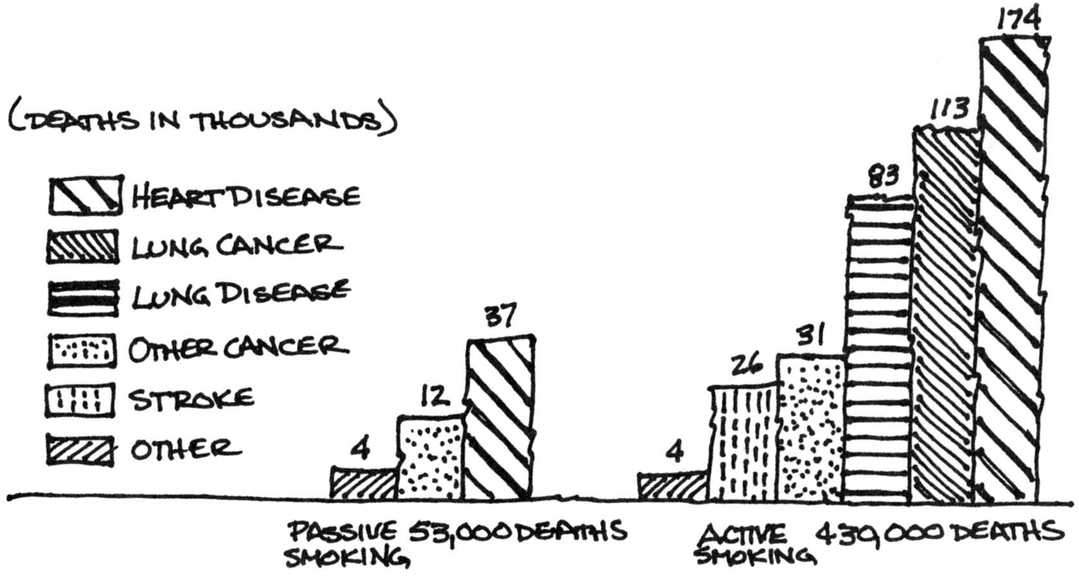

U.S. Deaths Attributed to Smoking in 1988
(DEATHS IN THOUSANDS)
HEART DISEASE
LUNG CANCER
LUNG DISEASE
OTHER CANCER
STROKE
OTHER
4
12
37
4
26
31
83
113
174
PASSIVE SMOKING 53,000 DEATHS
ACTIVE SMOKING 430,000 DEATHS

NAME ____________________

Blood Alcohol Content Wheel

Part I

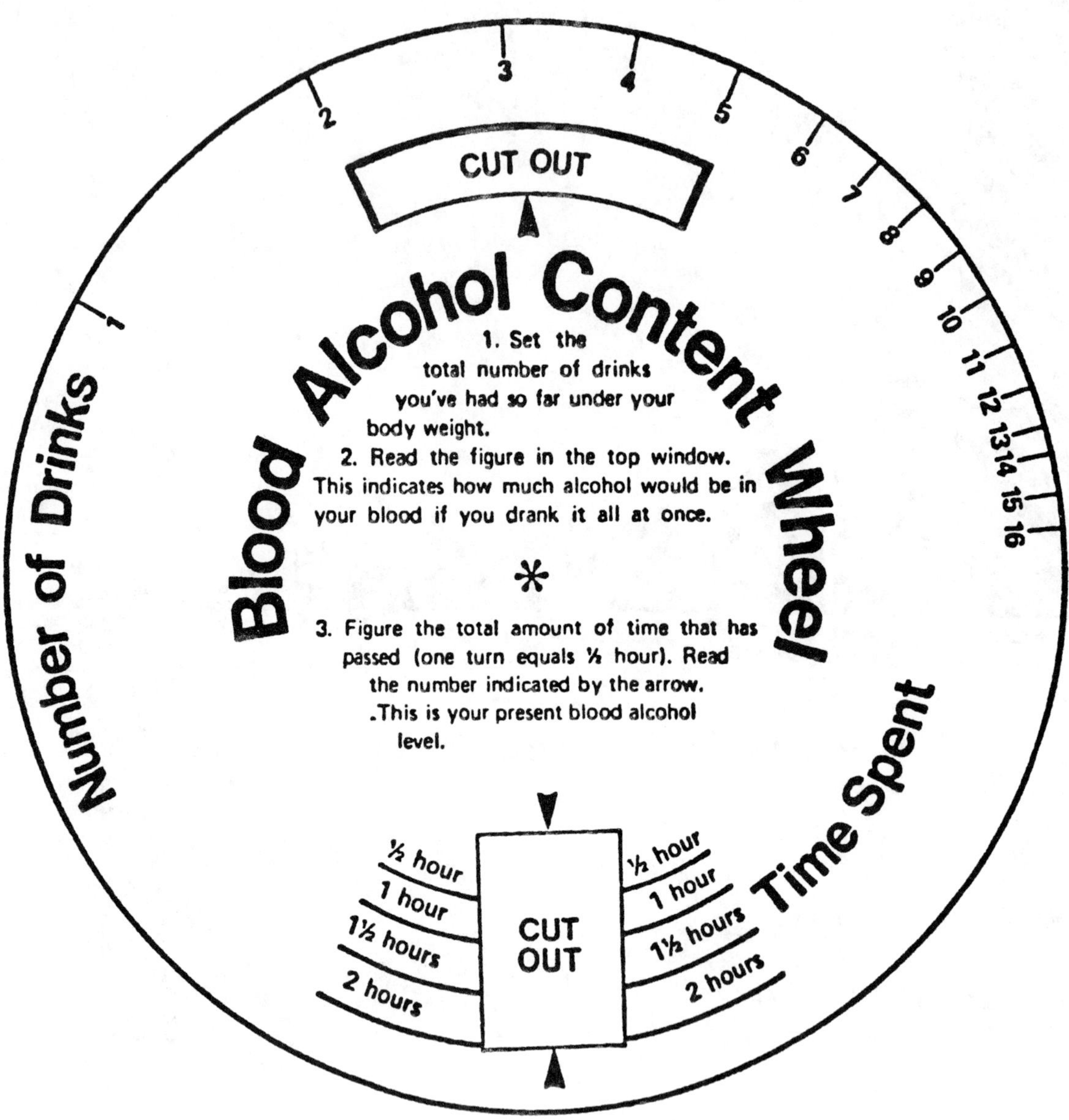

1. Paste each page onto cardboard or manila paper.
2. Trim around each circle.
3. Use a razor to cut the two sections marked "CUT OUT."
4. Put the smaller circle on top of the larger one, carefully fastening them together at the stars (centers) with a paper fastener.

Reprinted from *Alcohol and Alcohol Safety,* Volume 2, by Peter Finn and Judith Platt. U.S. Government Printing Office, 1972.

NAME ____________________

Blood Alcohol Content Wheel

Part 2

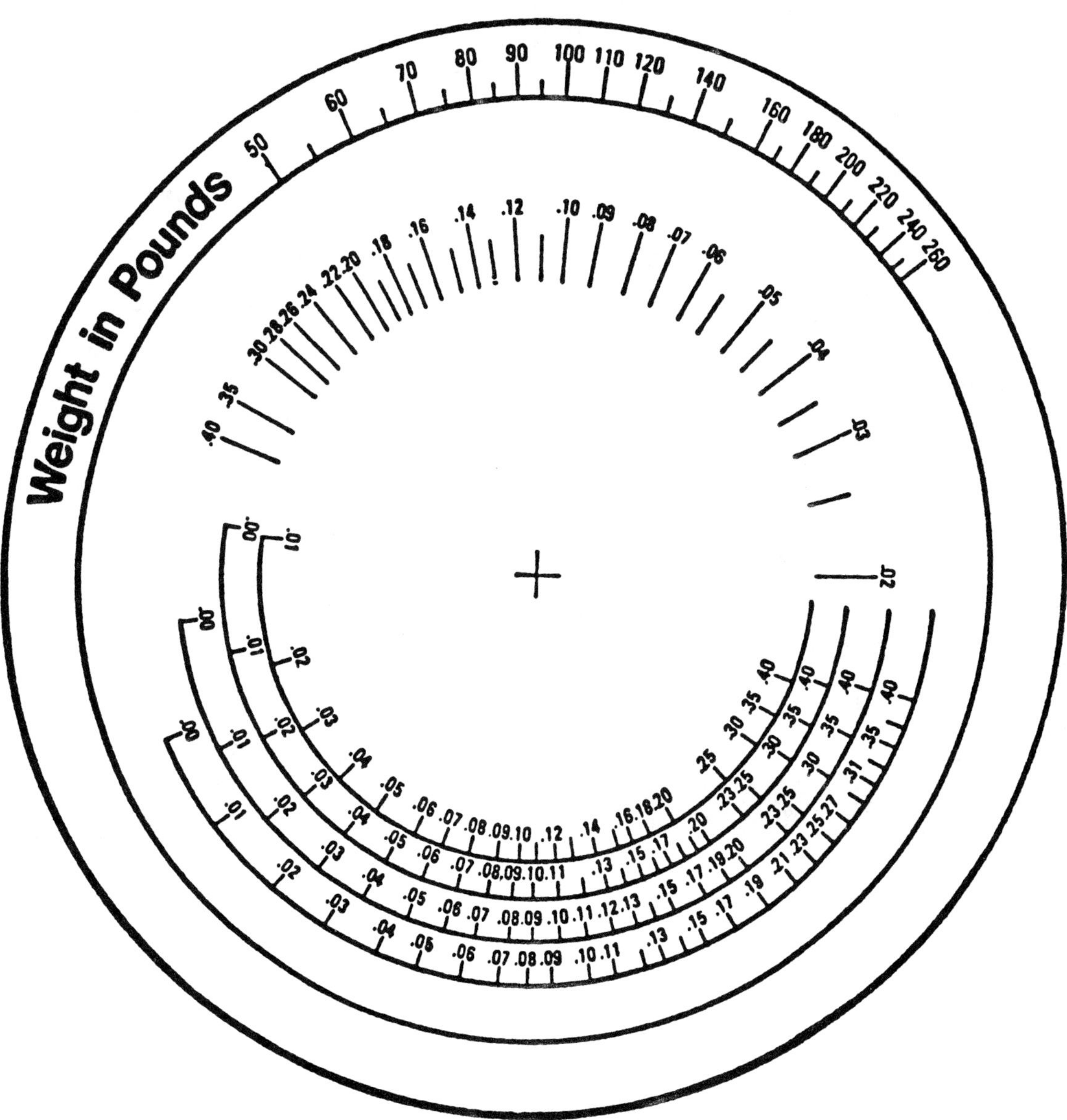

NAME ____________________

Levels of Intoxication

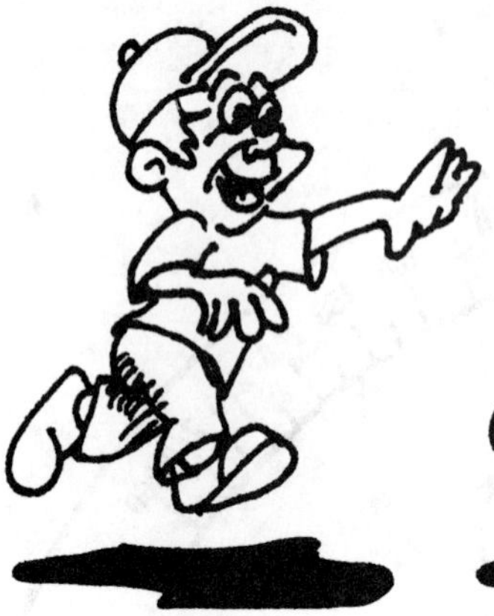

0.00–0.04
No apparent
change

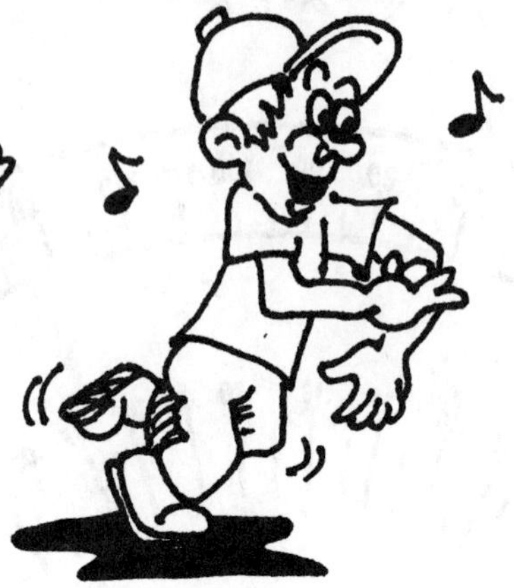

0.04–0.08
Slower reaction,
clumsy

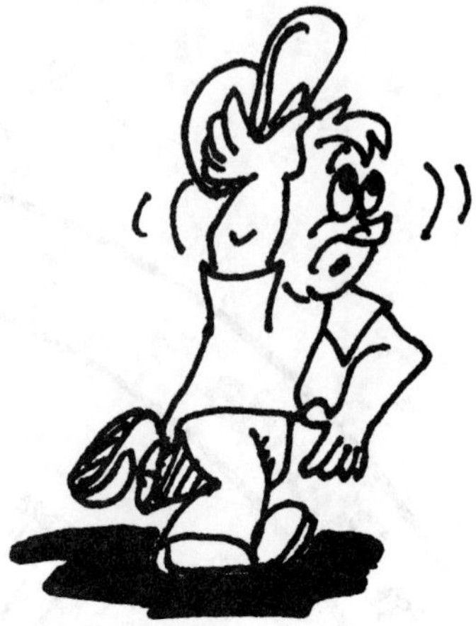

0.08–0.10
Legally drunk,
slurred speech

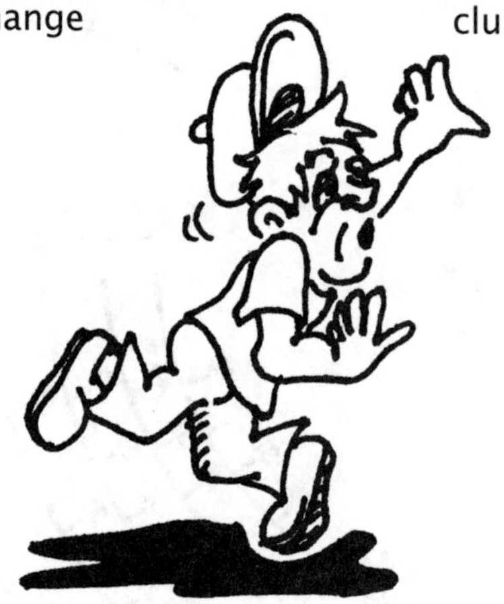

0.11–0.15
Irresponsible behavior,
poor balance

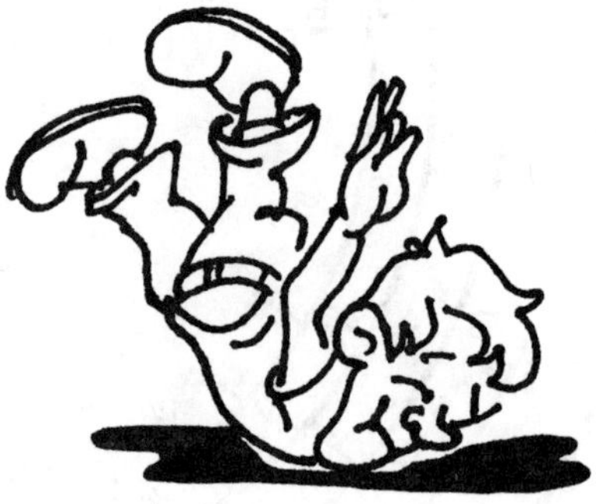

0.15–0.20
Lack of control,
mental confusion

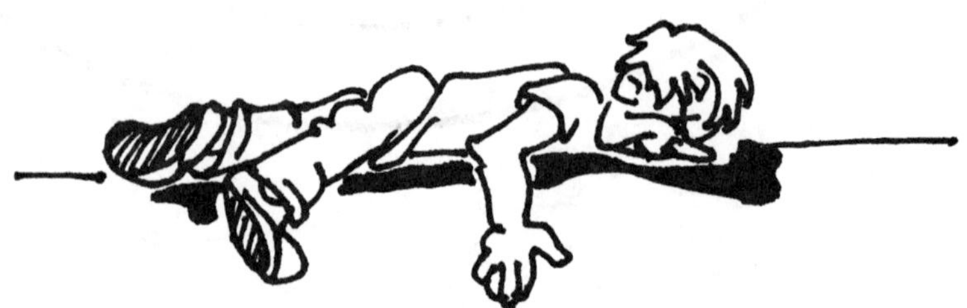

0.20–0.30
Unconsciousness,
all ability impaired

NAME ____________________

Questions Concerning Alcohol Consumption

Use the Blood Alcohol Content Wheel you made in class to answer the questions. Remember that a person is considered to be legally drunk in most states with a blood alcohol level of .10 (.08 in many states).

Questions about Alcohol:

1. Benjamin is a big guy weighing 200 pounds. He has had 7 shots of whiskey in an hour in a drinking contest. Is he considered legally drunk? __________

   If you subtract .01 for every 40 minutes that passes without Ben having a drink, how long will it take him to be *below* the legal limit of .10? __________

2. Sadie has had 2 drinks in an hour and weighs almost 100 pounds. Is she legally drunk? __________

3. Celia has only been drinking beer but has had 4 in 1 hour while dancing at a party. Celia weighs 100 pounds. Is Celia legally drunk? __________

4. How long would it take Celia to sober up enough to be *below* the legal limit of .10? __________

5. Johnna is 16. Is she able to legally drink alcoholic beverages in your state?

   ____

6. How many drinks can you have in one hour before reaching the legally drunk blood alcohol level? __________

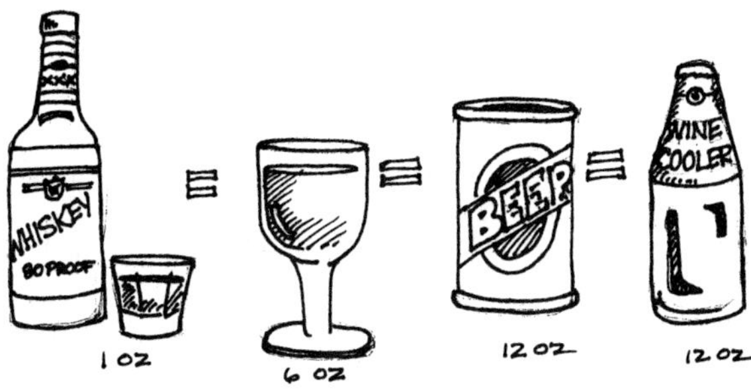

NAME ___________________________________

Refusal Role-Play

Read the following situation and write friendly refusals.

You and some friends are at a party where beer and hard liquor are being served although most of the kids are under the legal age. You have been to parties like this before and have never participated in the drinking. A very popular person of the opposite sex approaches you with a big smile. You start talking. You are really excited that you have finally been noticed and you want to build this into a friendship. The person offers you a beer.

Popular Person: You look like you need to relax a bit. Why don't you have a beer? I brought you a cold one . . .

Your Response:

Popular Person: Put the soda down. This is what's happenin'! Have a real drink. Join the crowd!

Your Response:

Popular Person: Oh, come on . . . everybody drinks! If you want to hang with my crowd you'll have to loosen up.

Your Response:

Popular Person: You don't seem to want to have any fun. You know you would love some beer.

Your Response:

Popular Person: I think you have a lot of potential. Relax a little.

Your Response:

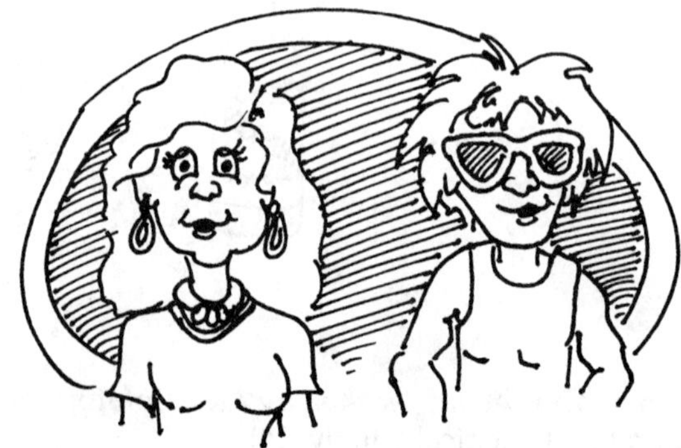

NAME ____________________

Practice Refusals

Below is a list of common ways that people try to pressure you into doing things that you don't really want to do. Think of ways to refuse their line. Try to remain friends as you refuse them.

"Come on! Everybody's doing it."

Your response:

"If you really love me, you'll have sex with me. Sex is part of love."

Your response:

"If you won't have sex with me, I don't want to see you anymore."

Your response:

"Try it! You'll like it. Be cool."

Your response:

"We had sex before. What is your problem this time?"

Your response:

"Try it. See what it's like. Aren't you curious?"

Your response:

"If you want to be popular . . . you will do it."

Your response:

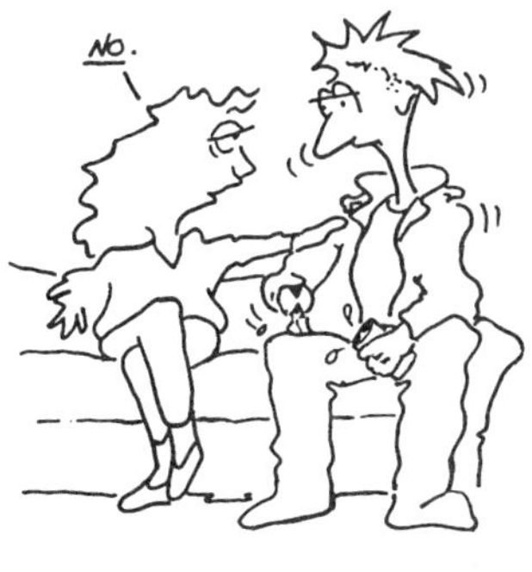

NAME ______________________________

Effects of Drugs on the Body

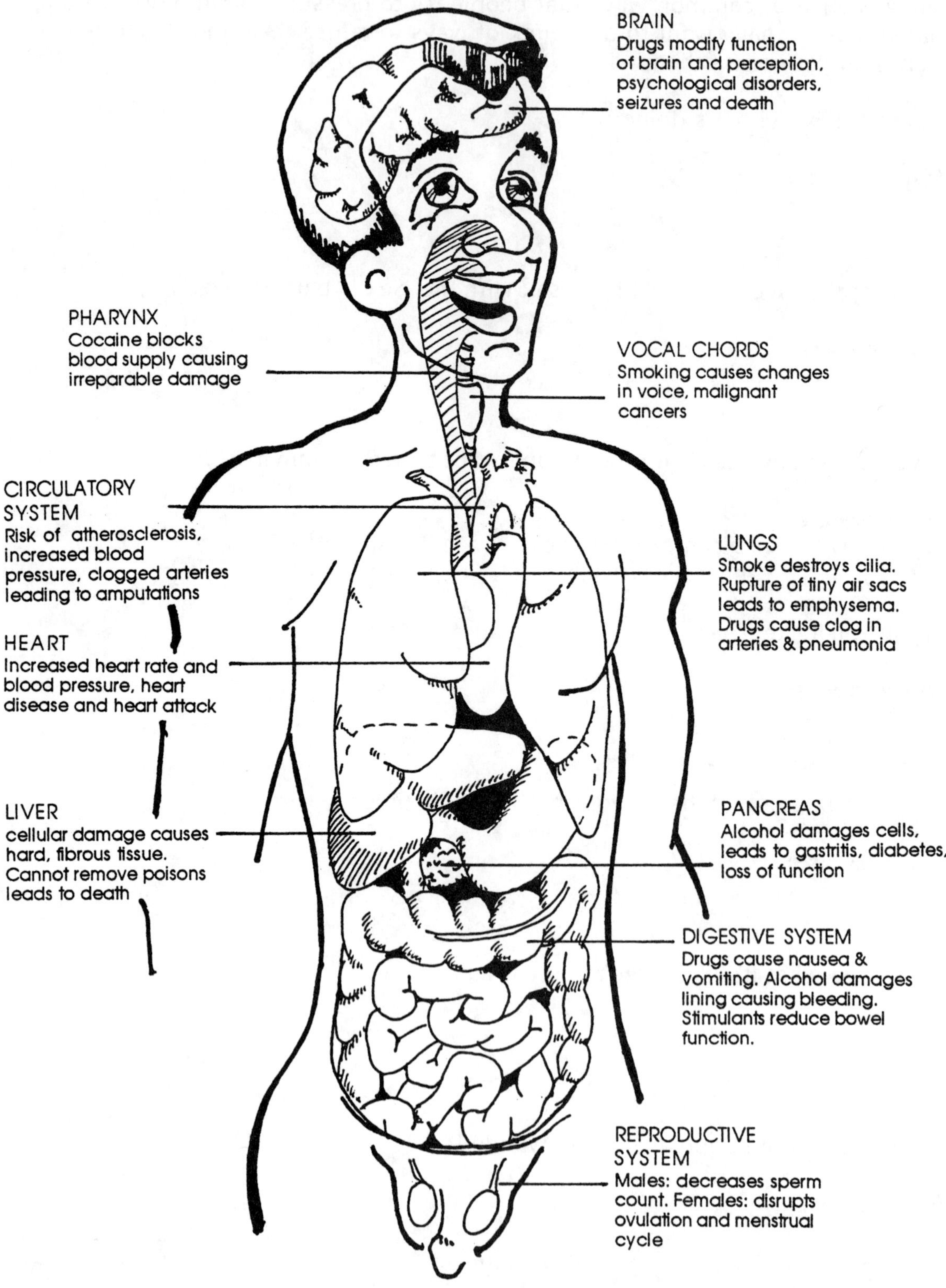

NAME ____________________

Drug Description

Cannabis:

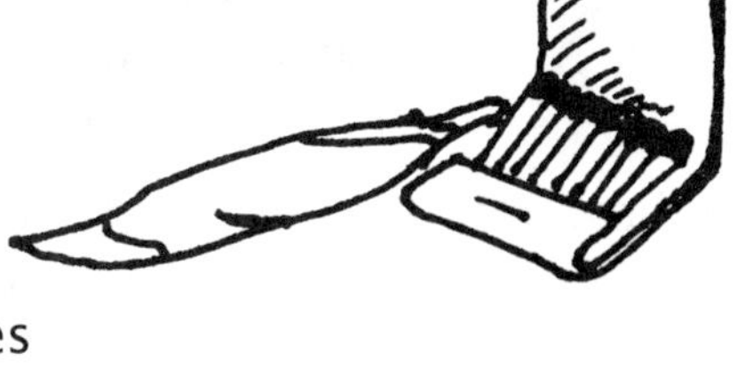

Drug: *Marijuana, Hashish*

Street names: pot, grass, weed, reefer, ganja, Acapulco Gold, joints, smoke

Method of use: smoked, eaten, or added to cigarettes

Medical use: reduce nausea and pain, treatment for glaucoma

Effects on the body: restlessness, euphoria, impaired short-term memory, lack of concentration and coordination, and, in high amounts, hallucinations and anxiety. Physical effects are red eyes and increased appetite.

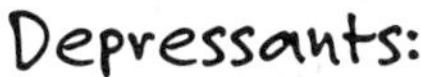

Depressants:

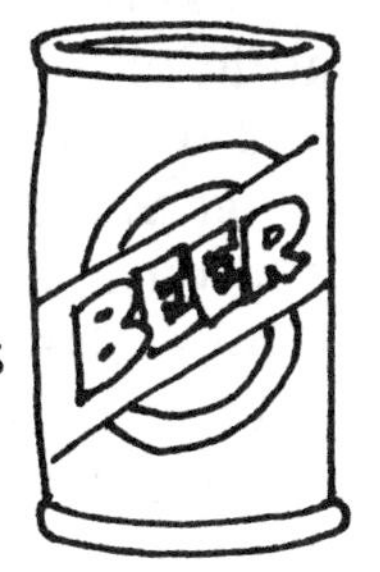

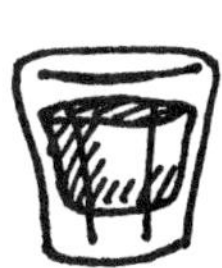

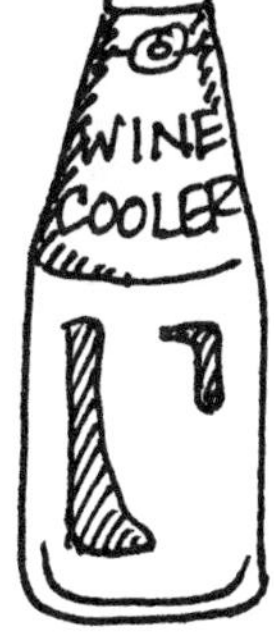

Drug: *Alcohol, Barbiturates*

Street names: *Alcohol*—booze
Barbiturates—downers, barbs, red devils, yellows, blue devils

Method of use: *Alcohol*—used in drinks and swallowed
Barbiturates—taken orally in pill form

Medical use: *Alcohol*—none
Barbiturates—sedative to induce sleep and control seizures

Effects on the body: *Alcohol*—euphoria, mood swings, impaired judgment, loss of coordination, blurred vision, dizziness, nausea, vomiting and, in large doses, loss of consciousness.
Barbiturates—drunken behavior and disorientation and an overdose can cause dilated pupils, shallow respiration, weak and rapid pulse, coma, or death.

Stimulants:

Drug: *Cocaine, Crack Cocaine, Amphetamines, Methamphetamine*

Street name: *Cocaine*—coke, blow, snow, snort, nose candy
Crack Cocaine—crack, rock, hubba
Amphetamines—speed, uppers, pep pills, black beauties, dexies
Methamphetamine—crystal, speed, crank, meth

NAME ______________________________

Method of use: *Cocaine*—inhaled through the nose, injected into veins, smoked
Crack Cocaine—smoked in small pipes
Amphetamines—pill form taken orally, inhaled through the nose, injected
Methamphetamine—injected, pill form taken orally, inhaled through the nose

Medical use: *Cocaine*—as a topical anesthetic on mucus membranes for eye surgery
Crack Cocaine—none
Amphetamines—improve mood, treat depression, suppress appetite, treat narcolepsy
Methamphetamines—same as amphetamines

Effects on the body: *Cocaine*—euphoria, increased alertness, and feelings of confidence and well being and an overdose can cause extreme agitation and death. Physical effects include dilated pupils, runny nose, and elevated heart rate and respiration.
Crack Cocaine—euphoria, high energy, insomnia, and appetite loss and the same physical effects as cocaine with the addition of irritability, depression, paranoia, convulsions and death if used over long periods.
Amphetamines and Methamphetamines—increased alertness, euphoria, appetite loss, increased heart rate, and dilated pupils. Use over long periods can cause dizziness, loss of coordination, and collapse. Overdose can result in high fever, stroke, or heart failure.

Hallucinogens:

Drug: *LSD, PCP, Mescaline, Psilocybin*

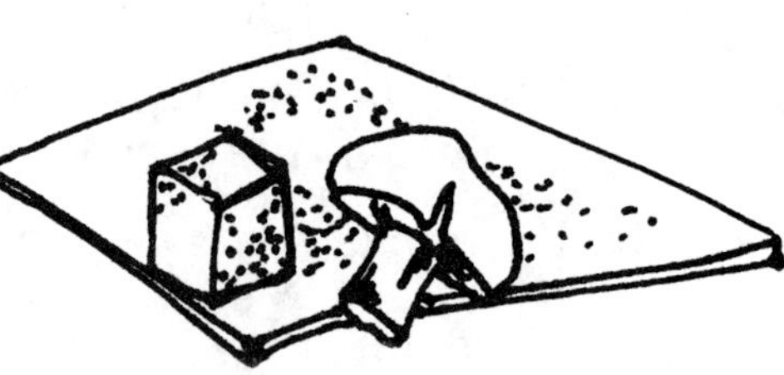

Street name: *LSD*—acid, icrodot, blotter acid
PCP—angel dust, supergrass, KJ, rocket fuel, killerweed, sherms
Mescaline—mesc
Psilocybin—shrooms, buttons

Method of use: *LSD*—taken orally or licked off paper
PCP—taken orally or smoked
Mescaline and Psilocybin—swallowed

Medical use: *LSD*—none today but once was used for treatment of mental and emotional problems
PCP—none
Mescaline and Psilocybin—no medical uses but approved for use by Native Americans in some religious ceremonies

NAME ______________________

Effects on the body: *LSD*—hallucinations, dilated pupils, high blood pressure, and fever. Hallucinations can result in confusion, panic, loss of control, flashbacks, and psychosis.
PCP—similar to LSD but with rapid eye movement and exaggerated walk. May experience extraordinary strength, sense of invulnerability, and image distortion.
Mescaline and Psilocybin—hallucinations, increased heart rate, confusion, anxiety, and flashbacks.

Inhalants:

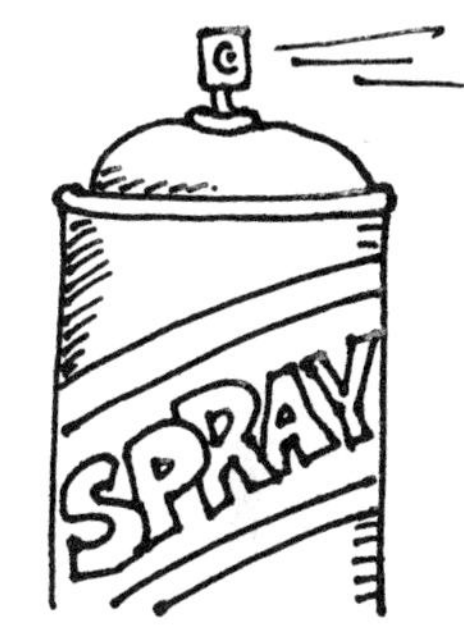

Drug: solvents, aerosols, glue and paint thinner

Street name: laughing gas, bullet, snappers, rush, bolt

Method of use: inhaled through the nose

Medical use: none

Effects on the body: hallucinations, decreased body temperature and blood pressure, confusion, nausea, sneezing, nosebleeds, fatigue, loss of coordination, brain damage, respiratory failure, and death.

Opiates or Narcotics:

Drug: heroin and heroin derivatives including codeine, morphine, methadone

Street name: smack, tar, mud, China white, Mexican brown

Method of use: injected into veins, inhaled through the nose, smoked, or the derivatives can be found in pill form and taken orally

Medical use: cough suppression, painkiller, and, in the case of methadone, as a substitute narcotic in the treatment of heroin addiction

Effects on the body: euphoria, drowsiness, constricted pupils, nausea, and vomiting. Overdose can result in slow and shallow breathing, convulsions, coma, and death.

NAME ____________________

Identifying the Signs of Dependency

Substance abuse:

__________ Do you think the substance is safe and not addictive?

__________ Do you look forward to using the substance?

__________ Do you seek out other people who use the substance?

__________ Do you feel more comfortable or more popular when using?

__________ Do you hide your use from other people?

__________ Are you beginning to avoid or distrust some people?

__________ Do you have health problems as a result of using?

__________ Do you get anxious if you run out of the substance?

__________ Do you avoid going places where you cannot use the substance?

__________ Has the use of the substance caused financial problems?

__________ Has your quality of work diminished; have your grades gone down?

__________ Has use of the substance interfered or caused changes in your sleep patterns?

__________ Do you have difficulty remembering things?

__________ Do you find that you don't care about things as much as you used to?

__________ Have you tried to stop using the substance and found reasons why you couldn't stop?

__________ Do you feel irritable or anxious if you stop using?

If you find yourself answering yes to many of these questions, you may have a problem with this drug or substance.

Behavioral addictions:

Workaholic or Perfectionist

__________ Do feel your work must be perfect?

__________ Do you find yourself working at the expense of leisure time?

NAME ____________________________

____________ Do you take work with you on trips or days off?

____________ Do you have a difficult time accepting criticism?

____________ Do you seem more critical of yourself than others are?

____________ Do you feel proud of the amount of work you accomplish and your lack of free time?

____________ Do you prefer work to socializing?

____________ Do you feel more comfortable relating to people in a work situation?

____________ Do you feel you have too much to do and not enough time to do it?

Compulsive Eating

____________ Do you turn to food when you are depressed or use it as a reward?

____________ Do you diet often?

____________ Do you think about food throughout the day?

____________ Do you eat when you feel rejected or lonely?

____________ Do you continue to eat, even when you are no longer hungry?

____________ Are you overweight?

____________ Do you feel anxious when you diet?

Note: There are eating disorders, like bulimia and anorexia, that are just as obsessive and addictive as overeating. These compulsions would focus more on lack of food but the individual is just as weight conscious and obsessed with food as the overeater.

If you answered yes to many of the questions about behavioral addictions, you may have a problem with that behavior. Remember, the questionnaire is not a scientific test but rather a tool for indicating a possible problem.

Where can you go for help?

National Drug Information and Referral Line	1-800-662-HELP
National Council on Alcoholism	1-800-NCA-CALL

NAME ______________________________

Reward

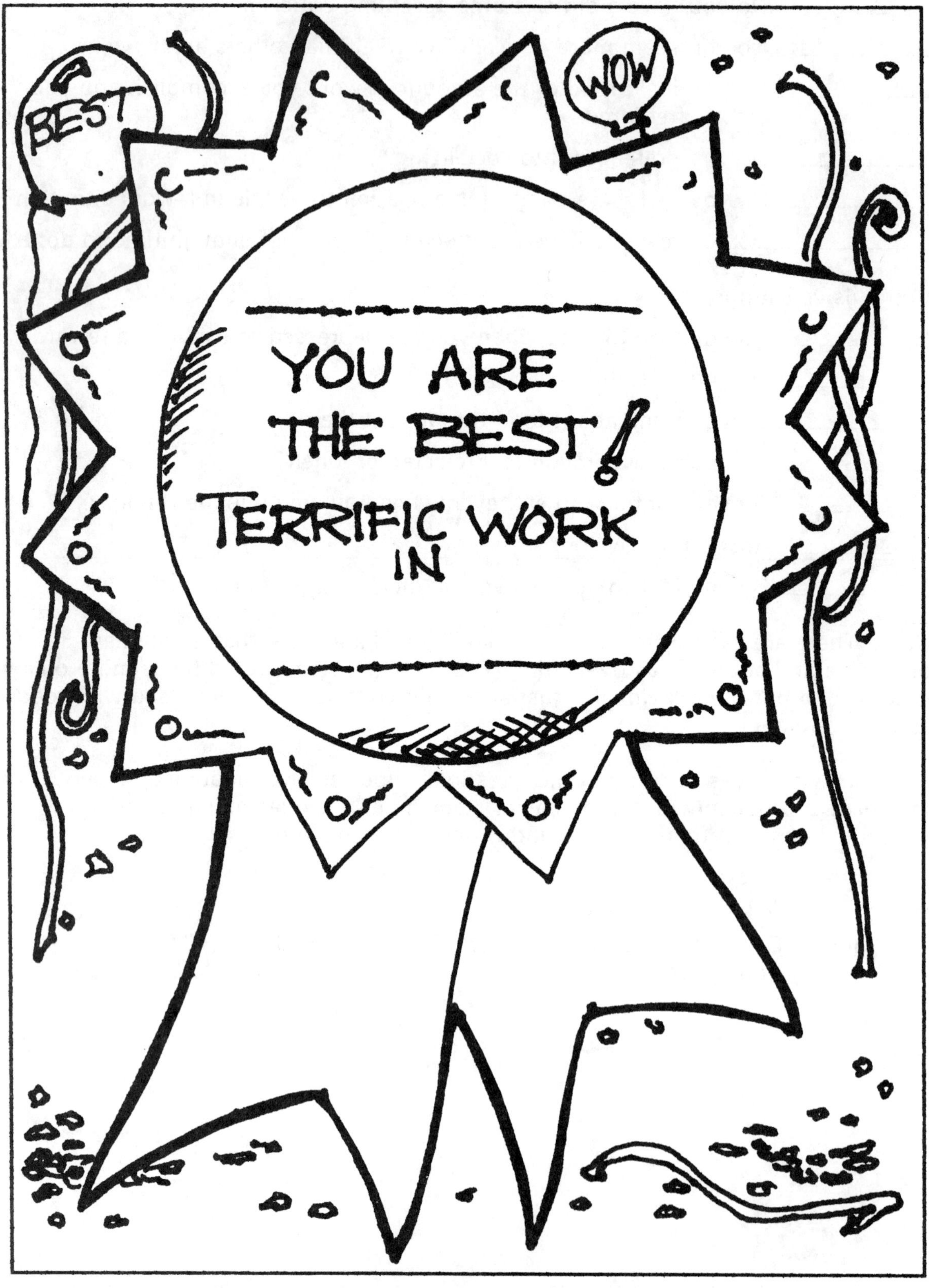

NAME ______________________________

Class Evaluation

Your opinions are important in preparing the activities and structure of the class for those students who follow you. Please be thoughtful and honest in offering your feelings in answering the questions below.

1. What was the most valuable part of this class for you? What things in this class—the seating arrangement, posters, activities—were most helpful to you in building a positive future?

____

____

____

____

____

2. What parts of this class were least valuable or unnecessary?

____

____

____

____

3. If you had all the money in the world to make this a better class and a more valuable experience for students following you, what would you do to improve the class?

____

____

____

____

4. What last thoughts or feelings would you like to share?

____

____

____

____

NAME ______________________________

Thoughts to Take with You

There are certain characteristics that successful people seem to have. Successful people:

- accept themselves as they are without criticism and yet have the desire to improve
- take risks
- set goals and work toward them
- know their strengths and use them
- look at the positive side of life
- see opportunities and challenges rather than obstacles
- do not dwell on failure—they see only lessons learned
- know how to play
- realize that respect must be earned

Success comes from within. It flows from your acceptance of and comfort in yourself. Belief and confidence in yourself is the single most important element of learning and life. People with high self-esteem achieve with integrity. What you believe about yourself, you can achieve.

Live your life each day as you would
climb a mountain. An occasional glance
toward the summit keeps the goal in mind,
but many beautiful scenes are to be
observed from each new vantage point.
Climb slowly, steadily, enjoying each
passing moment, and the view from the summit
will serve as a fitting climax
for the journey.

Harold V. Melchert

CREDITS

"Celebrate You" poem on p. xx is adapted from *Celebrate the Temporary* by Clyde H. Reid. Copyright © 1972 by Clyde H. Reid. Reprinted by permission from HarperCollins Publishers, Inc.

Activity 13 in Chapter 1, pp. 10–11, is from *TRIBES, a New Way of Learning and Being Together.* Copyright © 1995 Jeanne Gibbs, CenterSource Systems, Sausalito, CA 94965.

Activity 14 in Chapter 1, p. 11, is adapted from *How to Survive Teaching Health* by Kenneth G. Tillman and Patricia Rizzo Toner. Copyright © 1990. Reprinted by permission of the Center for Applied Research in Education/Prentice Hall.

Activity 21 in Chapter 1, pp. 15–16, is adapted with permission from *Prevention Skills for Youth,* ETR Associates Training Department. Santa Cruz, CA 1987–1998.

Activity 23 in Chapter 1, pp. 17–18, is from *Instructional Patterns: Curriculum for Parenthood Education,* "Birth Factors and Personality Traits," pp. 117–121, the California State Department of Education.

Activity 1 in Chapter 2, pp. 27–28, is adapted from *Substance Abuse Prevention Activities for Secondary Students* by Timothy and Patricia Gerne. Copyright © 1991. Reprinted with permission of the Center for Applied Research in Education/ Prentice Hall.

Activity 7 in Chapter 2, p. 33, is from *Instructional Patterns: Curriculum for Parenthood Education,* "Peer Pressure: An Outside Influence," p. 62, the California State Department of Education.

Activity 9 in Chapter 2, pp. 34–35, is from *TRIBES, a New Way of Learning and Being Together.* Copyright © 1995 Jeanne Gibbs, CenterSource Systems, Sausalito, CA 94965.

Activity 10 in Chapter 2, pp. 35–36, is inspired by *Instructional Patterns: Curriculum for Parenthood Education,* "Examining Family Relationships," pp. 141–142, the California State Department of Education.

Activity 3 in Chapter 3, p. 42, is reprinted with permission. Crisp Publications, Inc., 1200 Hamilton Court, Menlo Park, CA 94025; 800-442-7477 or 415-323-6100.

Activity 8 in Chapter 3, pp. 46–47, is adapted with permission from *Prevention Skills for Youth,* ETR Associates Training Department. Santa Cruz, CA 1987–1998.

Activity 13 in Chapter 3, pp. 49–50, is from Management Sciences for Health, Inc.

Activity 14 in Chapter 3, pp. 50–51, is adapted from *Substance Abuse Prevention Activities for Secondary Students* by Timothy and Patricia Gerne. Copyright © 1991. Reprinted with permission of the Center for Applied Research in Education/ Prentice Hall.

Activity 15 in Chapter 3, p. 51, is from Management Sciences for Health, Inc.

Activity 1 in Chapter 4, p. 53, is from *Building a Positive Self-Concept: 113 Activities for Adolescents* by Marjorie Jacobs, Blossom Turk, and Elizabeth Horn. Copyright © 1988 by J. Weston Walch, Publisher; Portland, Maine. Used with permission. All further reproduction prohibited.

Activity 3 in Chapter 4, p. 54, is from *Coping—Reacting to Stress, Coping—Coping with Stress,* by Corinne Sanders and Cynthia Turner. © Good Apple, a division of Frank Schaffer Publications, 23740 Hawthorne Boulevard, Torrance, CA 90505.

Activity 4 in Chapter 4, pp. 54–55, is from *Building a Positive Self-Concept: 113 Activities for Adolescents* by Marjorie Jacobs, Blossom Turk, and Elizabeth Horn. Copyright © 1988 by J. Weston Walch, Publisher; Portland, Maine. Used with permission. All further reproduction prohibited.

Activity 6 in Chapter 4, p. 56, is from *Coping—Reacting to Stress, Coping—Coping with Stress,* by Corinne Sanders and Cynthia Turner. © Good Apple, a division of Frank Schaffer Publications, 23740 Hawthorne Boulevard, Torrance, CA 90505.

Activity 9 in Chapter 4, pp. 57–58, is from Management Sciences for Health, Inc.

Activity 10 in Chapter 4, p. 58, is from *Guide to Adolescent Enrichment* by Monte Elchones, Ph.D. Monroe Press, Ventura, CA.

Activity 4 in Chapter 5, pp. 63–64, is from *Communicating—Speaking with Clarity, Communicating—Listening without Looking* by Mary Anne McElmorray. © Good Apple, a division of Frank Schaffer Publications, 23740 Hawthorne Boulevard, Torrance, CA 90505.

Activity 5 in Chapter 5, p. 64, is from *Communicating—Speaking with Clarity, Communicating—Listening without Looking* by Mary Anne McElmorray. © Good Apple, a division of Frank Schaffer Publications, 23740 Hawthorne Boulevard, Torrance, CA 90505.

Activity 4 in Chapter 6, p. 75, is from *Let's Talk About . . . s-e-x: A Read and Discuss Guide for People 9 to 12 and Their Parents,* by Gitchel and Foster, Planned Parenthood of Central California, 255 N. Fulton, Fresno, California, 93728.

Activity 11 in Chapter 6, pp. 83–84, is adapted with permission from *Prevention Skills for Youth,* ETR Associates Training Department. Santa Cruz, CA 1987–1998.

Activity 19 in Chapter 6, pp. 95–96, is from the California State Department of Education.

Activity 4 in Chapter 7, pp. 112–113, is adapted from *How to Survive Teaching Health* by Kenneth G. Tillman and Patricia Rizzo Toner. Copyright © 1990. Reprinted by permission of the Center for Applied Research in Education/ Prentice Hall.

Activity 1 in Chapter 8, pp. 126–127, is adapted from *Can I Handle Alcohol/Drugs? A Self-Assessment Guide for Youth,* 1987, Johnson Institute, Minneapolis, MN.

Activity 11 in Chapter 8, pp. 136–139, is adapted from *A Smoke-Free Generation,* "The Will to Be Healthy," Minnesota Coalition for a Smoke-Free Society 2000.